Preface

In this age of rapid technological advances, diagnostic imaging is commonly used in the diagnostic workup of sick or injured animals. Clients have come to expect higher-quality imaging and more accurate diagnoses. The best imaging plan is to no avail if the technical quality of the images does not allow complete disclosure of an animal's lesions. Simply stated, a radiographic diagnosis cannot be made without a diagnostic radiograph.

Our goal as instructors of diagnostic imaging for veterinary technicians was to develop a textbook that would provide both technicians and veterinarians basic technical knowledge in diagnostic imaging. Chapters 7-11 are designed to be used as a quick reference. It has been our experience that if radiographic procedures are performed infrequently and without a quick reference, the resulting images are often less than optimal.

The first 6 chapters deal with the fundamentals of radiology. More emphasis is placed on the variables involved in producing a diagnostic radiograph than on in-depth physics of x-ray production. References are provided for further study. Poor-quality intensifying screens and darkroom errors are probably responsible for ruining more radiographs produced in practice than all other reasons combined. Because of this, we describe darkroom techniques and artifacts, as well as other common artifacts that occur during exposure.

The next 5 chapters discuss patient positioning of both small and large animals with reference to the primary beam. Each radiographic projection contains a written description, a technical diagram of the positioning and an example of the finished radiograph. Also, we have described step-by-step procedures for contrast studies commonly performed in private veterinary practice.

Diagnostic ultrasound is quickly becoming a routinely used imaging tool in veterinary medicine. In Chapter 12, basic ultrasound physics, instrumentation, patient preparation and common artifacts are discussed to a depth that a practicing veterinarian or technician may understand how to maximize their ultrasound images.

We believe this unique guide will be useful to both veterinary technicians and veterinarians. By applying the principles and specific information presented here, a more accurate diagnosis can be made. Clients and their animals will be better served.

Connie M. Han, RVT
Cheryl D. Hurd, RVT

Acknowledgment

The authors gratefully acknowledge the assistance of all of the people involved with the publication of this book:

W.E. Blevins, W.R. Widmer and S. Jakoljevic for all their time, patience and encouragement in writing this book.

All of the veterinary students and veterinary technician students who helped position animals for the radiographic illustrations.

Mary Jo Carey and Mindy Brown for their patience and assistance with the radiographic illustrations.

Our husbands, Steve Han and David Hurd, for all their encouragement and assistance.

Dr. Paul Pratt and Liddie Stein, of American Veterinary Publications, for being so helpful during production of this book.

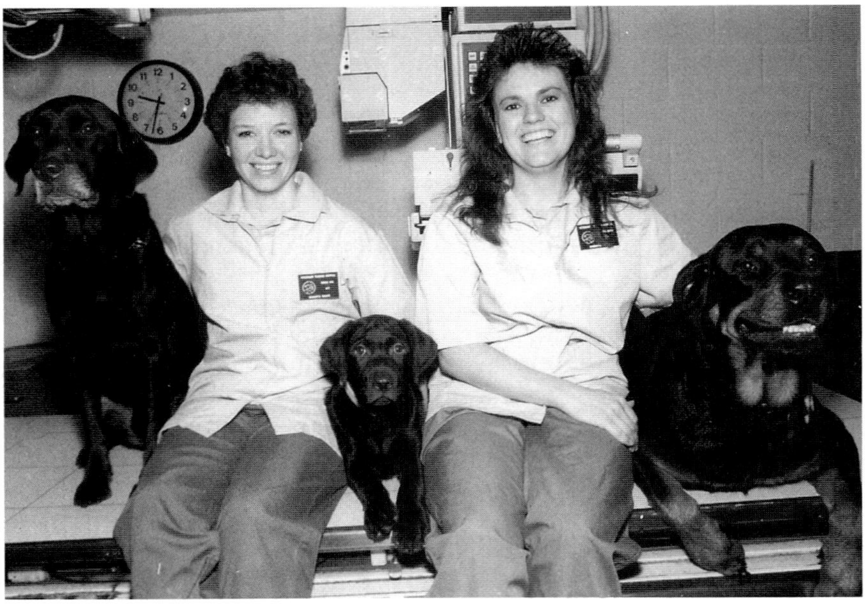

Left to right: Hershey (who posed for most of the radiographic illustrations), Connie, Buster Brown, Cheryl, Marta (who also posed for some of the radiographic illustrations).

Practical Guide to Diagnostic Imaging: Radiography and Ultrasonography

Connie M. Han, RVT
Cheryl D. Hurd, RVT
Lisa Kurklis, RVT
Purdue University
Veterinary Teaching Hospital
West Lafayette, IN 47907

Book Editor: Paul W. Pratt, VMD
Production Manager: Elisabeth S. Stein
Production Assistant: Matthew B. Davidson
Illustrations: Les Sealing, DVM

American Veterinary Publications, Inc.
5782 Thornwood Drive
Goleta, CA 93117

Library of Congress Catalog Card Number: 94-71186

ISBN 0-939674-54-8

Printed and Bound in the United States of America

Contents

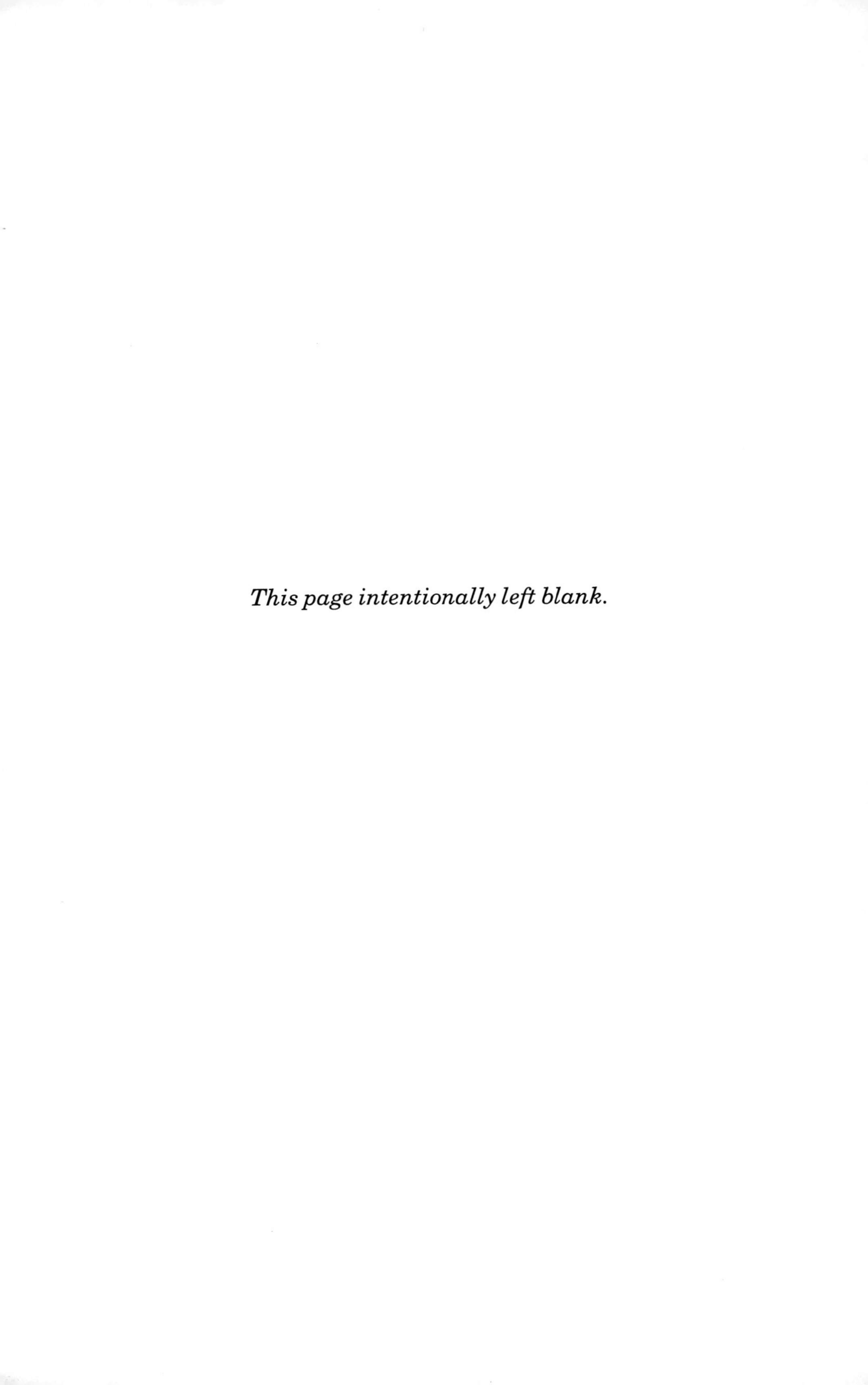

This page intentionally left blank.

1

X-Ray Generation

Production of X-Rays

X-rays are a form of electromagnetic radiation. Other forms of electromagnetic radiation include *gamma rays, radiowaves* and *visible light*. X-rays are similar to visible light with shorter wavelengths. A *wavelength* is the distance a wave can move in the time it takes to complete one cycle. The wavelength of x-rays is measured in nanometers (nm). A nanometer is equal to one-millionth of a millimeter. Medical x-rays are typically 0.05-0.01 nanometers. This short wavelength allows the x-rays to penetrate objects, whereas visible light is reflected or absorbed. Not only can x-rays be thought of as having wave form, but also they may be considered as representing small packets of energy called *quanta* or *photons*.

X-rays are generated when fast-moving electrons collide with any form of matter. The x-ray tube uses a stream of electrons directed toward a metal target. The energy of the electrons interacting with the atoms of the target is converted to heat (99%) and x-radiation (1%). Heat generation in the x-ray tube is a limiting factor in the production of x-rays. This is why higher-output x-ray machines have rotating anode x-ray tubes.

X-Ray Tube Anatomy

The x-ray tube contains a heated *filament* in the cathode where the electrons are generated and an *anode* containing a tungsten target where x-rays are generated. Both are enclosed in a vacuum-fitted glass envelope. A beryllium window in the glass envelope allows the x-rays to pass with minimal filtration. An aluminum filter is placed across the window to absorb the low-energy (soft) x-rays while allowing the more energetic and useful x-rays to form the x-ray beam. The entire tube is surrounded by oil, which acts as an electrical barrier while absorbing heat generated by the tube. The tube and oil are encased in a metal housing to prevent damage to the glass envelope and to absorb stray radiation (Fig 1).

At the *cathode* is a filament consisting of a tightly coiled tungsten wire. The cathode is housed within a *focusing cup* to focus the beam of electrons on the focal spot of the anode. As current is applied to the filament, electrons are "boiled off" and become available to be accelerated toward the anode and participate in the formation of x-rays. The hotter the filament, the more electrons that become available and, thus, more x-radiation is produced. The mA control on the machine affects the current to the cathode, and thereby controls the amount of radiation that is produced.

The anode contains a *tungsten metal plate* on which the electrons are focused. This is the site of x-ray generation. The focal spot is oriented at an 11- to 20-degree angle so that a relatively large focal

Figure 1. Anatomy of an x-ray tube. A. Cathode, B. Anode, C. Tungsten filament, D. Focusing cup, E. Accelerating electrons, F. Tungsten target, G. Glass envelope, H. Aluminum filter, I. Generated x-rays, J. Beryllium window.

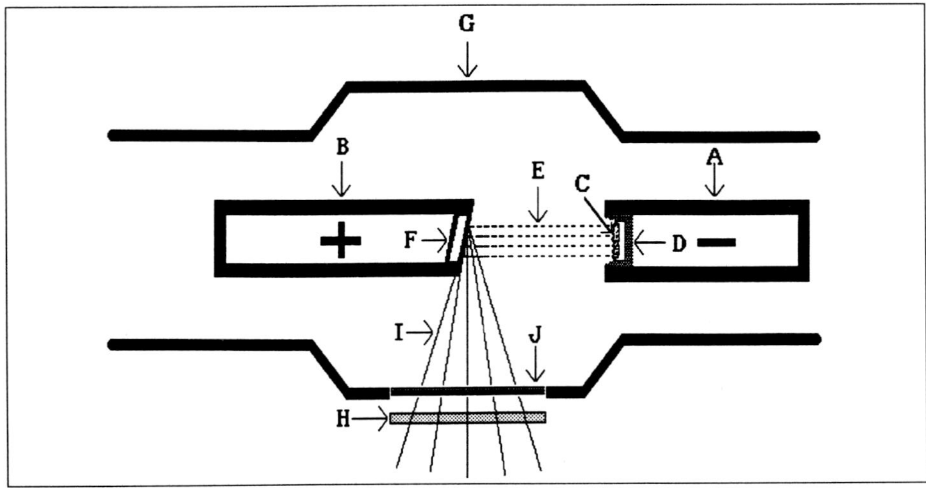

spot size is maintained while a relatively small effective focal spot size is used. This feature is inherent to the tube and cannot be changed by the operator. Small effective focal spots produce better resolution in the image but are less tolerant of heat. Remember that most of the energy used in producing x-rays is converted into heat.

The problem of heat production has caused the need for 2 types of anodes to be developed: *stationary* and *rotating. Stationary anodes* are used in low-output machines with low mA capabilities, *eg,* 5-50 mA. A block of tungsten is embedded into a block of copper on the anode side of the tube. The copper is not only a good conductor of electrical current but also helps conduct heat away from the tungsten target. A *rotating anode* is a disc-shaped piece of metal (usually molybdenum alloy) containing a tungsten insert around its periphery. This type of anode is used in higher-output machines with capabilities of 100-1200 mA. The anode rotates at a high speed during exposure to dissipate the heat over a greater surface area while maintaining a relatively small effective focal spot.

To produce x-rays, the filament in the cathode is heated to produce a cloud of electrons. The electrons are focused by the focusing cup onto the target in the focal spot area. Electrical potential is applied across the tube to accelerate electrons from the cathode and bombard the anode in the focal spot. The collision of electrons with the target causes heat and x-rays to be generated.

Transformers

High voltage potential is needed to accelerate the electrons from the cathode to the anode. The high voltage necessary on the anode side is produced by a *step-up transformer.* This transformer increases the incoming voltage (110-120 v in the case of a small portable machine and 440-880 v in a large stationary machine) up to the required 40-150 kilovolts (kv), depending on the machine. Relatively low voltage is required by the filament on the cathode side. A *step-down transformer* is used to decrease the incoming voltage but at the same time the amperage is increased to 5-1200 mA. Increasing the amperage in the filament circuit going to the cathode increases the number of electrons produced by the filament, increasing the number of x-rays produced. This means that there is a direct relationship between mA and the total number of x-rays produced.

Rectifiers

Electrical current used in the United States alternates at 60 cycles per second. The electrical potential oscillates in a positive direction for 1/120th of a second and negatively for 1/120th of a second. The complete cycle requires 1/60th of a second. Available electrical current may also be either *single phase* or *3 phase. Single-phase current* has only one flow of current cycling as described above. With *3-phase current,* 3 single-phase waves are superimposed over each other but out of synchronization by 120 degrees. The second wave starts after the first has cycled 120 degrees, then the third starts after the first has cycled 240 degrees. This overlapping pattern allows a more nearly constant maximum positive and negative oscillation of electrical current.

Electrons only flow from the cathode to the anode when positive potential (voltage) is applied across the tube. During one-half of the cycle, a negative potential is applied across the tube, resulting in no electron flow or x-rays being generated. Occasionally, rectifiers are placed in the high-voltage circuit to protect the anode from high negative voltages and the cathode from high positive voltages. Basically, the rectifers limit the electron flow to one direction, from the cathode to the anode. With low-output portable equipment, the x-ray tube itself acts as a rectifier, which is termed *self-rectification.*

There are 3 different ways that x-ray machines are rectified (Fig 2). The first method is *half-wave rectification* using single-phase current. This method allows the electrons to flow from the cathode to the anode only on the positive phase of the incoming alternating current. The disadvantage is that only the positive half of the cycle is used for x-ray production. Half-wave rectified units produce 60 pulses of x-rays per second, with each being 1/120th of a second long. Longer exposure times are necessary to produce an image. These units are found in low-output portable equipment.

The second is the *full-wave single-phase rectified unit.* With this unit not only is the positive phase used, but the negative phase is converted to a positive phase so it also can be used to produce x-rays. The full-wave rectified unit produces 120 pulses of x-rays per second. Faster exposure times can be used because twice the number of x-rays are generated per unit of time as compared with the half-wave rectified machine.

The third rectification method is the *3-phase rectified method* and is the most efficient. Using 3-phase current, a more nearly constant potential can be applied to the x-ray tube. Each phase of the current can be rectified so that 6 pulses of positive potential per cycle are used to generate x-rays. The result is a more continuous potential across the terminals of the tube, producing a higher energy of electrons and a more constant energy x-ray beam.

Tube Rating Charts

Tube rating charts prolong the life of the x-ray tube by helping the operator determine the maximum exposure characteristics that allow safe operation of the machine. The exposure characteristics are *kVp, mA, exposure time* and *focal spot size*. Extremely high and low exposure techniques should be checked on a chart provided by the x-ray tube manufacturer.

Figures 3 and 4 show tube rating charts for a 2-mm focal spot x-ray machine. The manufacturer provides a tube rating chart in one of these 2 styles. With Figure 3, plot the intersection of the kVp and the

Figure 2. Types of rectifiers. X-rays are generated only on the positive peak of the wave. A. Half-wave single-phase – 60 pulses/second, B. Full-wave single-phase – 120 pulses/second, C. 3-phase – almost continuous x-ray production.

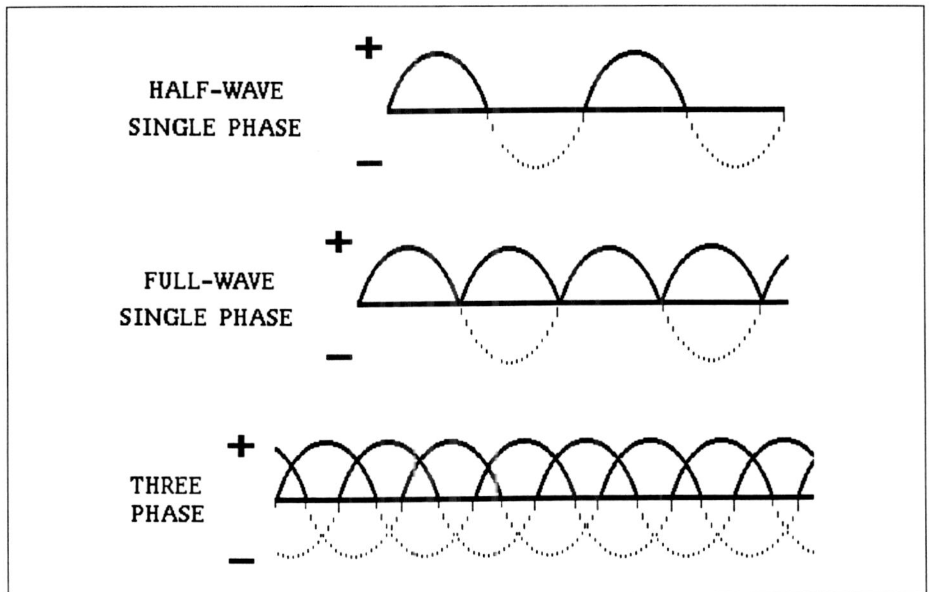

exposure time to be used. If that point falls below the mA value curve, then that exposure setting can safely be used with that machine. With Figure 4, plot the intersection of the mA and exposure time to be used. The kVp curve directly above that point represents the maximum kVp setting for that mA and exposure time.

Two types of damage may occur from an improperly set exposure technique. The first is *tube overload*. This occurs when the combined kVp and mAs are too high for the machine. Too much heat is created, causing the anode to crack. The second is *tube saturation*. This happens when there is not enough positive potential (voltage) between the cathode and anode to pull all the electrons across the tube. The extra electrons build up on the glass envelope. This "electroplating" of the glass envelope may cause it to be nearly as attractive to the electrons as the anode during a high kVp exposure. If the electrons "short" to the glass envelope and tube housing, the tube will crack and be destroyed.

Manufacturers of the larger x-ray generators usually build in tube protection circuits to protect the tube. These protection circuits usually only protect against tube overload and only extreme tube satu-

Figure 3. One type of tube rating chart provided by an x-ray tube manufacturer.

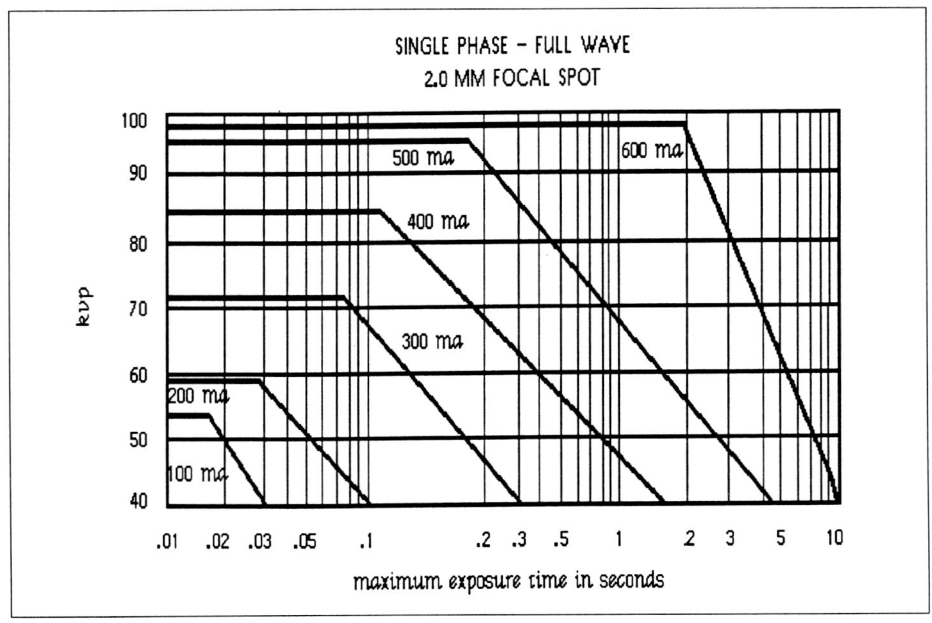

ration conditions. To protect against tube saturation, it is wise to not use mA settings over 500 with 60 kVp or less.

Another condition that contributes to electroplating of the glass envelope is an overly long time between starting the rotating anode and making the exposure. When the x-ray machine is on but no exposures are being made, there is a very low current applied to the filament in the cathode. When the rotating anode is started, the current is boosted up to the full mA that is selected. Electrons are boiled off from the filament and made available for the exposure. If an excessive filament boost is used and a low kilovoltage is selected, all of the electrons that are produced are not attracted to the anode. The excess electrons contribute to the electroplating of the glass envelope.

Anode Heel Effect

The *anode heel effect* is the unequal distribution of the x-ray beam intensity emitted from the x-ray tube. Tubes with lower target angles, *eg,* 11 degrees, have a distribution of x-ray beam intensity that decreases rapidly on the anode side of the tube (Fig 5). This is caused

Figure 4. Another type of tube rating chart provided by an x-ray tube manufacturer.

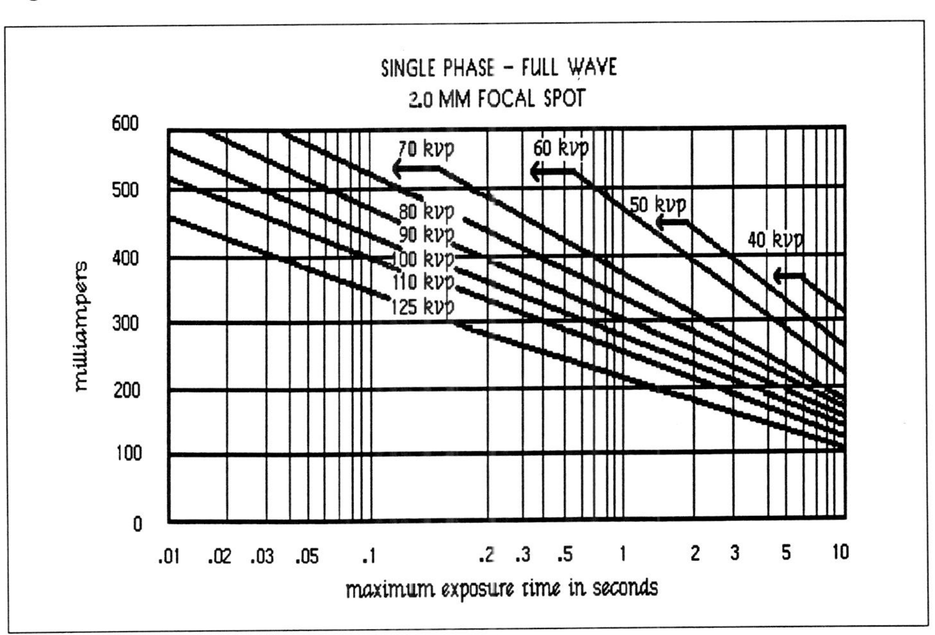

by absorption of the x-ray beam by target and anode material. This can be advantageous when radiographing areas of unequal thickness, such as the thorax or abdomen. By placing the patient's head toward the anode side, the part of the x-ray beam with the higher intensity (cathode side) is directed to the thickest area. This produces a more even film density. The heel effect is most noticeable when large films and short focal-film distances are used.

Summary

By understanding how the x-ray machine works in a general way, it is much easier to understand how the x-ray machine controls may be used to produce high-quality radiographs. There are 3 basic controls on an x-ray machine that the user routinely must adjust for proper exposure. They are kVp, mA and exposure time. Think of kVp as controlling mainly the *quality* of the x-ray beam. The higher the kVp, the more potential is applied across the terminals of the x-ray tube. The electrons hit the target "harder" and produce a more energetic (more penetrating) x-ray. Think of mA and exposure time both affecting the *quantity* of x-rays produced. If you double the mA,

Figure 5. The anode heel effect. The x-ray beam intensity decreases toward the anode side because of absorption by the target and anode material.

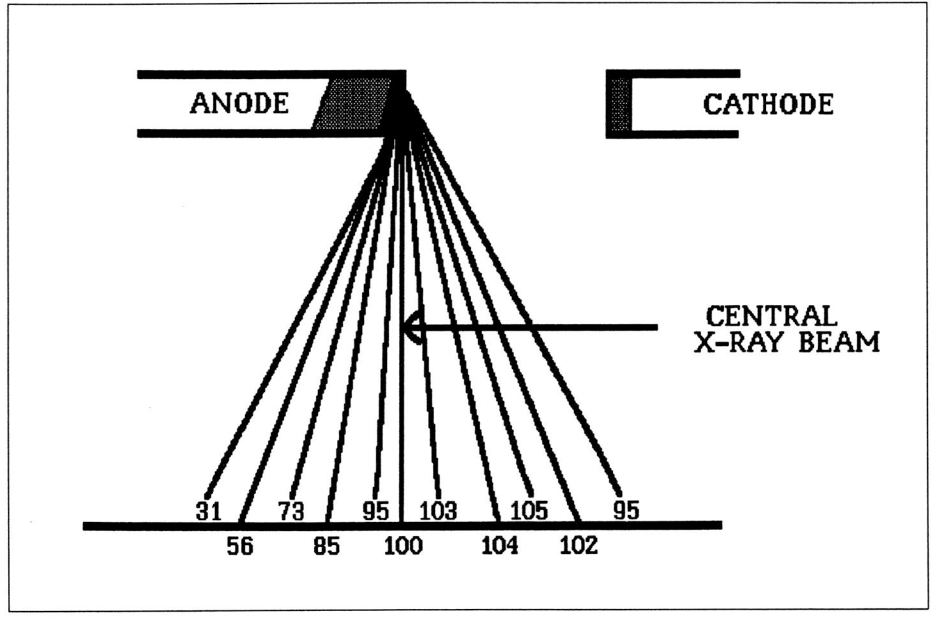

you double the amount of electrons boiled off at the filament and double the number of x-rays produced. If you double the exposure time, you also double the number of x-rays produced because the electrons have more time to bombard the target and produce x-rays.

Both mA and exposure time work together, as will be explained later in this text. They have a linear effect on film density. For example, if you double the mA or the time, the film density is doubled. Conversely, if you halve the mA or time, the film density is half as much.

Recommended Reading

Curry TS III *et al: Christensen's Physics of Diagnostic Radiology.* 4th ed. Lea & Febiger, Philadelphia, 1990. pp 10-60.

Douglas SW *et al: Principles of Veterinary Radiography.* 4th ed. Bailliere Tindall, London, 1987. pp 3-18.

Eastman Kodak: *The Fundamentals of Radiology.* 12th ed. Eastman Kodak Company, Rochester, NY, 1992. pp 5-13.

Morgan JP and Silverman S: *Techniques of Veterinary Radiography.* 3rd ed. Veterinary Radiology Associates, Davis, 1982. pp 1-24.

Ticer JW: *Radiographic Technique in Veterinary Practice.* 2nd ed. Saunders, Philadelphia, 1984. pp 3-11.

Notes

Notes

2

Achieving Radiographic Quality

Radiographic Density

Radiograph density is the degree of blackness on a radiograph. The dark areas are made up of black metallic silver deposits on the finished radiograph. These deposits occur in areas where x-rays have penetrated the patient and exposed the emulsion of the film (Fig 1). Radiographic density can be increased either by increasing the mA or the exposure time. Both increase the number of x-rays produced by increasing the number of electrons in the electron cloud or the amount of time the electrons are allowed to travel from the cathode to the anode. A higher kVp produces more radiographic density by increasing the penetrating power of the x-ray beam.

Radiographic Contrast

Radiographic contrast is defined as the differences in radiographic density between adjacent areas on a radiographic image. Radiographs that show a long scale of contrast have a few black and white shades, with many shades of gray. On the other hand, with a short scale of contrast there are black and white shades with only a few shades of gray in between. For most studies a long scale of contrast is desired.

The amount of radiographic contrast depends on 4 factors: subject density, kVp level, film contrast and film fogging.

Subject density is the ability of the different tissue densities to absorb x-rays. X-rays penetrate the various tissues, depending on the differences in atomic number and thickness. These tissues are listed from least dense to most dense: air, fat, water/muscle, bone, metal (Fig 2). Bone containing mainly calcium and phosphorous has a high average atomic number as compared with muscle, which contains mainly hydrogen and nitrogen. Bone absorbs more x-rays than muscle and appears whiter on the finished radiograph. The thickness of the area also affects the amount of x-rays that are absorbed. If you radiograph an area that ranges from 3 cm to 15 cm in thickness, the area measuring 15 cm in thickness absorbs more x-rays than the 3-cm area.

Radiographic contrast can be increased or decreased by increasing or decreasing the kVp. The higher the kVp, the longer the scale of contrast (the more grays that can be visualized). Radiographs made with a high kVp have more exposure latitude. Minor errors in technique still produce a diagnostic radiograph.

Figure 1. Image 1 displays more radiographic density than Image 5. This means Image 1 was exposed with a higher mAs.

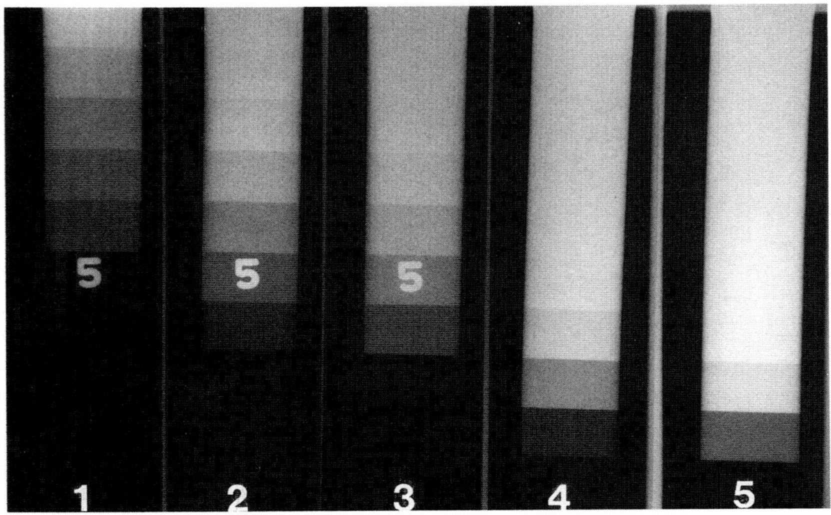

Film contrast is also a factor that affects the radiographic contrast. Some types of film have an inherent capability of producing a long scale of contrast or long latitude. Long-latitude film allows for more variation in technique while still producing a diagnostic radiograph. The scale of contrast can be shortened by changing the exposure technique when using long-latitude film. However, the scale of contrast cannot be lengthened when using contrast film (film that produces a short scale of contrast).

Film fogging can greatly decrease the radiographic contrast by decreasing the differences in densities between 2 adjacent shadows (Fig 3). Care must be taken in the storage and handling of the film to prevent fogging. Films can become fogged from low-grade light leaks into the darkroom, scatter radiation, heat and improper processing.

Radiographic Detail

A diagnostic radiograph is one with good radiographic detail. Good radiographic detail is characterized by sharp tissue and organ inter-

Figure 2. Subject densities: 1. air, 2. fat, 3. water/muscle, 4. bone, 5. metal. Air is the least dense, allowing the x-rays to penetrate and expose the film. Metal is the most dense, absorbing most of the x-rays and allowing only a few to penetrate, exposing the film.

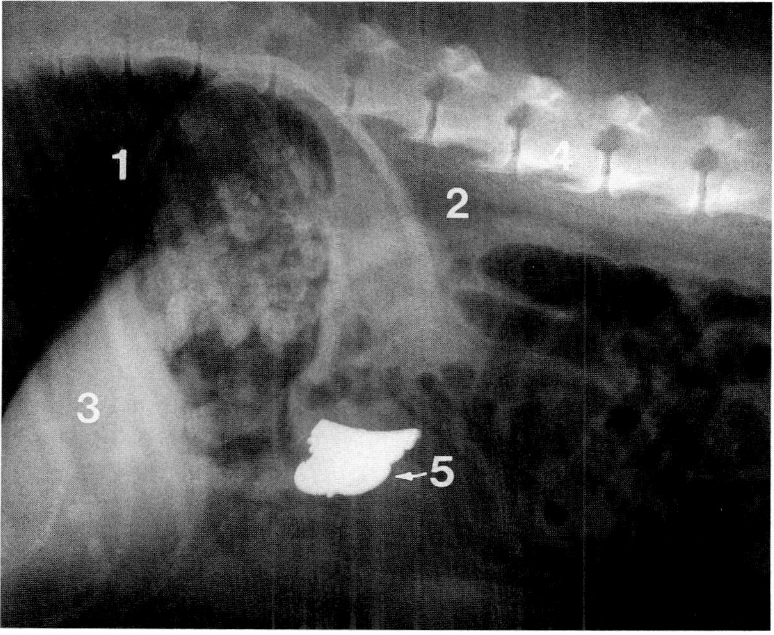

faces. Many factors can affect the detail on a radiograph. Two of the most common are patient motion and the penumbra effect.

Patient motion causes loss of detail because of blurred interfaces. It is generally a result of a long exposure time combined with motion of the patient (Fig 4). This can be controlled by using the shortest possible exposure time. If that is not adequate, then sedation of the patient is recommended.

A loss of detail is also caused by the *penumbra effect*. Excessive penumbra causes blurring at the edges of the shadows cast by the x-ray exposure. There are 3 main factors in the amount of penumbra on a radiograph. Changes in these factors increase or decrease the radiographic detail.

The first is the *size of the focal spot*. The larger the focal spot, the more pronounced the penumbra effect (Fig 5). Decreasing the focal spot size decreases the penumbra; however, this is not something that can be changed on most equipment. Manufacturers design the focal spot size as small as possible without losing the ability to dissipate heat effectively.

Figure 3. This radiograph was fogged from scatter radiation. This decreases the differences in densities between 2 adjacent shadows.

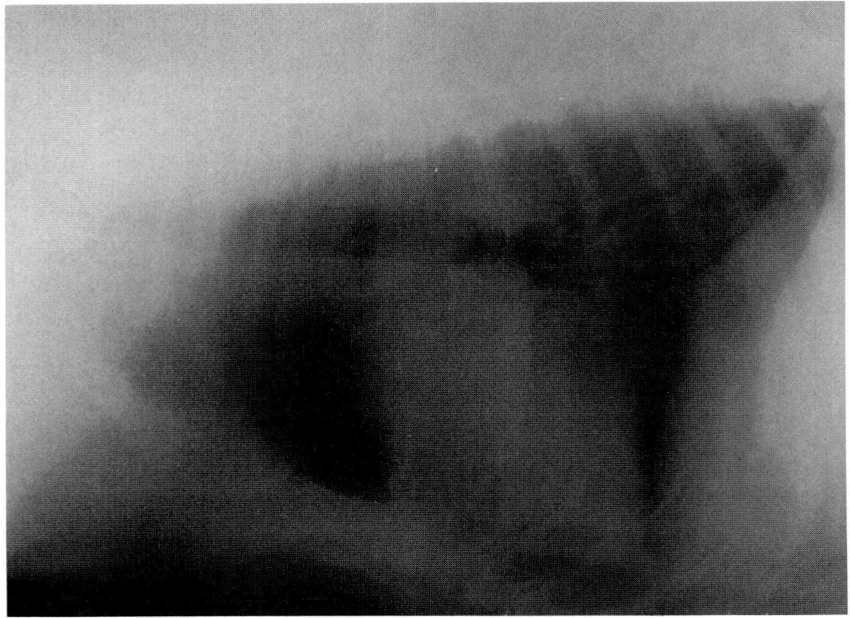

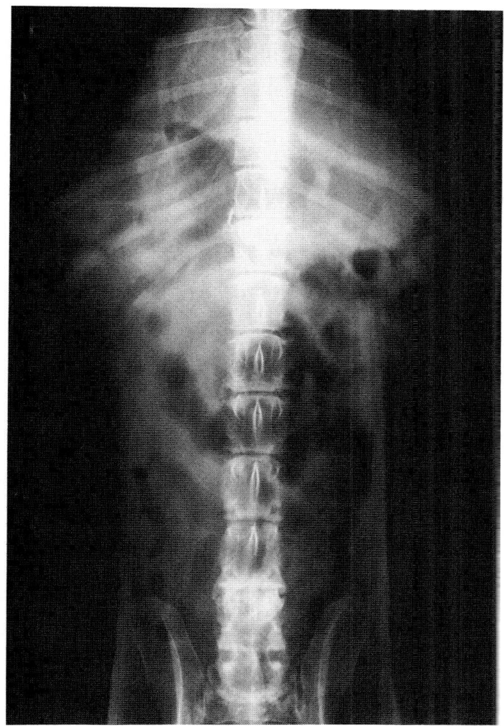

Figure 4. A long exposure time with an animal that is panting causes a decrease in detail because of blurring from patient motion.

Figure 5. Increasing the size of the focal spot increases the amount of penumbra, decreasing radiographic detail.

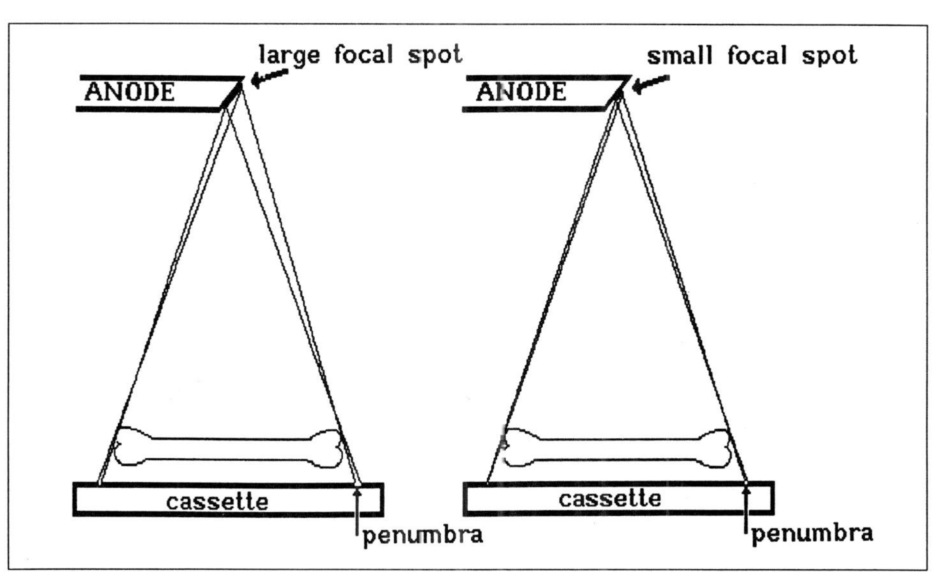

Another factor that affects the amount of penumbra is the *focal-film distance* (FFD). This is the distance from the target to the film. The penumbra effect can be decreased by increasing the FFD (Fig 6). There is a limit to this because of what is stated in the Inverse Square Law. The intensity decreases at a rate inverse to the square of the distance. In simpler terms, if the FFD is doubled, the mAs must increase 4 times to maintain the radiographic density. In most cases this is not practical because the shortest possible exposure times are necessary to counteract patient motion. A FFD of 36-40 inches is sufficient to minimize the penumbra effect.

The third factor affecting penumbra is the *object-film distance* (OFD). This is the distance between the object that is being imaged and the film. The penumbra is decreased by keeping the OFD as short as possible (Fig 7). By using a combination of these factors, the penumbra is minimized and good radiographic detail can be achieved.

Distortion

A diagnostic radiograph must accurately record the size, shape and location of the anatomic structures of the patient. Distortion occurs when there is a misrepresentation of these factors. Therefore it is

Figure 6. Increasing the focal-film distance (FFD) decreases the amount of penumbra, increasing radiographic detail.

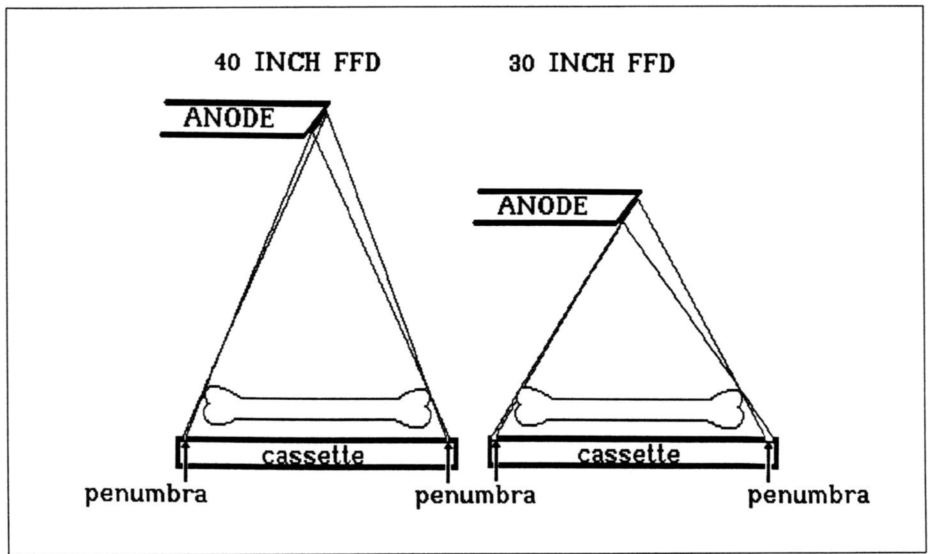

important to understand how the x-rays project anatomic structures on the film.

Foreshortening occurs when the object is not parallel to the recording surface. This distorts the size of the object by shortening the length of the object (Fig 8). This occurs mainly when imaging long bones, such as the humerus or femur. If one end of the bone is farther away from the recording surface than the other, the bone appears shorter.

Not only must the object be parallel to the recording surface, but also the OFD must be as short as possible. Increasing the OFD increases the penumbra and greatly magnifies the size of the object (Fig 9). The amount of magnification increases as the distance to the recording surface increases.

It is important to accurately project areas between a series of radiodense and radiolucent objects. The vertebral column is a good example. The vertebrae must be parallel to the recording surface. When radiographing the cervical vertebrae in lateral recumbency, if the patient is allowed to lie naturally, the mid-cervical vertebrae tend to sag. This produces a false narrowing of the intervertebral disk spaces (Fig 10). A small amount of padding brings the vertebral

Figure 7. Increasing the object-film distance (OFD) increases the amount of penumbra, decreasing radiographic detail.

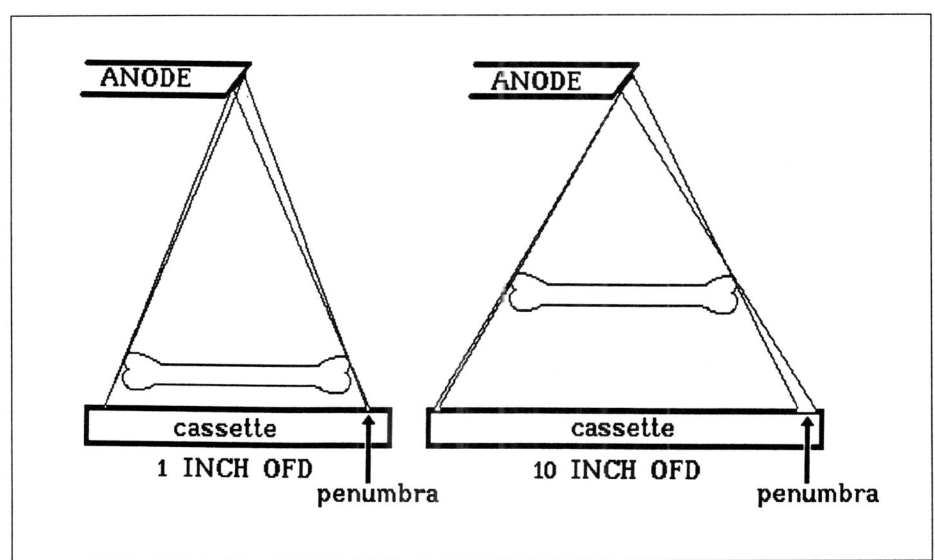

column parallel the recording surface (Fig 11). Care must be taken not to use too much padding because this elevates the column, also producing a false narrowing of the intervertebral disk spaces.

Distortion can occur when the x-ray beam is not perpendicular to the recording surface. The x-rays in the center of the primary beam penetrate perpendicular to the intervertebral disk spaces. As the distance from the center of of the primary beam increases, the x-rays strike the intervetebral disk spaces at an increasing angle. A false narrowing of the intervertebral disk space occurs because of this increase in distance from the center of the primary beam (Fig 12). Sometimes it is necessary to make multiple images of the vertebral column, centering the primary beam over multiple areas. This type of distortion is also apparent when radiographing complex joints, such as the stifle and elbow. When imaging these areas, the primary beam should be centered directly over the joint.

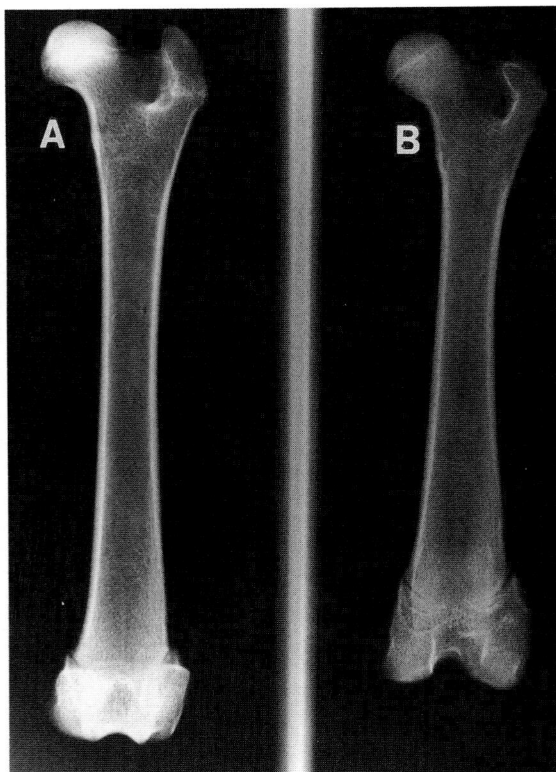

Figure 8. Foreshortening. The same femur was used for both images. With Image A the femur was parallel to the cassette. With Image B the distal end of the femur was elevated 5 inches, placing the femur at a 45-degree angle to the cassette. Notice Image B appears shorter than Image A.

Scatter Radiation

When an x-ray photon strikes an object, it does 1 of 3 things. It penetrates the object, it is absorbed by the object or it produces scatter radiation (Fig 13). *Scatter radiation* does not contribute to formation of the useful image. It fogs the film, greatly decreasing contrast. It also is a safety hazard to the patient and personnel. Scatter radiation

Figure 9. Magnification. The same skull was used for both images. With Image A the skull was placed directly on the cassette (0" OFD). With Image B the skull was elevated 10" (10" OFD). Notice that Image B is larger and there is decreased detail, especially around the tympanic bulla and carnassial tooth.

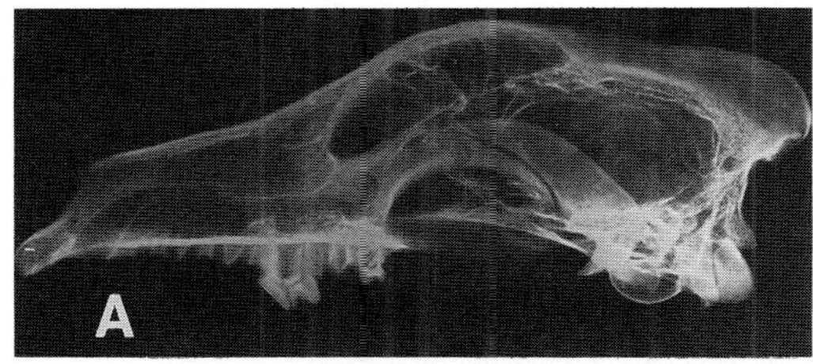

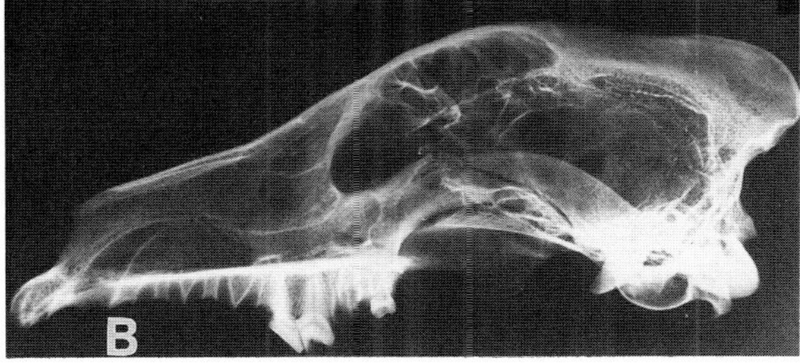

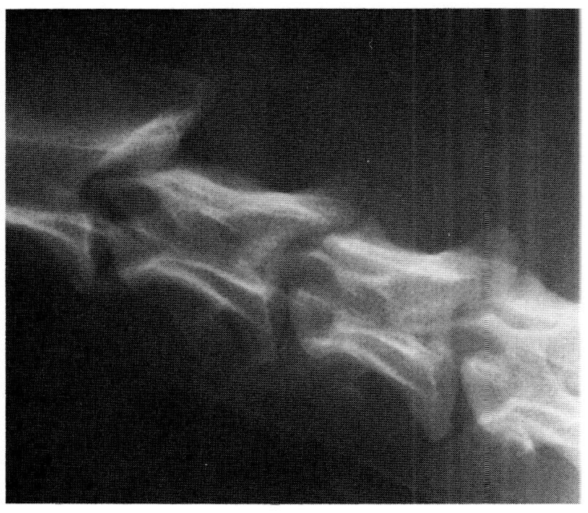

Figure 10. A false narrowing of the intervertebral disk spaces occurs when the vertebrae are not parallel to the recording surface.

has a longer wavelength than the primary beam and is projected in all directions. Because it has a long wavelength and is less energetic, it is likely to be absorbed by the next object it strikes, whether it is the patient, personnel or the cassette.

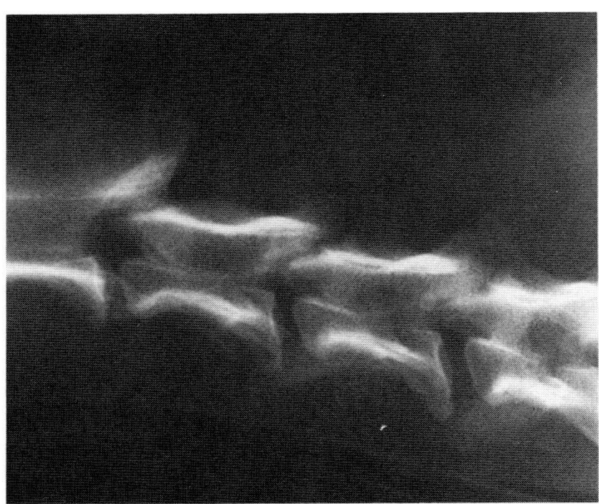

Figure 11. The vertebrae are placed parallel to the recording surface by padding under the neck. Notice the size of the intervertebral disk spaces when compared with Figure 10.

Figure 12. The intervertebral disk spaces appear narrow toward the edges of the radiograph when compared with the disk spaces in the center of the radiograph.

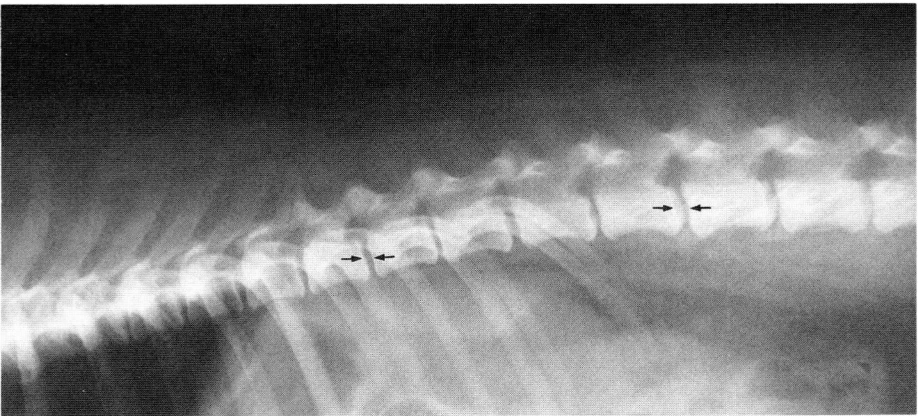

Exposure techniques using a high kVp produce more scatter radiation. The thickness of the area being imaged dictates the amount of kVp needed. Objects greater than 9 cm thick produce enough scatter radiation to significantly decrease the detail on the radiograph.

Beam-limiting devices are commonly used to decrease scatter radiation. These devices confine the primary beam to the area being examined. There are several types of beam-limitation devices available. *Cones* are lead cylinders of fixed size and are placed over the collimator on the x-ray tube head. A cone restricts the primary beam to the size of the cone being used.

Diaphragms are sheets of lead with rectangular, square or circular openings. They have a fixed size and fit on the tube head near the tube window. They limit the size of the primary beam to the size of the diaphragm being used.

Collimators consist of lead shutters installed in the tube head of the x-ray machine. They are adjustable and have a light that allows visualization of the actual size of the primary beam field.

Finally, *filters* are used to absorb the less penetrating or soft x-rays as they leave the tube head. They are made of a thin sheet of aluminum and are placed over the tube window.

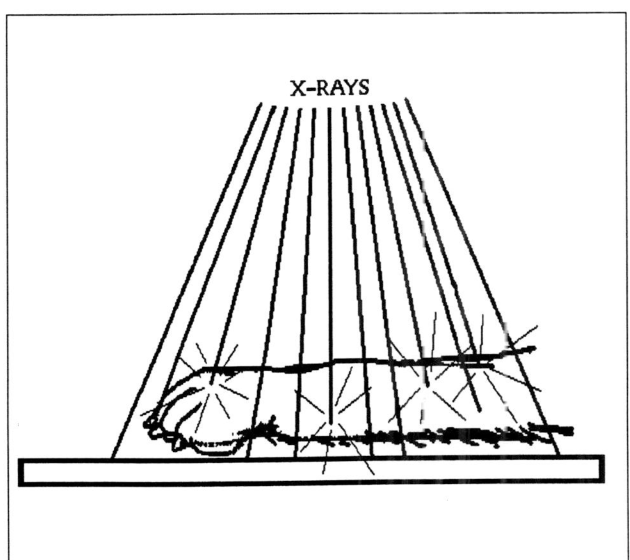

Figure 13. X-ray photons penetrate the object, are absorbed by the object, and produce scatter radiation.

Grids

Grids are used to decrease scatter radiation and increase the contrast on the radiograph. As the thickness of the area being imaged increases, the amount of kVp required also increases. The higher the kVp, the more scatter radiation that is produced. To eliminate the increase of scatter radiation, grids are necessary when imaging objects with a thickness of 9 cm or greater (Fig 14).

A grid is a series of thin, linear strips made of alternating radiodense and radiolucent material. The radiodense strips are made of lead, while the radiolucent interspacers are plastic, aluminum or fiber. The grid is placed between the patient and the cassette. X-rays that penetrate the patient and pass in perfect alignment between the lead strips expose the film. Scatter radiation diverges in all directions and is more likely to be absorbed by one of the lead strips.

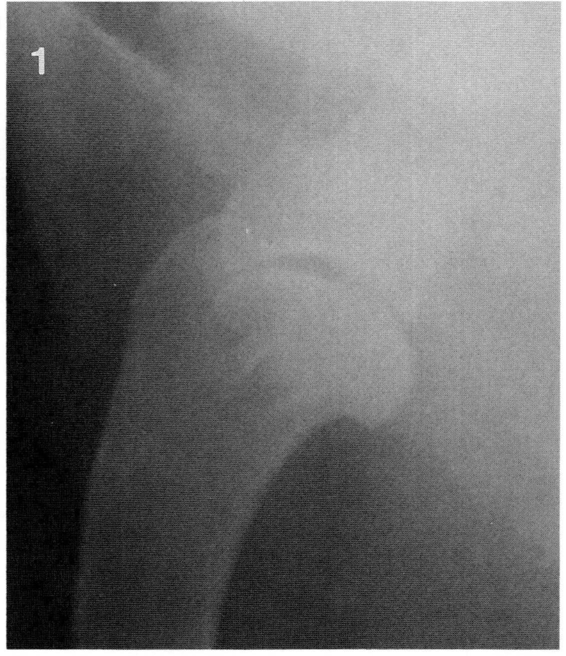

Figure 14. Non-grid vs grid technique. Both images are of the same subject measuring 12 cm. Image 1 was exposed using a tabletop technique. Image 2 was exposed using a grid. Notice the increase in contrast and decrease in scatter with Image 2.

The grid also absorbs a portion of the usable x-rays. To compensate for this loss, the number of x-rays generated must be increased by increasing the mAs. Depending on the type of grid used, the increase may be up to 6.6 times the mAs that was required for the tabletop exposure.

Grid Ratio

Grid efficiency is dependent on *grid ratio*. The grid ratio is the relationship of the height of the lead strips to the space between them. For example, a grid with lead strips that are 2.5 mm high and 0.5 mm apart has a 5:1 grid ratio. The higher the grid ratio, the more efficient the grid is in absorbing scatter radiation. Therefore, a grid with a 5:1 ratio is less efficient than a 10:1 grid ratio. However, grids with high ratios not only absorb more scatter, they also absorb more of the

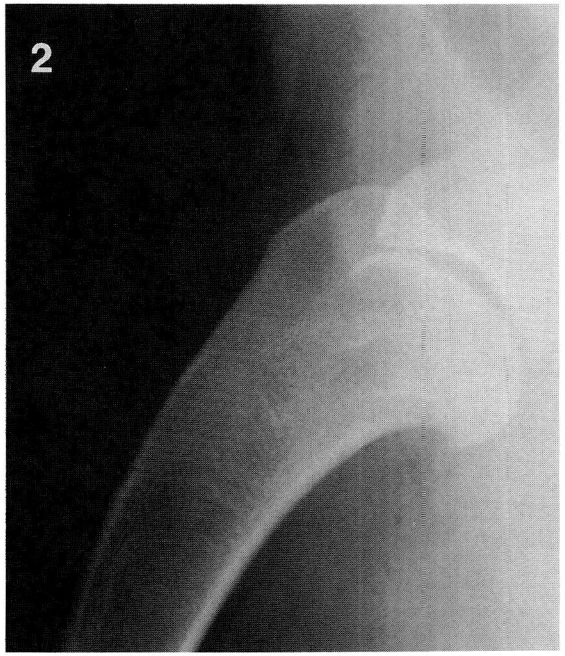

Figure 14, continued.

available x-rays. Therefore, a greater increase in mAs is necessary with the more efficient high-ratio grids.

Types of Grids

Grids are manufactured with either parallel or focused lead strips. These 2 types are made with a crossed or a linear configuration (Fig 15).

Parallel grids have the lead strips placed perpendicular to the grid surface. The x-rays and scatter radiation that interact with the lead strips are absorbed, while the ones that interact with the interspacers pass through to expose the film. A disadvantage of a parallel grid is that the x-ray beam diverges at increasing angles and is absorbed at the periphery of the grid. This decreases the amount of x-rays reaching the film nearer the grid edges, commonly called "grid cutoff." The higher the grid ratio, the more pronounced the grid cutoff.

Focused grids have the lead strips placed at progressively increasing angles to match the divergence of the x-ray beam (Fig 16). By angling the lead strips, the cutoff of the primary beam is eliminated and the density of the radiograph is uniform. For the focused grid to be effective, there is distance or "window" of distances set up by the manufacturer called the *grid focal distance*. Setting the FFD outside of the grid's focal distance produces primary beam cutoff on the

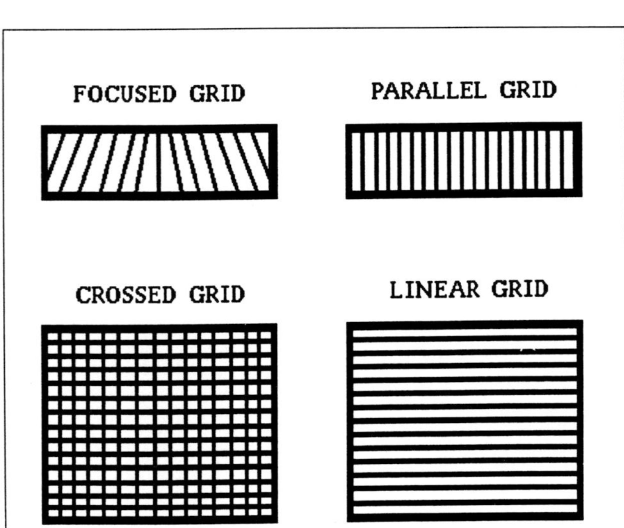

Figure 15. Grids are manufactured with parallel or focused lead strips. These 2 types are made with linear or crossed configurations.

periphery of the radiograph. Cutoff of the primary beam also occurs if the grid is not perpendicular to or centered with the x-ray tube (Fig 17).

Linear grids have the lead strips placed parallel to each other. The grid is placed so the lead strips are parallel with the length of the

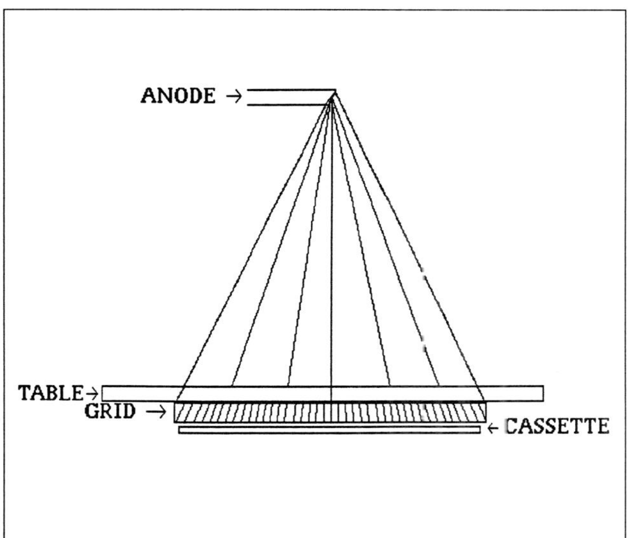

Figure 16. Focused grids contain lead strips placed with progressively increasing angles to match the divergence of the x-ray beam.

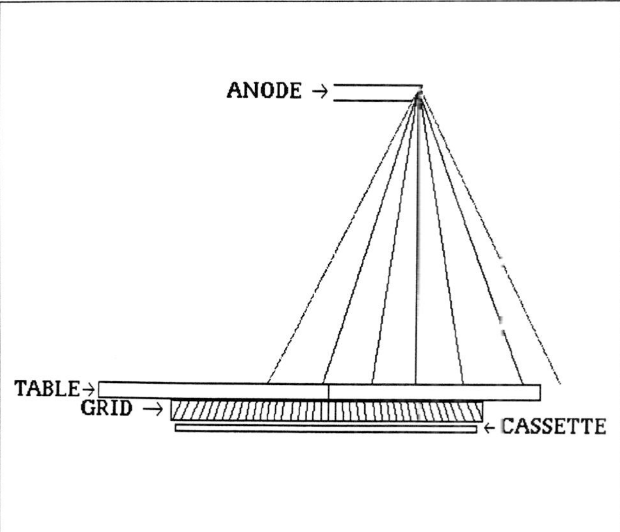

Figure 17. When a grid is not centered with the x-ray tube, grid cutoff occurs. This produces visible grid lines more prominently on one end of the film and an overall decrease in radiographic density.

table. With linear grids the primary x-ray beam can be angled along the length of the grid without absorption of x-rays by the lead strips.

Crossed grids have 2 linear grids placed on top of one another. The lead strips on the top grid cross those on the bottom grid. This type of grid removes more scatter radiation than the linear grid. However, the tube cannot be tilted without producing cutoff. Because crossed grids contain more lead, more x-rays are absorbed, requiring a higher mAs than used with linear grids.

Eliminating Grid Lines

Grids produce thin white lines on the finished radiograph. Visibility of the grid lines can be decreased 3 ways. First, they can be decreased by making the lead strips as thin as possible while retaining their ability to effectively absorb scatter radiation. The thinner the lead strips, the thinner the white line produced on the radiograph.

The second way is to increase the number of lines per inch, making the individual lines less visible. To increase the lines per inch and keep the thickness of the lead the same, the width of the radiolucent strips must be decreased. This produces a grid with more lead in it, which absorbs more of the primary beam and requires a higher mAs. A grid with 80-100 lines per inch is sufficient to make the grid lines less visible.

The third way is by using a *Potter-Bucky diaphragm,* also called a Bucky. This device sets the grid in motion, blurring the white grid lines on the radiograph. The distance and speed of travel are sufficient so that the lines are not seen on the film. The Bucky is placed in a cabinet beneath the x-ray table with a tray to hold the cassette. When using a grid in combination with a Bucky, fewer lines per inch are necessary. This allows for a lower mAs. One disadvantage of using a Bucky mechanism in veterinary medicine is the noise and vibration that it produces. Some animals may object to this and struggle or move during the x-ray exposure.

Air Gap Technique

Scatter radiation can also be reduced with use of the *air gap technique.* This method is most useful in large animal radiography, for which use of a grid cassette may not be possible. With this technique the FFD is increased to 6 feet and the OFD is increased to 6 inches. By increasing the OFD, the amount of scatter radiation reaching the cassette is decreased. Increasing the FFD decreases the penumbra and magnification that occurs with a greater OFD. The air gap acts somewhat like a grid by allowing the scatter radiation to bypass the cassette (Fig 18).

Figure 18. Air gap technique. By increasing the object-film distance to 6 inches, the scatter is allowed to pass by the cassette, not affecting the film. Then, increasing the focal-film distance to 72 inches decreases the magnification and penumbra that occurred from increasing the object-film distance.

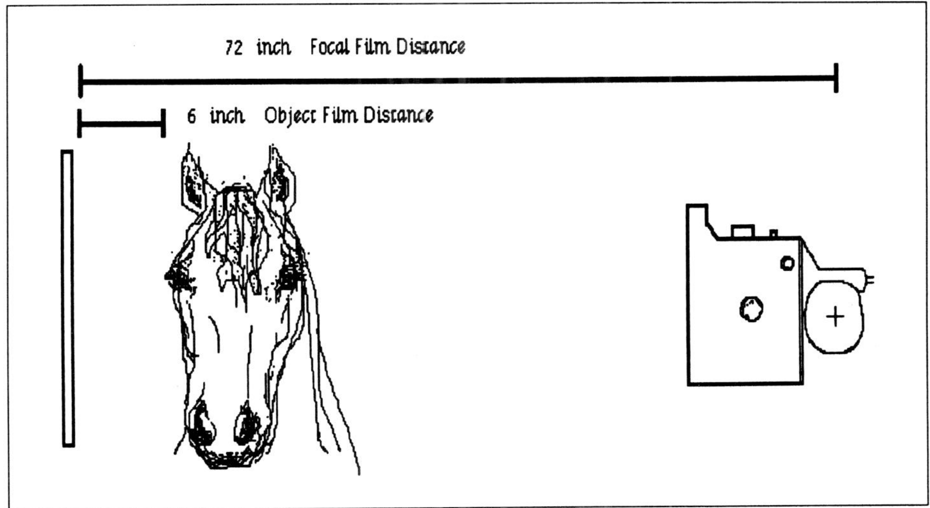

Recommended Reading

Curry TS III *et al: Christensen's Physics of Diagnostic Radiology.* 4th ed. Lea & Febiger, Philadelphia, 1990. pp 61-117.

Douglas SW *et al: Principles of Veterinary Radiography.* 4th ed. Bailliere Tindall, London, 1987. pp 42-54, pp 69-70.

Eastman Kodak: *The Fundamentals of Radiogrcphy.* 12th ed. Eastman Kodak, Rochester, NY, 1992. pp 17-33.

Liebel-Flarsheim: *Characteristics and Applications of X-ray Grids.* Liebel-Flarsheim, Cincinnati, 1989.

Morgan JP and Silverman S: *Techniques of Veterinary Radiography.* 3rd ed. Veterinary Radiology Associates, Davis, 1982. pp 36-53.

Myer W: Radiography review: radiographic density. *J Am Vet Radiol Soc* 18:138-140, 1977.

Ticer JW: *Radiographic Technique in Veterinary Practice.* 2nd ed. Saunders, Philadelphia, 1984. pp 12-28.

Wrigley RH and Borak TB: The effect of kVp on the dose equivalent from scattered radiation by radiography personnel. *Vet Radiol* 24:181-182, 1983.

28

Notes

3

Exposure Variables

Four exposure factors control the radiographic density, contrast and detail. These are *mAs, kVp, focal-film distance* and *object-film distance*. Changing one of these factors usually requires adjustments in another factor in order to maintain the same radiographic density.

mAs

The mAs is a product of the milliamperage and the exposure time. The *milliamperage* controls the number of electrons in the electron cloud generated at the filament of the cathode. This is done by controlling the temperature of the cathode filament. When the milliamperage (mA) is increased, the temperature of the filament is increased, producing more electrons to form the electron cloud. Increasing the mA increases the amount of radiographic density because more x-rays are generated.

The other factor is the *time* the electron current is allowed to flow from the cathode to the anode. By varying the exposure time, the total number of x-rays generated is controlled. Using a longer exposure time allows the electrons more time to cross from the cathode to the anode, generating more x-rays.

mA and exposure time are inversely related. The higher the mA, the shorter the exposure time required to maintain the desired number of x-rays generated. Many different combinations of mA and time can produce the same mAs. For example,

$$300 \text{ mA at } 1/60 \text{ sec} = 5 \text{ mAs}$$
$$200 \text{ mA at } 1/40 \text{ sec} = 5 \text{ mAs}$$
$$100 \text{ mA at } 1/20 \text{ sec} = 5 \text{ mAs}$$

When faced with a choice of which mAs to use, always choose the one with the highest mA and the fastest exposure time. The mAs can be used to adjust the radiographic density by following these rules:

- *To double the radiographic density, double the mAs.*
- *To halve the radiographic density, halve the mAs.*

kVp

The *kilovoltage peak* (kVp) is the voltage applied between the cathode and the anode. It is used to accelerate the electrons toward

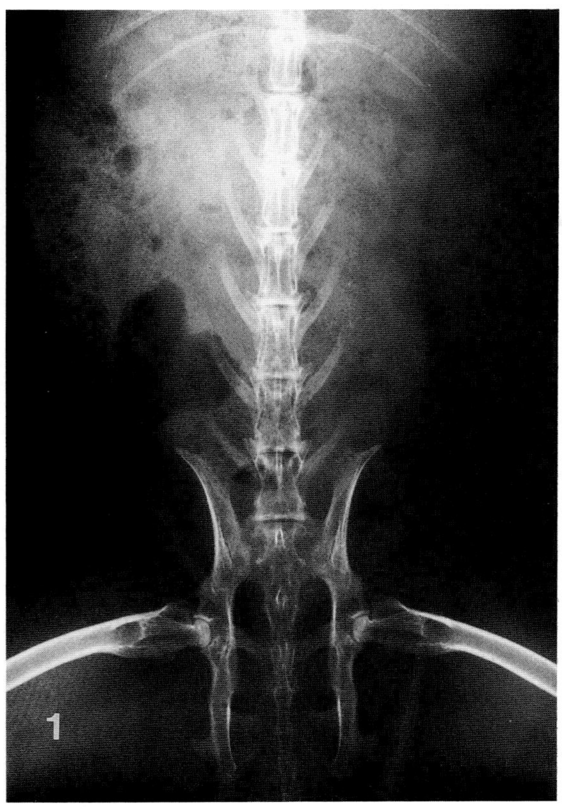

Figure 1. The radiographic density can be doubled by doubling the mAs or halved by halving the mAs. Image 1 (left) was exposed at 8 mAs and 56 kVp. Image 2 (next page) was exposed at 16 mAs and 56 kVp. Image 2 has more radiographic density than Image 1 because the mAs was double that of Image 1.

the target. The negatively charged electron cloud is on the cathode side. Increasing the kVp increases the positive charge on the anode. This causes the electrons to move across faster, increasing the force of the collision with the target. The result is a shorter-wavelength x-ray beam, with more penetrating power.

The correct kVp setting is determined by the thickness of the part being imaged. The thicker the part, the higher the kVp setting required because more penetration is needed. A higher kVp gives a longer scale of contrast and more exposure latitude. A greater exposure latitude allows for more variation in exposure factors that would still produce a diagnostic radiograph.

As with mAs, there are rules when changing the radiographic density with kVp:

- *To double the radiographic density, increase the kVp by 20%.*

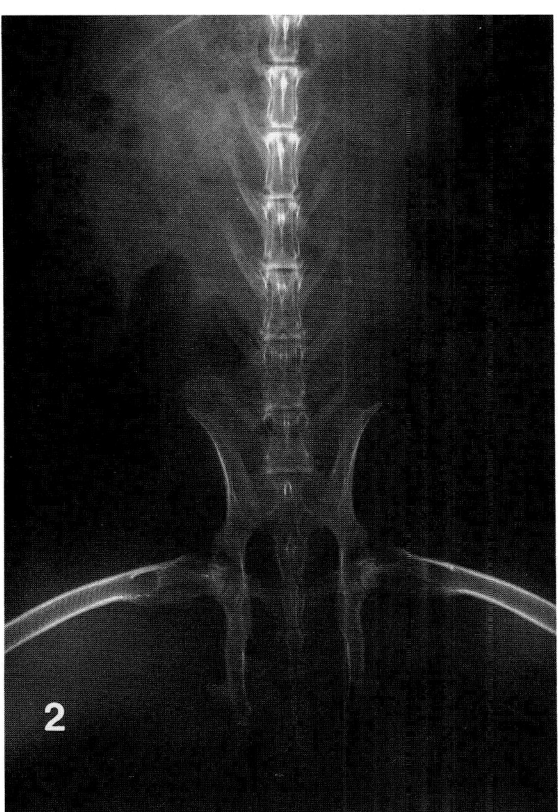

Figure 1, continued.

- *To halve the radiographic density, decrease the kVp by 16%.*

Focal-Film Distance

Focal-film distance (FFD) is the distance from the target to the recording surface (cassette). For most radiographic procedures this distance is held constant, around 36-40 inches. There may be situations where the FFD must be changed. This requires changing one of the other factors to maintain the radiographic density.

The Inverse Square Law states that the intensity of the x-ray beam is inversely proportional to the square of the distance from the source of the x-ray. This means that if the FFD is doubled, the mAs must be increased 4 times to maintain radiographic density. The same number of x-rays must diverge, covering an area that is 4 times as large.

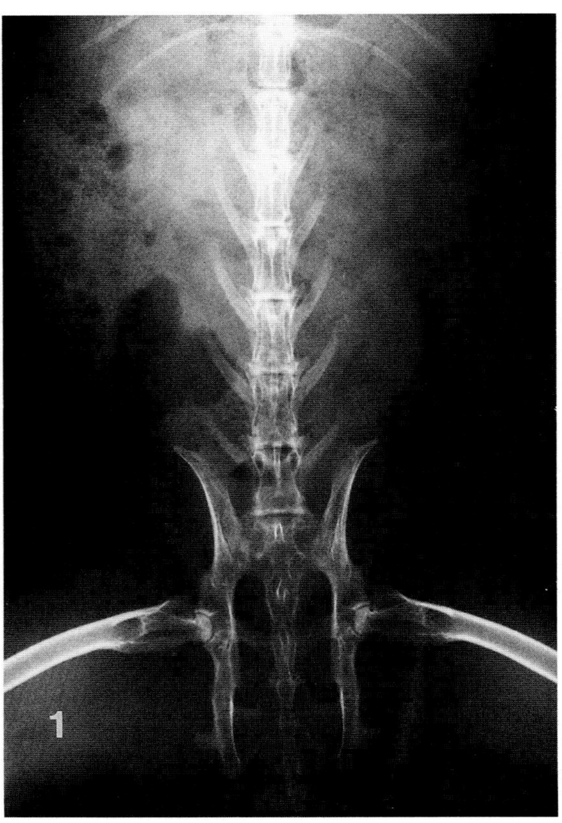

Figure 2. The radiographic density can be doubled by increasing the kVp 20% or radiographic density can be halved by decreasing the kVp 16%. Image 1 (left) was exposed at 8 mAs and 56 kVp. Image 2 (next page) was exposed at 8 mAs and 64 kVp. The kVp was increased 20% from Image 1 to Image 2, while the mAs remained constant. Image 2 has double the radiographic density of Image 1.

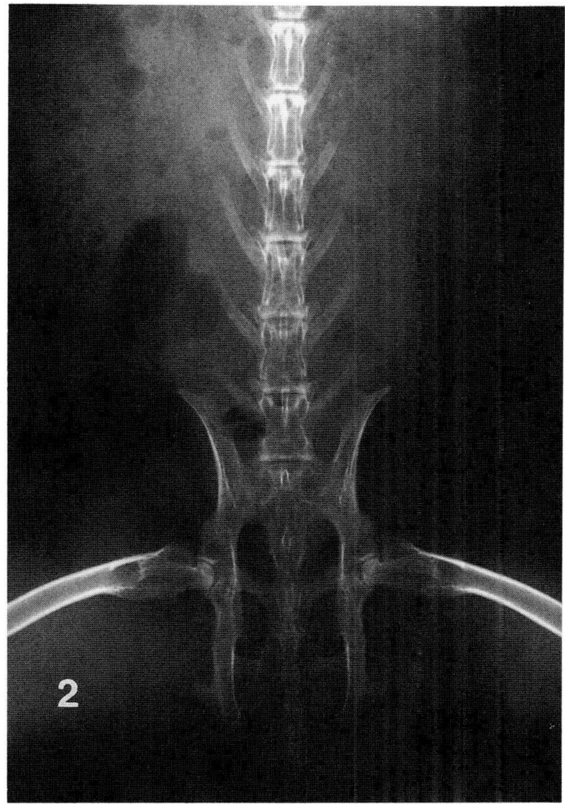

Figure 2, continued.

Changing the FFD does not affect the penetrating power of the x-ray beam, so kVp remains constant.

Object-Film Distance

The *object-film distance* (OFD) is the distance from the object being imaged to the recording surface (film). This distance should be as short as possible to minimize the penumbra effect and the magnification that occurs with a large OFD.

Recommended Reading

Curry TS III *et al: Christensen's Physics of Diagnostic Radiology.* 4th ed. Lea & Febiger, Philadelphia, 1990. pp 29-35.

Eastman-Kodak: *The Fundamentals of Radiology* 12th ed. Eastman Kodak, Rochester, NY, 1992. pp 14-19.

Ticer JW: *Radiographic Technique in Veterinary Practice.* 2nd ed. Saunders, Philadelphia, 1984. pp 55-59.

34

Notes

4

Recording the Image

When x-rays generated by an x-ray tube are directed toward an object, part of the x-rays interact with the object and part are deflected or absorbed. Some pass through the object. Use of x-ray film and intensifying screens provides a method of recording an image created by varying degrees of x-ray penetration within the patient.

X-Ray Film

X-ray film consists of several layers: a thin protective layer, an emulsion containing silver halide crystals, and a polyester film base (Fig 1).

The first layer is a thin, clear *gelatin* that acts as a protective coating. This protective material helps to decrease damage to the sensitive film emulsion.

Figure 1. Layers of the x-ray film.

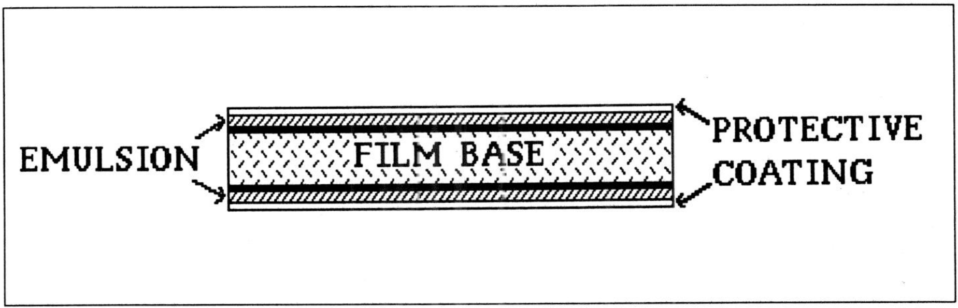

The second layer is the *emulsion,* which contains finely precipitated silver halide crystals in a gelatin base. The emulsion coats both sides of the film base. This gives the film greater sensitivity, increasing the speed, density and contrast. By increasing the speed of the film, the exposure required to produce an image can be decreased, thus decreasing exposure to the patient and personnel. The silver halide emulsion is 90-99% silver bromide crystals and 1-10% silver iodide crystals. The gelatin that suspends the silver halide crystals is a colloid. It liquefies in high temperatures and remains solid at cool temperatures. When placed in the chemicals, the emulsion swells, allowing the chemicals to act on the exposed or sensitized crystals without actually losing the crystals. Once it is dry, it hardens again, trapping the black metallic silver.

The *film base* is in the center of the film, giving it support. It does not produce a visible light pattern or absorb the light, though a blue tint has been added to ease eye strain.

When the silver halide crystals are exposed to electromagnetic radiation, they become more sensitive to chemical change. These sensitized crystals are what make up the *latent image.* When the film is placed into the developer, the latent image is reduced to black metallic silver. The removal of the remaining silver halide crystals occurs in the fixer. The results are varying shades of black metallic silver and the clear film base.

Film is sensitive to all types of electromagnetic radiation. Some of them are gamma, particulate radiation (alpha and beta), x-rays, heat and light. Film is also sensitive to excessive pressure, so care must be taken when handling and storing the film.

Film Types

The 2 types of film used in veterinary radiography are screen-type film and direct-exposure film.

Screen-Type Film: Screen-type film is most sensitive to the light produced by intensifying screens. There are 2 types of screen-type films: blue-sensitive film and green-sensitive film. *Blue-sensitive film* is most sensitive to the light emitted from screens containing blue light-emitting phosphors. Calcium tungstate and some rare-earth phosphors are the most common blue light-emitting phosphors. They emit light in the ultraviolet, violet and blue light range. *Green-sensi-*

tive film is most sensitive to the light from green light-emitting phosphors. Rare-earth phosphors are the most common green light-emitting phosphors.

Direct-Exposure Film: Direct-exposure film is more sensitive to direct x-rays than it is to light. Because it does not use the intensifying effect of the screens, it requires a higher mAs than screen film. General anesthesia or heavy sedation may be necessary to prevent motion artifact on the radiograph because of the higher mAs. Direct-exposure film is mainly used for extremities or the rostral mandible or maxilla, where high detail is needed. It comes packaged in a paper folder enclosed in a stout light-proof envelope. Care must be taken when handling this film because it is only protected by paper. Pressure artifacts can easily occur. Some direct-exposure film can only be manually processed because of the thickness of the emulsion. However, there is direct-exposure film available that can be used with an automatic processor.

Film Speeds

Film speeds are rated as *high* (regular or fast), *average* (par), and *slow* (detail). The faster the film speed, the more sensitive it is and the lower mAs it requires. High-speed film requires less exposure than slow-speed film to produce a given radiographic density.

Film speed is changed by increasing the size of the silver halide crystals. High-speed film has larger silver halide crystals than average- or slow-speed film. The drawback to using high-speed film is that, with the larger crystal size, the image has a more granular appearance. This decreases the detail considerably. Average-speed (par) film should be used for most veterinary radiography.

Film Latitude

Another important feature in x-ray film is *film latitude*. This is the film's inherent ability to produce shades of gray. Film with a long or increased latitude can produce images with a long scale of contrast (many shades of gray). Long-latitude film is desirable, as it allows for greater exposure errors while still producing a diagnostic radiograph.

Film Storage and Handling

Proper storage and handling of film is important to ensure a good diagnostic radiograph. Unexposed film should be stored in a cool dry place, away from strong chemical fumes. A base fog can occur if film is kept under adverse conditions over a long period. Film is pressure sensitive, so it should be stored on end and not laid flat on its side.

Intensifying Screens

Intensifying screens contain fluorescent crystals bound to a cardboard or plastic base. When exposed to x-rays, they emit foci of light. Placing the film in direct contact with the screens accurately records any x-rays that penetrate the patient and irradiate the screens. Approximately 95% of the film's radiographic density is caused by fluorescence of the intensifying screens, while only 5% is related to direct x-ray exposure. With each x-ray photon the screen absorbs, it emits 1000 light photons, amplifying the photographic effect of the x-rays. The film is sandwiched between 2 screens mounted inside a light-proof cassette. The cassettes hold the film in close uniform contact with the screens.

The screens are supported by a plastic or cardboard base. Next to the base is a thin reflecting layer that reflects the light back toward the film side or front of the screen.

The third component is the phosphor layer. The 2 most common phosphors used are calcium tungstate and compounds containing rare earth elements. Calcium tungstate is a blue light emitter. Some of the rare-earth phosphors also emit blue light. Lanthanum oxybromide and gadolinium oxysulfide are 2 rare-earth phosphors that emit green light. All the rare-earth phosphors differ from calcium tungstate in the respect that they have an increased ability to absorb x-rays and convert them into light energy. Rare-earth screens allow a reduction in exposure technique as compared with a calcium tungstate screen of the same thickness. Over the phosphor layer is a thin waterproof protective coating. This coating serves 3 functions: it prevents static when loading and unloading, it provides physical protection and it provides a surface that can be cleaned.

Screen Speeds

Intensifying screens come in 3 different speeds: high (regular), par (medium) and slow (detail or fine). High-speed screens require less exposure as compared with the par or slow speeds, but also detail is decreased. With shorter exposure times, the high-speed screens are ideal for soft tissues with unavoidable movement, such as the thorax and abdomen. Better detail can be achieved with slow-speed screens requiring a longer exposure time. When changing from a high-speed to a par-speed screen, the mAs must be increased 2 times. When changing from high speed to slow speed, the mAs must be increased 4 times to maintain the radiographic density.

There are 3 methods for changing the speed of screens. The first is to increase the thickness of the phosphor layer. A thicker layer absorbs more x-ray energies than a thin layer emitting more light. The disadvantage of increasing the thickness is that it allows the light to diffuse, causing the image to be blurred (Fig 2). Another way the speed is changed is to increase or decrease the size of the phosphor crystals. Larger phosphor crystals can absorb more x-rays and emit a larger area of light (Fig 3). High-speed screens have larger crystals than par-speed or slow-speed screens. This means that high-speed screens require lower mAs than the others, but the image has a grainier appearance. Light-absorbing dyes are sometimes incorporated into the phosphor layer. These dyes absorb the lateral spreading light that blurs the image. The amount of light that reaches the film is decreased but the increase in detail is helpful. By combining the factors of thickness, crystal size and dyes, a good balance of speed and detail can be achieved.

Figure 2. The thicker the phosphor layer, the faster the screen. However, a thick phosphor layer allows for more light diffusion, giving the image a more grainy appearance.

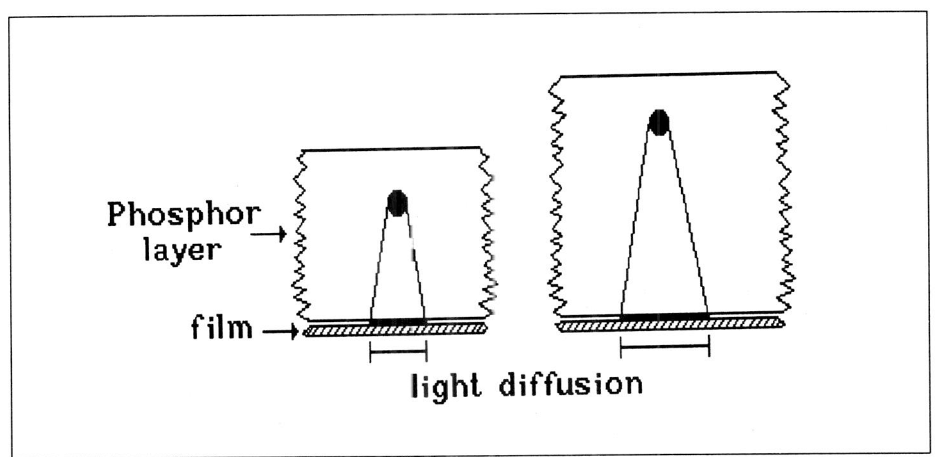

Care of Screens

Proper care of intensifying screens is very important in veterinary radiography. Regular cleaning is necessary to ensure that the screens are free from dirt and foreign material. Such material can prevent the light emitted from the screens from reaching the film, leaving it unexposed. The result is a white area on the film in the likeness of the foreign material. Labeling the screens on the inside and on the outside of the cassette allows the dirty cassette to be retrieved and cleaned.

Processing chemicals can permanently damage the screens' surface if it is not promptly cleaned. The screens should be cleaned with a soft lint-free cloth and an intensifying screen cleaning solution. If a commercial cleaner is not available, warm water is the next best thing. Do not use denatured alcohol or abrasive products, as they can damage the protective coating and phosphor layer. Be sure to allow the screen to completely dry before reloading.

The cassettes are precision instruments and should be handled that way. Do not drop them or set heavy objects on them. This can lead to poor film-screen contact and an area of the image that is blurred.

To check the film-screen contact of your screens, place paper clips over the surface of the cassette. Use enough to completely cover every area. Expose the cassette using 50-60 kVp and half the mAs you

Figure 3. Increasing the size of the phosphor crystals increases the speed of the screen. However, the image appears more grainy.

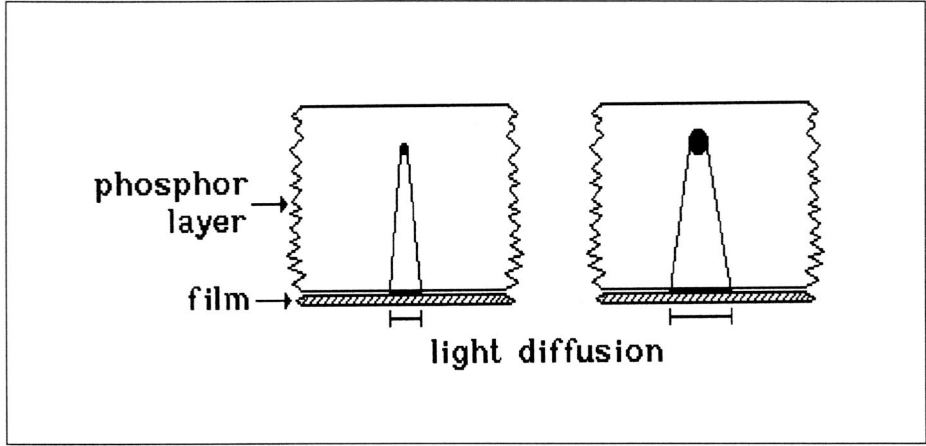

would use for non-grid extremity. Process the film and view it dry. Any areas with poor film-screen contact have a blurred image of the paper clips (Fig 4).

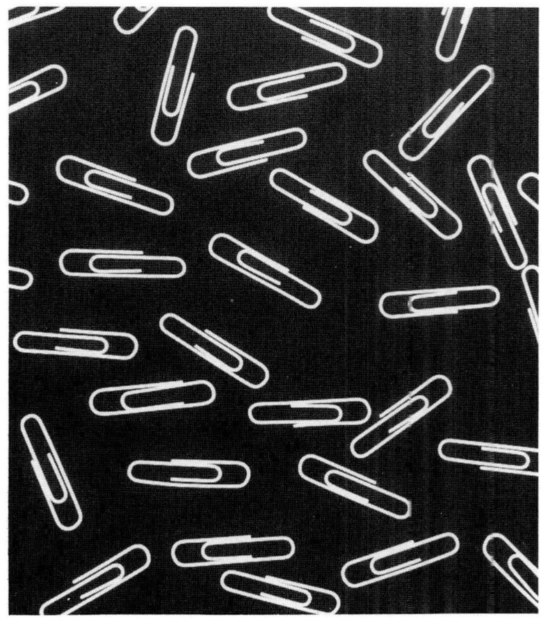

Figure 4. Radiograph exposed to check the film-screen contact. Poor film-screen contact results in decreased detail on the finished radiograph.

Recommended Reading

Curry TS III *et al: Christensen's Physics of Diagnostic Radiology.* 4th ed. Lea & Febiger, Philadelphia, 1990. pp 118-164.

Douglas SW *et al: Principles of Veterinary Radiography.* 4th ed. Bailliere Tindall, London, 1987. pp 55-68.

Eastman Kodak: *The Fundamentals of Radiology.* 12th ed. Eastman Kodak, Rochester, NY, 1992.

Koblik PD *et al:* Rare earth intensifying screens for veterinary radiography: an evaluation of two systems. *Vet Radiol* 21:224-232, 1980.

Morgan JP and Silverman S: *Techniques of Veterinary Radiography.* 3rd ed. Veterinary Radiology Associates, Davis, CA, 1982. pp 54-66.

Skucas J and Gorski J: Application of modern intensifying screens in diagnostic radiology. *Med Radiol Photographer* 56(2):25-36, 1980.

Ticer JW: *Radiographic Technique in Veterinary Practice.* 2nd ed. Saunders, Philadelphia, 1984. pp 29-34.

Notes

5

Darkroom Techniques

It is essential that, along with a good technique chart, proper darkroom techniques be followed to ensure radiographs of consistent quality. Properly exposed radiographs can quickly become non-diagnostic with poor film handling and darkroom techniques.

Darkroom Layout

Bench Areas

For most veterinary practices, the darkroom does not need to be large or fancy, as long as the layout is designed for efficiency. The room must be just large enough to provide a "dry bench" area away from the "wet bench" area (Fig 1). The dry bench area is used to unload and load cassettes and for film storage. The wet bench is for film processing and drying. These areas must be separated to prevent processing chemical splashes from damaging the dry films or sensitive intensifying screens. In a small room this can be achieved by placing a partition between the 2 areas. Also, an adequate amount of electrical outlets should be provided to supply the safelights, viewboxes and labeling equipment.

Light Proofing

The most important feature of a darkroom is that it must be light proof. White light that leaks in around the door, through a blackened window, or around ventilation fans can fog the film. Film is more sensitive after it has been exposed to x-rays, so even low-grade light leaks decrease the quality of the finished radiograph.

When checking for light leaks, stand in the darkroom for at least 5 minutes to allow your eyes to adjust to the darkness. Look around the door frame, ventilation fan or blackened windows for any signs of white light. When performing this test, vary the intensity of light outside the door. Because the work in the darkroom is done with a limited amount of light, painting the walls and ceiling in colors that reflect the available light helps greatly.

Ventilation

The darkroom should have adequate ventilation to prevent accumulation of volatile chemical fumes in the room. These fumes can cause fogging of the film, damage to electrical equipment and health problems for personnel. A light-proof ventilation fan installed in the ceiling helps remove the fumes and also controls the temperature and humidity in the room. The exhaust from automatic processors and

Figure 1. Schematic drawing of a darkroom. Notice the dry bench has been separated from the wet bench by a partition.

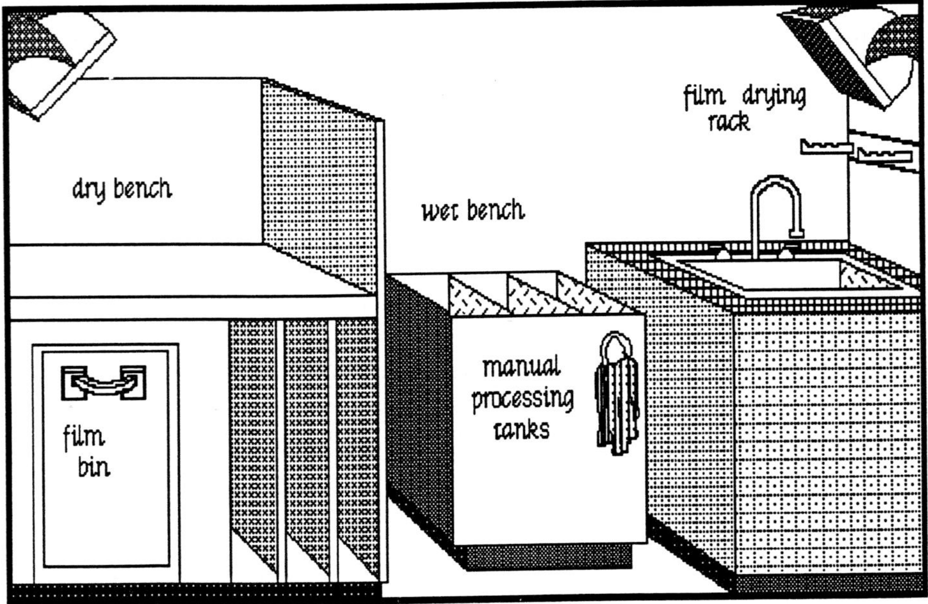

film dryers should also be vented away from the darkroom, as they contain volatile chemical fumes.

Cleanliness

Cleanliness is important in the darkroom because intensifying screens and film are exposed to this area. Dirt and hair on countertops can fall into cassettes, causing white artifacts on subsequent radiographs from that cassette. Chemical spills also cause artifacts on the radiographs and damage the intensifying screens. Keeping both wet and dry areas of the darkroom clean prevents these problems. Film hangers for manual processing should also be cleaned regularly. Chemicals that remain on the hanger clips drip down the next film to be processed, causing an artifact.

Film Identification

Permanent labeling is necessary for all radiographs. Each film must be identified before the film is processed for legal purposes and for certification organizations. Labeling can be done during the exposure or after the exposure but before the film is processed. The label should include the clinic name, date, owner's name and address, and patient's name, species, sex and age.

There are several methods for film identification. One method is the *photo labeler.* This uses a cassette containing a leaded window that protects the area during exposure. During identification, the window slides back to expose the information from a card to the protected area. This forms a latent image of the information on the film.

Manual printers are similar to photo labelers except they use a flash of light through an information card to produce a latent image on the film. The manual printer is placed in the darkroom and the film is taken out of the cassette to be identified.

Other methods use lead letters or radiopaque tape. These are placed on the cassette before exposure of the radiograph.

Safelights

Safelight illuminators are important for darkroom processing. The purpose of a safelight is to provide a sufficient amount of light to the room without fogging of the film. Safelights can be mounted to provide light directly or indirectly. For direct lighting, the safelight is mounted at least 48 inches above the workbench and directed toward the workbench. Indirect lighting has the safelight directed toward the ceiling and uses the reflected light to illuminate the room. With indirect lighting, the safelight can be mounted closer to the bench but should be as high as possible (Fig 2).

There are many types of safelight filters available to filter out light in different areas of the light spectrum. The type of film used dictates which filter is necessary. Film that is blue light sensitive requires a safelight that filters out blue and ultraviolet light. This can be done with a Wratten series 6B filter. Film that is green light sensitive requires a safelight to filter both green and blue light. A filter like the Kodak GS-1 can accomplish this. This filter can also be used with blue light-sensitive film. *A red light bulb should never be used to replace a safelight filter.* It does not filter the light, it only colors it. A white frosted 7- to 10-watt bulb is recommended for most safelight filters.

Figure 2. Direct and indirect safelight illumination.

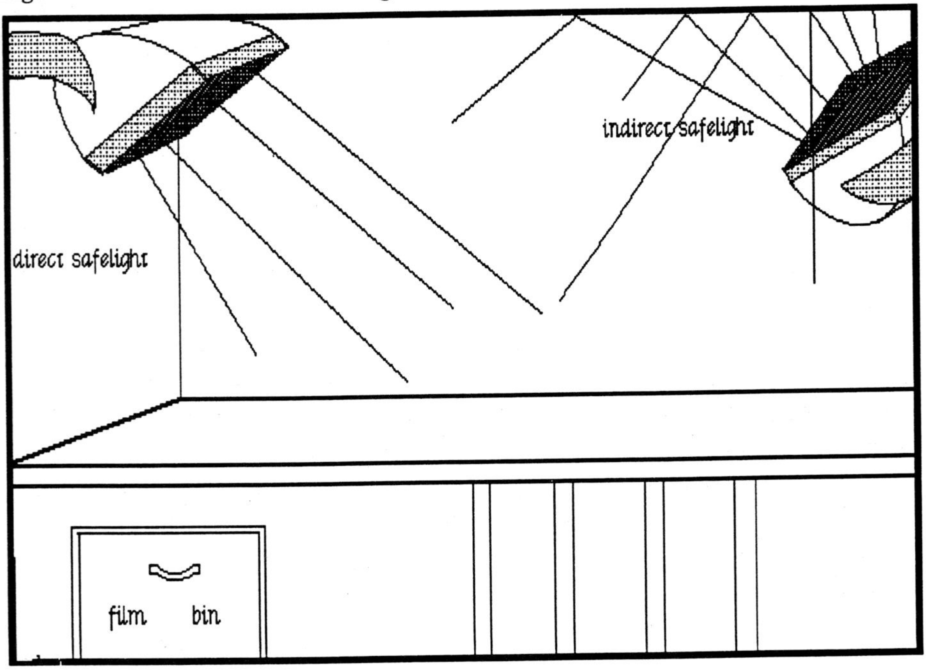

A periodic check of the safelight filter is recommended. This procedure is done by first making a moderate exposure on a film using approximately 1-2 mAs and 40-50 kVp. Film that has been exposed to x-rays is more sensitive to low-grade light, producing an overall fogged appearance. Cover two-thirds of the film with black paper or cardboard and allow the remaining one-third to be exposed to the safelight for 30 seconds. This is a little longer than it would take to place the film in an automatic processor or place the film on a hanger and into the manual tanks. After 30 seconds, uncover another one-third of the film and wait 30 more seconds. Repeat the process for the final one-third and develop the film. This test exposes portions of the film to the safelight for 30, 60 and 90 seconds. Once the film is dry, look for areas of increased film density. If an increase in density is detected, a close check of the darkroom is necessary. Improper safelight distance, a cracked safelight filter, and light leaking around the filter can all cause film fogging.

Manual Processing

Equipment

Manual processing tanks are usually made from stainless steel and are large enough to accept 14 x 17-inch film hangers. Tanks with a 5-gallon capacity are sufficient. Plastic or wooden lids are needed to cover the developer and fixer tanks. This helps to decrease the rate of evaporation and oxidation of the chemicals. Stirring rods for the developer and fixer are used to mix the chemicals before processing. Also, an accurate timer and a floating thermometer should be available.

Developer

The developer's main function is to change the sensitized silver halide crystals into black metallic silver. The sensitized silver halide crystals are those that have been exposed to electromagnetic radiation, making them susceptible to chemical change. The developer contains 5 ingredients: solvent, reducing agents, restrainer, activator and preservative.

Water is used as the solvent to keep all the ingredients in solution. It also causes the film emulsion to swell so that the reducing agents can penetrate reaching the sensitized crystals. The *reducing agents* are responsible for changing the sensitized silver halide crystals into black metallic silver. The most common reducing agents are a combination of hydroquinone and metol. The *restrainers* are used to protect the unexposed silver halide crystals by preventing the reducing agents from affecting the unsensitized crystals. Potassium bromide and potassium iodide are the most common restrainers. Bromide ions are produced during the exchange between the reducing agents and the sensitized crystals. In a fresh solution, the bromide ions are not available. They are added as a starter solution but are not placed in replenishing solutions. Too many bromide ions inhibits the reducing agents. The *activator* helps to soften and swell the film's emulsion so that the reducing agents can work effectively. The reducing agents cannot function in an acidic or neutral solution. The activators, usually a carbonate or hydroxide of sodium or potassium, provide an alkaline pH in the range of 9.8 to 11.4. The *preservative* prevents the solution from rapidly oxidizing. Sodium or potassium sulfite is the most commonly used preservative.

Developing chemicals are manufactured in 2 forms, liquid and powder. The liquid form requires dilution with water. The powder form requires dissolving and mixing to form a solution. The powder form should never be mixed in the darkroom. The chemical dust contaminates unprotected films, causing artifacts. Always mix in a bucket outside the darkroom and then finish the dilution in the darkroom.

Developing x-ray film is a chemical process that is dependent upon not only the chemicals but also on time and temperature of the chemicals. The recommended time for development is 5 minutes. This allows just enough time for the reducing agents to convert the sensitized silver halide crystals. The temperature of the chemicals is also important. The warmer the temperature, the more the emulsion swells and the faster the chemicals work. Cold temperatures also affect the chemicals by decreasing their ability to penetrate the film's emulsion.

Manufacturers generally recommend a temperature for the chemicals they produce. Most use 68 F (20 C), with 5 minutes of developing time. In some cases this may not be possible, so the time can be adjusted to compensate for the increase or decrease in temperature. The time can be decreased by 30 seconds for every 2-degree increase in temperature. Also, the time can be increased by 30 seconds for every 2-degree decrease in temperature. This applies only between 65 F (18 C) and 74 F (23 C).

Rinse Bath

The rinse bath removes the developer from the film, preventing any from being carried over into the fixer tank. Agitating the film in the running water bath for 30 seconds adequately removes the developer. The rinse water should be continually exchanged to prevent accumulation of developer. The temperature of the incoming rinse water can often be used to regulate the temperature of the developer and fixer tanks.

Fixer

The fixer removes the unchanged silver halide crystals from the film emulsion, leaving varying shades of black metallic silver. It also hardens the film emulsion, decreasing the susceptibility to scratches. The fixer contains 5 ingredients: solvent, fixing agent, acidifier, hardener and preservative.

Like the developer, the *solvent* is water. It keeps the ingredients in solution and causes the film emulsion to swell, allowing the fixing agents to reach the silver halide crystals that have not been changed in the developer. The *fixing agents* are either sodium or ammonium thiosulfate and are responsible for clearing the remaining silver halide crystals from the film's emulsion. The *acidifier* is acetic or sulfuric acid and is used to neutralize any alkaline developer remaining on the film. Ammonium chloride is used as a *hardener.* It hardens and prevents excessive swelling of the film's emulsion, shortening the drying time. The final ingredient is the *preservative.* As with the developer, sodium sulfite is used to prevent decomposition of the fixing agents.

Fixer chemicals are manufactured in 2 forms, liquid and powder. The liquid form requires dilution with water. It is more expensive than the powder form but is more efficient. The powder form requires dissolving and mixing to form a solution. It should never be mixed in the darkroom. The chemical dust contaminates unprotected films, causing artifacts. Always mix in a bucket outside the darkroom and then finish the dilution in the darkroom. Also, it requires a longer clearing time than the liquid form.

Fixing is a chemical process that depends on time and the temperature of the chemicals. The standard temperature is 68 F (20 C). The fixing time is double the developing time. The temperature also affects the time the film is left in the fixer. The warmer the chemicals, the shorter the fixing time needed. The film can be removed from the fixer after 30 seconds and viewed with white light. However, it must be placed back into the fixer for the remainder of the time. The clearing time increases as the thickness of the emulsion increases. Direct-exposure film has a thicker emulsion and requires a longer time in the fixer.

Final Wash

The purpose of the final wash is to rinse away the processing chemicals. Failure to rinse the film completely results in a film that eventually becomes faded and a brown color. This is caused by oxidation of the chemicals remaining in the film's emulsion. The wash tank should have fresh circulating water to decrease the time needed for the final wash. Generally, the wash time is at least 30 minutes.

Maintaining the Tanks

There are 2 methods for maintaining manual processing tanks. The first is the *exhausted method*. With this method the chemicals are allowed to drain back into their respective tanks and not into the wash tank. This permits the exhausted chemicals to remain in the tank, maintaining the chemical levels.

The second method is the *replenishing method*. The chemicals are not allowed to drain back into their respective tanks, but are placed in the wash tank. The chemical levels are maintained with replenishing chemicals that are more concentrated than the starting solutions. In this way the activity and levels of the chemicals can be preserved. With both methods the chemicals should be changed every 3 months.

Steps for Manual Processing

Things To Do Daily

1. Check the chemical temperature. Optimal chemical temperature is 68 F (20 C).

2. Stir both of the chemicals.

3. Check the chemical levels.

4. Clean countertops.

5. Turn on water flow to the wash tank.

Processing Individual Films

1. Locate the proper size of hanger(s).

2. Set the timer.

3. Turn on the safelight.

4. Turn off the white lights.

5. Unload the cassette and place the film on the hanger.

6. Immerse the film in the developer. The optimal time is 5 minutes at 68 F (20 C).

7. Gently agitate the film to dislodge any air bubbles that may cling to the film's surface.

8. Reload the empty cassette.

9. After 5 minutes of developing time, place the film in the wash tank and agitate for 30 seconds.

10. Lift the film out of the wash tank, allowing the excess water to drain back into the wash tank.

11. Place the film into the fixer tank and agitate gently to dislodge air bubbles that cling to the surface.

12. White lights can be turned on without causing problems after 30 seconds of clearing time in the fixer.

13. Remove the film from the fixer tank after 10 minutes or double the developing time.

14. Place the film in the wash tank for 30 minutes or longer, depending on the amount of water replenishing.

15. After washing the film, let it hang till dry.

Every 3 Months

1. Completely drain all 3 tanks.

2. Clean the tanks with a 1:32 solution of chlorine bleach and water.

3. Rinse the tanks well.

4. Refill the tanks with fresh chemicals.

Automatic Processing

Use of an automatic processor has some advantages over manual processing. Automatic processors are faster. They can process and dry a film in 90-120 seconds. Also, automatic processors consistently process high-quality radiographs. This eliminates the need for retakes because of processing errors.

Automatic processors move the film through the developer, fixer wash bath and dryers at a uniform rate of speed. Chemicals and film are specially manufactured to withstand the high temperatures that are necessary to provide a rapid transit. The chemical temperatures are kept at temperatures around 95 F (35 C), depending on the type of film and equipment used. Automatic processing film emulsion is harder, preventing scratches from the roller. This film can also be manually processed in case of mechanical problems with the automatic processor.

Small tabletop automatic processors are easily maintained in most veterinary practices. The equipment should be completely cleaned every 3 months. This includes draining and cleaning the tanks. A 1:32 solution of bleach helps to reduce growth of algae and to remove chemical buildup. The rollers can be cleaned with a mild detergent and a soft sponge. When any cleaning solution is applied to the tanks or rollers, they should be rinsed thoroughly before replacing the chemicals. Also check the springs and gears for signs of wear and replace if necessary. The feed tray and top rollers should be wiped each day with a clean soft sponge. This helps to remove dirt, debris and chemical residue between the routine maintenance procedures.

Silver Recovery

When an exposed film is placed in the developer, the exposed silver halide crystals are changed to black metallic silver. The remaining silver halide crystals are removed from the film in the fixer. Over time, the fixer solution becomes rich with silver that can be reclaimed. Silver recovery systems can be attached to automatic processors to filter and store the silver that would otherwise be discarded down the drain. The black metallic silver found in the radiographs can also be recovered.

The manual processing fixer solution, silver recovery systems and old radiographs can be sold to companies that reclaim the silver. These companies are usually listed in the Yellow Pages under the headings of "Gold and Silver Refiners and Dealers."

Recommended Reading

Douglas SW *et al: Principles of Veterinary Radiography.* 4th ed. Bailliere Tindall, London, 1987. pp 75-94.

Eastman Kodak: *The Fundamentals of Radiology.* 12th ed. Eastman Kodak, Rochester, NY, 1992. pp 93-106.

Morgan JP and Silverman S: *Techniques of Veterinary Radiography.* 3rd ed. Veterinary Radiology Associates, Davis, CA, 1982. pp 73-88.

Ticer JW: *Radiographic Technique in Veterinary Practice.* 2nd ed. Saunders, Philadelphia, 1984. pp 35-54.

Notes

Notes

6

Radiation Safety

Ionizing radiation is a difficult concept to grasp because at diagnostic levels it cannot be seen, felt or heard by the patient or operators. Why is radiation safety important? Radiation ionizes intracellular water. This action releases toxic products that can damage critical components of the cell, such as DNA.

Radiation can do any of 4 things when it comes in contact with the cells of living tissue:

- Pass through with no effect
- Produce cell damage that is repairable
- Produce cell damage that is *not* repairable
- Kill the cell

Effects of Radiation

Radiation damages the body in several ways. It may have carcinogenic effects, which means that cancer may occur in any of the body's systems. The effects on the body may be somatic, occurring only within the lifetime of the individual, or they may be genetic, occurring in future generations. The organ systems that are most sensitive to ionizing radiation are systems that have rapidly growing or reproducing cells.

The reproductive organs may suffer from temporary or permanent infertility, decreased hormone production, or mutations. The hematopoietic (blood-forming) cells are relatively sensitive to ionizing radiation. The lymphocytic series is the most sensitive. Damage to these cells can cause lowered resistance to infection, and clotting disorders. The thyroid gland, intestinal epithelium and the lens of the eye are also radiosensitive tissues. There may be an increased incidence of squamous-cell carcinoma with chronic low-level skin exposure. Radiodermatitis (reddened, dry skin) can be an indicator of excessive, chronic low-level radiation exposure.

The developing fetus is sensitive to the effects of ionizing radiation. The degree of sensitivity depends on the stage of pregnancy and the dose received. The preimplantation period (0-9 days) is the most critical time for the embryo regarding intrauterine lethality. Organogenesis (10 days to 6 weeks) carries the greatest risk of congenital malformation in the fetus, as this is the critical development period for fetal organs. The fetus may have skeletal or dental malformations. Other abnormalities include microphthalmia and overall growth retardation. A fetal dose of greater than 25 rads (0.25 Gray) is the reported threshold for significant damage to the fetus. The fetal period (6 weeks to term) is the least sensitive time for the fetus; however, growth and mental retardation may still occur. Irradiation after 30 weeks is less likely to cause abnormalities because the sensitivity of the fetus approaches that of the adult.

Exposure Terminology

Following is a brief description of the terminology used when describing doses of radiation. *REM* stands for *roentgen equivalent man*. It is the amount used to express the dose equivalent that results from exposure to ionizing radiation. REM takes into account the quality of the radiation, so doses from different kinds of radiation can be compared. *Sievert* or *SV* is the current terminology used to define a REM (1 SV = 100 REM). A *millirem* or *MREM* is equal to 0.001 REM or 1/1000th REM. A *RAD* is the *radiation absorbed dose*. Current terminology is *Gray* or *GY* (1 GY = 100 RAD).

Because we are dealing with x-rays only and not other types of radiation, RADs are equivalent to REMs. Other types of radiation must have a quality factor figured in to determine the dose. *MPD* is the *maximum permissible dose*. This may be figured by the following equation, MPD in REM = 5 x (n-18), where n is the current age.

The National Council on Radiation Protection and Measurements (NCRP) recommends that the maximum permissible dose (MPD) per year for occupational persons not exceed 0.5 REM per year. An occupationally exposed individual is one who normally performs work in a restricted-access area, and has duties that involve exposure to radiation. *ALARA* stands for *as low as reasonably attainable*. The MPD for nonoccupational persons is 10% of the MPD, or 0.5 REM per year. This is known as the ALARA MPD.

It is also recommended that a fetus not receive more than 0.5 REM for the entire gestation period. A pregnant employee who chooses to continue working around radiation-producing devices should wear an additional badge at waist level, underneath the lead gown, to monitor the fetal dose. This badge should not receive exposure above 0.05 REM per month.

Minimizing Exposure

There are 3 important ways to minimize exposure to occupational radiation. They are use of lead shielding, increased distance, and reduced time of exposure.

Lead Shielding

Lead shielding should be a requirement for all personnel remaining in the room while exposures are being made. Lead gowns, gloves and thyroid shields should all contain at least 0.5 mm of lead. Lead-based glasses can also be worn to protect the lens of the eye.

Lead apparel is very expensive, so it should be handled appropriately. Lead aprons should be draped over a rounded surface, without folds or wrinkles, so as to prevent cracks in the lead. Lead gloves can be stored with open-ended soup cans inserted to prevent cracks and provide air circulation to the liners. Lead gloves should be radiographed every 6 months, and lead gowns every 12 months to screen for holes and cracks in the lead. A commonly used technique for this procedure is 5 mAs and 80 kVp. This can be adjusted as needed to attain the proper density in your radiographs.

Increased Distance

Personnel exposure may also be decreased by increasing the distance from the primary beam. The Inverse Square Law states that x-ray beam intensity decreases to one-fourth if the distance between the x-ray source and the operator is doubled. The personnel restraining the animal should make a point of remaining as far as possible from the x-ray source. During exposure, the restrainers should lean back and look away from the beam to protect the lenses of their eyes (Fig 1). Employees should wear lead apparel properly to obtain full protection, unlike the personnel in Figure 2. Placing a glove over a hand for protection does not protect from scatter radiation. The scatter can come from any direction, including from beneath the tabletop.

Reduced Time

Reduced time of exposure is also an important factor in reducing radiation exposure. Using the fastest film-screen combinations reduces exposure of the patient and personnel. Proper darkroom practices and technique charts allow for consistently high-quality films, which reduce the number of retakes. It is very important to collimate the beam down to the area of interest, because this reduces scatter radiation exposure to personnel. Cones and diaphragms may also be attached to the tube window to increase detail and reduce scatter

Figure 1. Proper safety practices. The restrainers have increased their distance from the primary beam by leaning back. They are also protecting the lenses of their eyes by looking away.

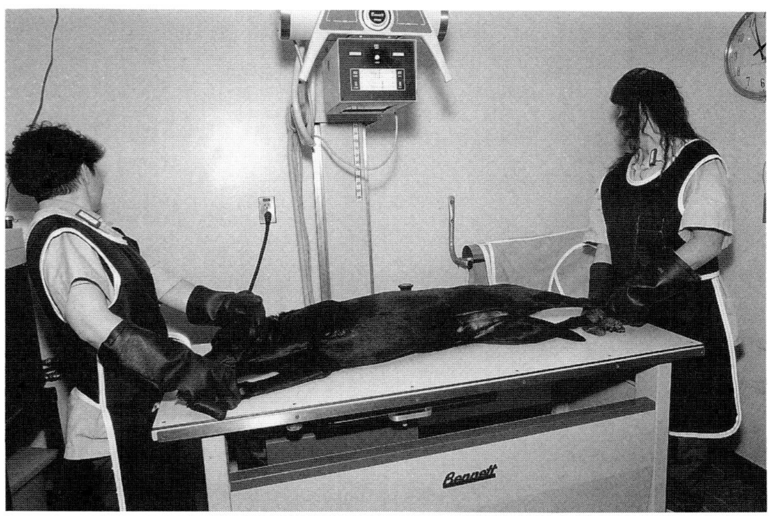

radiation. A 2-mm aluminum filter is used at the tube window to filter out soft rays that are too weak to penetrate the patient. If these rays are not filtered out, they scatter about the room, fogging the film and striking personnel.

Radiation Protection Supervisor

Each clinic should have a Radiation Protection Supervisor. This role can be filled by a veterinary technician. The responsibilities include educating personnel on radiation safety, monitoring those safety practices, and maintaining a radiologic badge system. The supervisor also maintains the x-ray equipment, darkroom facilities and radiographic records.

A good radiation control program consists of safe x-ray equipment, low exposure techniques, shielding, and monitoring personnel radiation exposure. The x-ray equipment is usually under control of state government (*ie,* State Board of Health). Regulations vary between states; check with your state government about their policy regarding radiation-producing devices.

Figure 2. Improper safety practices. The restrainers are leaning in and looking at the patient. Also, one hand is not properly gloved.

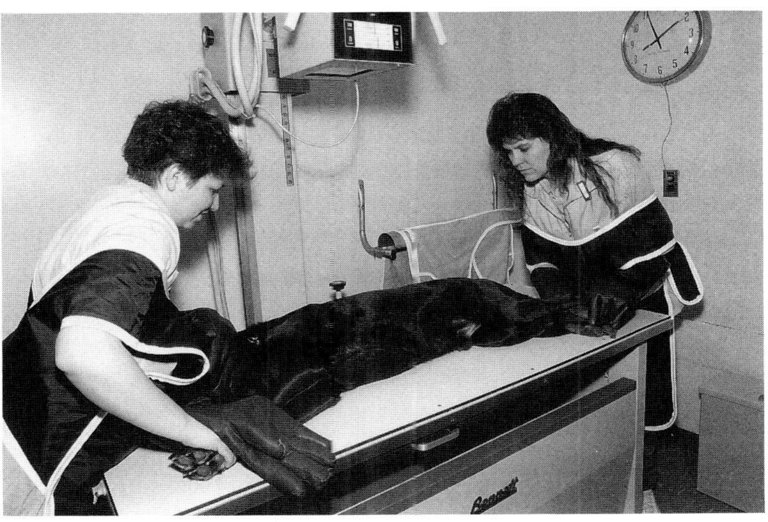

General Radiation
Safety Rules

- *Always wear lead gloves and lead aprons when remaining in the room during radiography or fluoroscopy.* Lead gowns and lead gloves *must* be worn by all individuals involved in restraint of the animal.

- *Always wear a radiation-monitoring device on your collar, outside the apron, when working around x-ray equipment. Note:* Badges should not be exposed to sunlight, dampness or extreme temperatures. This could cause falsely high readings.

- *Never allow any part of your body to be exposed to the primary beam.* Lead clothing does not protect against primary beam exposure.

- *Always look away from the x-ray beam during an exposure,* to protect the lens of your eye. Lead-based glasses may be worn for protection.

- *Use alternative methods of restraint* (drugs, tape, sandbags, etc) *when using high-power radiographic techniques.*

- *Pregnant women and persons under the age of 18 should not be involved in radiographic procedures.*

- *Only the minimum number of people required for restraint should remain in the room when an exposure is being made.*

Recommended Reading

Frankel R: *Radiation Protection for Radiologic Technologist.* McGraw-Hill, New York, 1976. pp 25-69.

Hendee WR and Edwards MF: Trends in radiation protection of medical workers. *Hlth Phys* 58:251-257, 1990.

Kleine LJ: Radiation control program. *Anim Hlth Tech* 4:172-177, 1983.

Morgan JP and Silverman S: *Techniques of Veterinary Radiography.* 3rd ed. Veterinary Radiology Associates, Davis, CA, 1982. pp 121-133.

Noz ME and Maguire GQ: *Radiation Protection in the Radiologic and Health Sciences.* 2nd ed. Lea & Febiger, Philadelphia, 1985.

Pizzarello DJ and Witcofski RL: *Medical Radiation Biology.* 2nd ed. Lea & Febiger, Philadelphia, 1982.

Ryan GD: *Radiographic Positioning of Small Animals.* Lea & Febiger, Philadelphia, 1981. pp 1-13.

Ticer JW: *Radiographic Technique in Veterinary Practice.* 2nd ed. Saunders, Philadelphia, 1984. pp 70-77.

Widmer WR *et al:* Radiation biology and radiation safety. *Compend Cont Ed* 11:1237-1248, 1989.

Wrigley RH and Borak TB: The effect of kVp on the dose equivalent from scattered radiation by radiography personnel. *Vet Radiol* 24:181-182, 1983.

Notes

Notes

7

Developing a Small Animal Radiographic Technique Chart

One of the most valuable pieces of information in a radiology department is a radiographic technique chart. A technique chart allows you to produce radiographs of consistent quality, with a reduced number of repeat exposures, which reduces radiation exposure to the patient and personnel. The construction of a technique chart is very simple when following these step by step procedures.

Preparation

Some important factors must be considered before starting. The animal to be used for the technique chart development should not be overweight or underweight. A dog weighing approximately 40 pounds is ideal. The dog should be anesthetized when performing the chart development. The process will progress quicker if the animal does not have to be restrained.

You must eliminate the variables that can affect the radiographic density. The first variable is the film processing chemicals. They should be fresh and not months old. Also, the same brand of chemicals should be used after the technique chart has been established. Use consistent processing times and chemical temperatures. Increasing or decreasing either affects the radiographic density.

A standard focal-film distance of 36-40 inches should be maintained, as well as a consistent film-screen combination. Finally, check the safelights and darkroom for light leaks. This eliminates possible film fogging, decreasing the quality of the radiograph. Once the technique has been established, if any of these variables changes, then adjustments in the technique chart will be necessary.

Establishing the Baseline mAs Chart

Step 1: Construct an mAs matrix chart using the mA stations and exposure times available on the x-ray machine (Fig 1).

Step 2: With the dog in lateral recumbency, measure the thickness of the abdomen in centimeters at the widest point, usually over the liver area. This measurement should be 10-20 cm. Also it is used to establish the kVp chart (see Fig 4).

Set the kVp for the 3 trial exposures according to the following measurements:

<10 cm = 60 kVp

10-20 cm = 70 kVp

>20 cm = 80 kVp

Step 3: Divide a 14 x 17-inch cassette with lead blockers into 3 sections to make 3 trial exposures (Fig 2). Center each exposure over the caudal thoracic and the liver area. Using one 14 x 17-inch cassette conserves film and reduces processing variables. A high-speed screen is used or the fastest-speed screen available for soft tissues. The cassette is placed on the tabletop for this first series of exposures, regardless of the thickness of the area.

Set the mAs for the 3 trial exposures at:

1 mAs for the first exposure

3 mAs for the second exposure

6 mAs for the third exposure

If these exact mAs choices are not available, use numbers that are as close as possible and the fastest times available.

Step 4: Process the film.

Step 5: Choose the technique that allows the best visualization of the soft tissue structures. If you are not satisfied with any of the exposures, adjust the mAs accordingly and make exposures of the entire abdomen. The technique chosen will be used as the tabletop abdominal technique. Also, it will be a baseline mAs for the remainder of the technique chart.

Step 6: Using the selected mAs value as the tabletop abdominal technique, with the following conversion factors, develop the remainder of the mAs chart (Fig 3).

High-Speed Screens*

Tabletop abdomen	selected value
Grid abdomen	3 times tabletop abdomen
Tabletop thorax	1/2 tabletop abdomen
Grid thorax	3 times tabletop thorax

Slow-Speed Screens*

Tabletop bone	4 times tabletop abdomen
Grid bone	3 times tabletop detail

*High-speed screens to slow speed = 4 times the high-speed mAs. High-speed screens to par speed = 2 times the high-speed mAs.

Step 7: Prepare a kVp chart using the following rules: (Fig 4).

Rule 1. Subtract 2 kVp from the initial kVp used for each centimeter of decrease from the initial measurement.

Rule 2. Add 2 kVp to the initial kVp used for each centimeter of increase from the initial measurement. This is done up to 80 kVp.

Rule 3. Add 3 kVp for each centimeter of increase between 80 and 100 kVp.

Rule 4. Add 4 kVp for each centimeter of increase above 100 kVp.

Step 8: Make one exposure for each of the calculated techniques (tabletop abdomen, grid abdomen, tabletop thorax, grid thorax, tabletop bone, grid bone) using the mAs and kVp charts. If adjustments are necessary, adjust the mAs, leaving the kVp as it is. Also test the techniques on large dogs, small dogs, and cats.

Example of Technique Chart Development

Develop the mAs chart using the available mA stations and exposure times. Multiply each mA station and exposure time together to chart the mAs values that are available for that x-ray machine (Fig 1).

Figure 1. mAs matrix chart.

Time (sec)	mA				
	50	100	150	200	300
1/120	0.42	0.83	1.25	1.67	2.5
1/60	0.83	1.67	2.5	3.3	5
1/40	1.25	2.5	3.75	5	7.5
1/30	1.67	3.3	5	6.6	10
1/24	2.08	4.2	6.2	8.3	12.5
1/20	2.5	5	7.5	10	15
7/120	3	5.8	8.7	11.7	17.5
1/15	3.3	6.7	10	13.3	20
1/12	4.2	8.3	12.5	16.7	25
1/10	5	10	15	20	30
2/15	6.67	13.3	20	26.67	40
1/6	8.3	16.67	25	33.3	50

When choosing an mAs, always use the mAs with the highest mA station and the fastest time. This technique chart is calculated using an anesthetized 40-pound dog that measures 15 centimeters over the liver area.

Figure 2. Exposures using a 14 x 17-inch cassette.

Exposure #1	Exposure #2	Exposure #3
1.7 mAs 70 kVp	3.3 mAs 70 kVp	5.0 mAs 70 kVp

Exposure #2 with 3.3 mAs and 70 kVp was chosen as the best tabletop abdominal technique. An mAs chart is calculated using 3.3 mAs as the tabletop abdomen mAs (Fig 3). If the exact mAs values are not available on the x-ray unit, use the nearest choice giving the highest mA station and the shortest exposure time. The kVp chart is calculated using 70 kVp at 15 cm (Fig 4).

kVp Charts for Machines with Maximum Capacity of 90 kVp

With low-output machines, the previous technique chart is not possible because the maximum kVp output is 90. A kVp chart can be developed that does not exceed 90 kVp. Because both mAs and kVp can affect the radiographic density, the mAs can be increased to maintain the radiographic density while the kVp is reduced.

Figure 3. mAs chart established after tabletop abdomen technique has been chosen.

Technique	mAs
Tabletop abdomen	3.3
Grid abdomen	9.9
Tabletop thorax	1.6
Grid thorax	4.8
Tabletop bone	13.2
Grid bone	39.6

Figure 4. kVp chart.

	cm	kVp		cm	kVp
	1	42		16	72
	2	44		17	74
	3	46	Rule 2	18	76
	4	48		19	78
	5	50		20	80
	6	52		21	83
Establishing	7	54		22	86
kVp	8	56	Rule 3	23	89
Rule 1	9	58		24	92
	10	60		25	95
	11	62		26	98
	12	64		27	102
	13	66	Rule 4	28	106
	14	68		29	110
	15	70		30	114

kVp-Radiographic Density Relationship

Increase the kVp by 20% = Double the radiographic density

Decrease the kVp by 16% = Halve the radiographic density

mAs-Radiographic Density Relationship

Double the mAs = Double the radiographic density

Halve the mAs = Halve the radiographic density

This low-output kVp chart is calculated using the same anesthetized dog measuring 15 centimeters over the liver area as in the previous example (Fig 5). The mAs chart is figured the same way (Fig 6). The best tabletop abdominal technique was 3.3 mAs and 70 kVp.

Figure 5. kVp chart with maximum 90 kVp output.

cm	kVp	cm	kVp
1	42	16	72
2	44	17	74
3	46	18	76
4	48	19	78
5	50	20	80
6	52	21	83
7	54	22	86
8	56	23	89
9	58	24*	77
10	60	25*	79
11	62	26*	82
12	64	27*	85
13	66	28*	88
14	68	29**	76
15	70	30**	78

* At 24 cm, adding another 3 kVp to 89 will exceed the maximum kVp limits of the machine. The kVp is lowered to 77 by subtracting 16% of 92. Consequently, this decreases the radiographic density by one-half. To compensate for the loss of density, the mAs must be doubled to return the radiograph to its original density.

** Again, adding 3 kVp will exceed the maximum 90 kVp limit. The kVp is once more decreased by 16%, resulting in one-half the radiographic density. To compensate, the mAs is doubled again.

Examples using the mAs and kVp chart for equipment with a maximum 90 kVp output are as follows:

Exposure technique for a thorax measuring
20 cm = 5 mAs and 80 kVp

Exposure technique for a thorax measuring
26 cm = 10 mAs and 82 kVp

Exposure technique for a thorax measuring
30 cm = 20 mAs and 78 kVp

mAs Chart When Detail Screens Are Not Available

Some veterinary practices image with only one speed of intensifying screens. Most of those practices use high-speed screens.

The same 40-pound anesthetized dog is used. As in the previous example, the best tabletop abdominal technique was 3.3 mAs and 70 kVp. The mAs chart is figured in the same way as the other examples except the tabletop bone technique is 1 mAs greater than the tabletop abdomen mAs (Fig 7). That value is multiplied by 3 to establish the

Figure 6. The method of establishing the mAs chart does not change when working with a machine of maximum capacity 90 kVp.

Technique	mAs
Tabletop abdomen	3.3
Grid abdomen	9.9
Tabletop thorax	1.6
Grid thorax	4.8
Tabletop bone	13.2
Grid bone	39.6

Figure 7. mAs chart for use without detail screens.

Technique	mAs
Tabletop abdomen	3.3
Grid abdomen	9.9
Tabletop thorax	1.6
Grid thorax	4.8
Tabletop bone	4.3
Grid bone	12.9

grid bone mAs. The kVp chart is unaffected by having only one speed of intensifying screens and is set up the same as the first example.

Recommended Reading

Liebel-Flarsheim: *Characteristics and Applications of X-ray Grids.* Liebel-Flarsheim, Cincinnati, 1989.

Mendenhall A and Cantwell HD: *Equine Radiographic Procedures.* Lea & Febiger, Philadelphia, 1988. pp 8-11.

Ticer JW: *Radiographic Technique in Veterinary Practice.* 2nd ed. Saunders, Philadelphia, 1984. pp 59-68.

Notes

Notes

8

Radiographic Artifacts

An artifact is any unwanted density in the form of blemishes arising from improper handling, exposure, processing or housekeeping. Artifacts can mimic or mask a disease process or distract from the overall quality of the film.

Before radiographing an animal, check for external changes. Remove any dirt or mats from the animal's haircoat. If the haircoat is wet, try to dry it as much as possible. Remove any collars and leashes. Bandage material is visualized on radiographs, so it should be removed if at all possible. The following discussion will help identify possible artifact problems.

Artifacts Occurring Before Processing

Fogged Film
(Overall Gray Appearance)

- The film was exposed to excessive scatter radiation. A grid is necessary when radiographing areas greater than 9 cm thick.

- The film was exposed to radiation during storage.

- The film was stored in an area that was too hot or humid.

- The film was exposed to a safelight filter that was cracked or inappropriate for the type of film being used.
- The film was exposed to a low-grade light leak in the darkroom.
- The film has expired.

Black Crescents or Lines

- Rough handling of the film either before or after exposure (Fig 1).
- Static electricity caused by low humidity.
- Scratching the film surface before or after exposure.
- Fingerprints caused by excessive pressure during handling before or after exposure.

Black Areas

- Black irregular border on one end of the film, caused by light exposure while still in the box or film bin.

Figure 1. Black crescent from rough handling of the film before or after exposure.

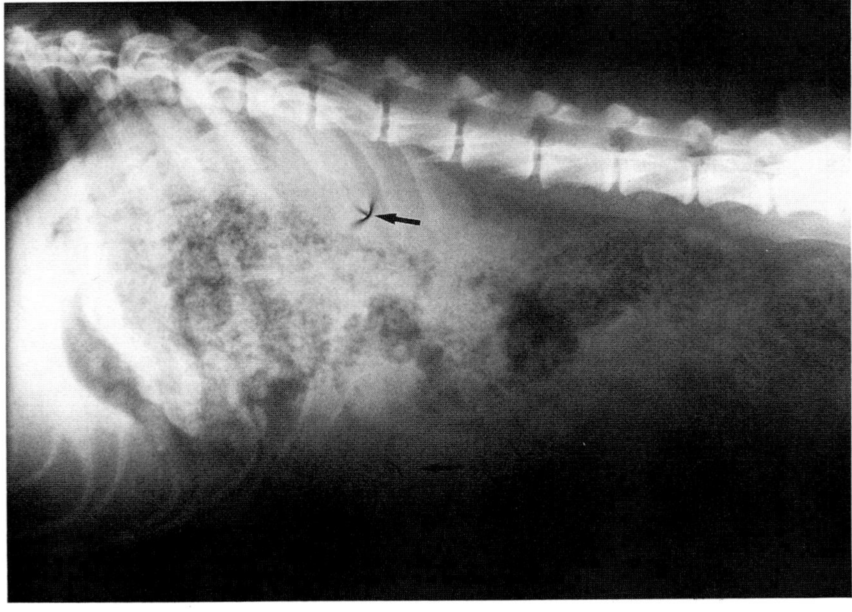

- Black irregular border occurring on multiple sides of the film, caused by felt damage in the cassette.

White Areas

- Foreign material between the film and screen (Fig 2).
- Chemical spill on the screen, causing permanent damage to the phosphor layer.
- Contrast medium on the patient, table or cassette.
- White fingerprints on the film, caused by contamination of fingers with oil or fixer before processing.

Visible Grid Lines

- Grid lines on the entire film related to the focal-film distance not in the range of the grid's focus.

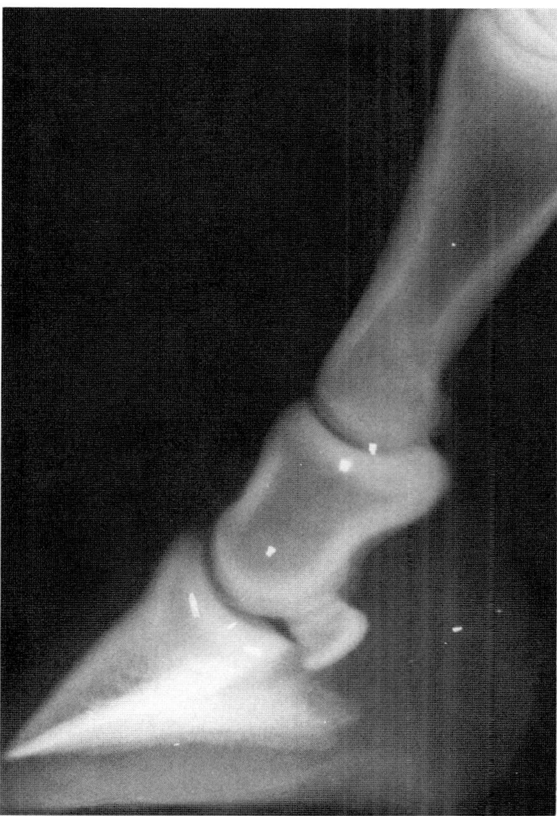

Figure 2. Foreign material between the film and screen blocking the light from the intensifying screen from exposing the film.

- Grid lines more visible on one end of the film and an overall decrease in radiographic density, caused by the grid's not being centered within the primary beam (Fig 3).
- Grid lines on the entire film, caused by the grid's not being perpendicular to the center of the primary beam.
- Grid lines visible in some areas more than others, related to damage to the grid.

Decrease in Detail

- Patient motion (Fig 4).
- Poor film-screen contact.
- Increased object-film distance.
- Decreased focal-film distance.

Figure 3. Grid cutoff from the grid's not being centered within the primary beam.

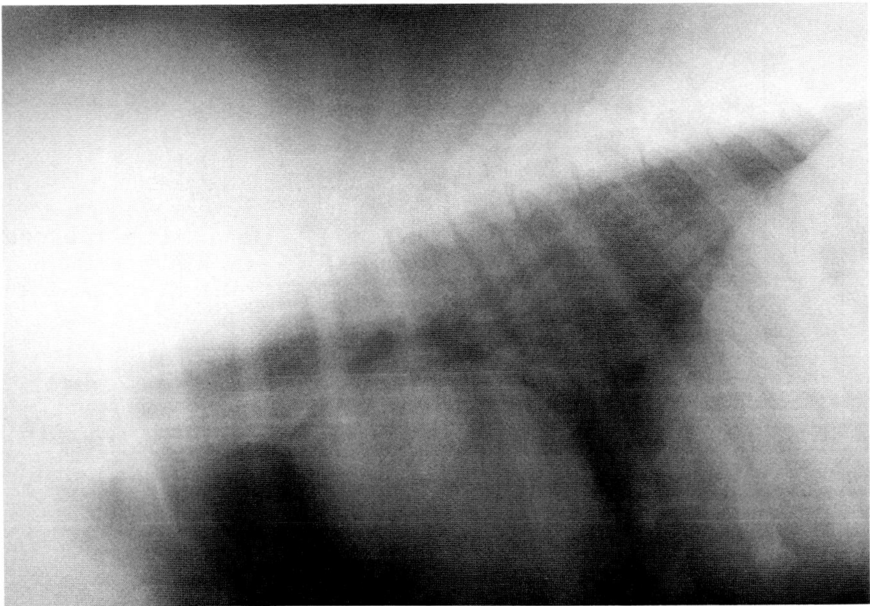

Artifacts Occurring
During Processing
(Manual and Automatic Processing)

Increased Radiographic Density
With Poor Contrast

- The film was overdeveloped (longer than chemical's manufacturer recommends).
- The film was developed in chemicals that were too hot. Correct temperature: manual tanks 68 F (20 C), automatic processor 95 F (35 C).
- The film was overexposed.

Decreased Radiographic Density
With Poor Contrast

- The film was underdeveloped (shorter than the chemical's manufacturer recommends).

Figure 4. Lack of patient cooperation or a panting patient combined with a long exposure time results in a blurred image.

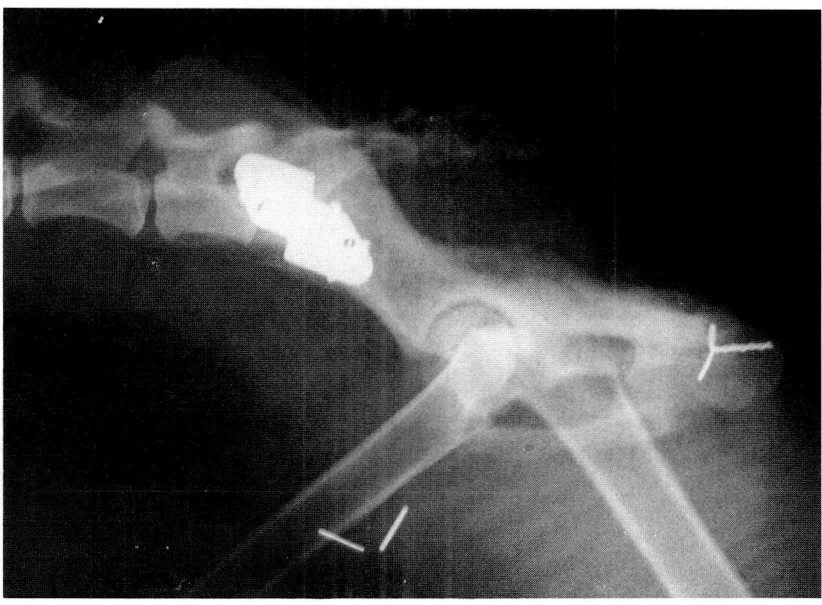

- The film was developed in chemicals that were too cold. Correct temperature: manual tanks 68 F (20 C), automatic processor 95 F (35 C) (Fig 5).
- The film was processed in chemicals that are old or exhausted (Fig 5).
- The film was underexposed.

Uneven Development

- Lack of stirring allows chemicals to settle to the bottom of the tank.
- Periodically pulling the film from the solution to check the film to determine the development time.
- Uneven chemical levels.

Black Areas, Spots or Streaks

- Identical black areas occurring on 2 films that were processed together are caused by the films' being stuck to one another in the fixer and not cleared properly.

Figure 5. The radiograph was processed in chemicals that were too cold (<68 F/20 C) or in chemicals that were old and exhausted.

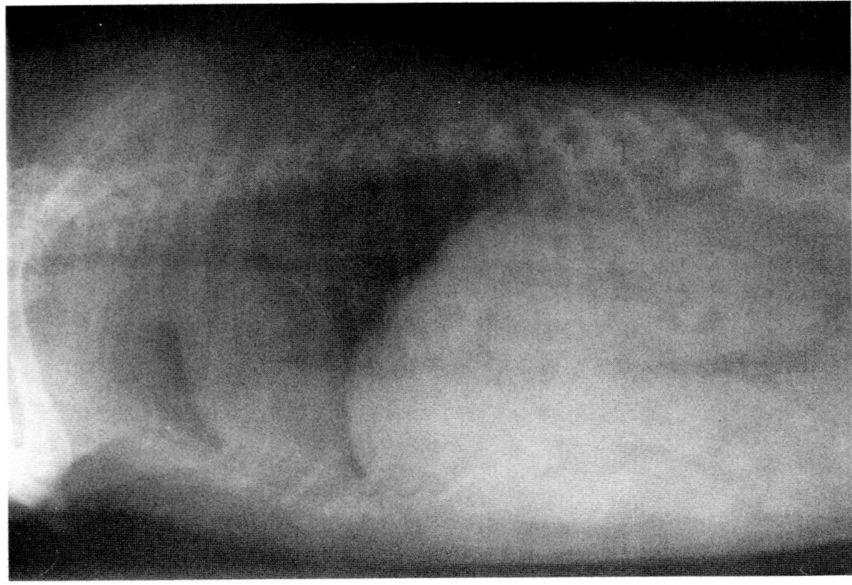

- Black area occurring on one film is caused by sticking to the side of the tank.
- Well-defined spots or streaks are caused by developer splash before processing.
- Linear black lines along the full length of the film and an equal distance apart are caused by pressure from rollers in the processor.

Defined Areas of Decreased Radiographic Density

- Identical light areas on 2 films that were processed together are caused by the films' sticking together in the developer.
- Light area on one film is caused by sticking to the side of the tank during development (Fig 6).

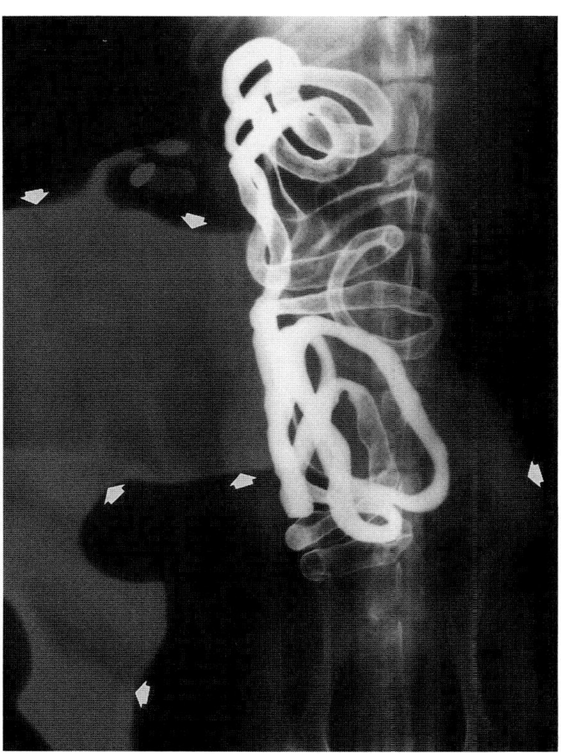

Figure 6. This radiograph stuck to the side of the manual tank while in the developer. The arrows outline the artifact. A light image can still be seen because the film has emulsion on both sides of the film base. One side developed normally.

- Air bubbles clinging to the film during development.
- Well-defined spots or streaks are caused by fixer splash before processing.

Clear Areas or Spots

- Streaks where the emulsion has been scratched away.
- Large areas of the film are clear because the film has been left in the final wash too long and the emulsion is sliding off the film base.

Entire Film Clear

- No exposure.
- Film placed in the fixer before being placed in the developer.

Film Turns a Brown Color

- Improper final wash.

Recommended Reading

Morgan JP and Silverman S: *Techniques of Veterinary Radiography.* 3rd ed. Veterinary Radiology Associates, Davis, CA, 1982. pp 92-98.

Ryan GD: *Radiographic Positioning of Small Animals.* Lea & Febiger, Philadelphia, 1981. pp 35-47.

Ticer JW: *Radiographic Technique in Veterinary Practice.* 2nd ed. Saunders, Philadelphia, 1984. pp 40-54.

Notes

9

Small Animal Radiographic Positioning

Proper patient positioning is as important as the radiograph itself. Misinterpretations can result from inaccurate positioning. The following is a reference for the radiographic procedures that are conducted in a veterinary hospital.

Terminology

A basic knowledge of directional terminology is essential when describing radiographic projections. The American College of Veterinary Radiology (ACVR) has standardized the nomenclature for radiographic projections, using the currently accepted veterinary anatomic terms. The projections are described by the direction the central ray enters and exits the part being imaged (Fig 1).

Ventral (V): Situated toward the underside of quadrupeds. Opposite of dorsal.

Dorsal (D): Situated toward the back or topline of quadrupeds. Opposite of ventral.

Medial (M): Situated toward the median plane or midline.

Lateral (L): Situated away from the median plane or midline.

Cranial (Cr): Situated toward the head (formerly anterior).

Caudal (Cd): Structures or areas situated toward the tail (formerly posterior).

Rostral (R): Areas on the head situated toward the nose.

Palmar (Pa): Situated on the caudal aspect of the front limb, distal to the antebrachiocarpal joint.

Plantar (Pl): Situated on the caudal aspect of the rear limb, distal to the tarsocrural joint.

Proximal (Pr): Situated toward the point of attachment or origin.

Distal (Di): Situated away from the point of attachment or origin.

Oblique Projections

Oblique projections are used to set off an area that would normally be superimposed over another area. Some rules should be followed when deciding what type of oblique projection is needed and how it is identified.

- *The area of interest should be as close to the cassette as possible.* This decreases magnification and increases detail.

- *Place a marker on the cassette before exposure to indicate the direction of entry and exit of the primary beam.*

Figure 1. Veterinary anatomic terminology.

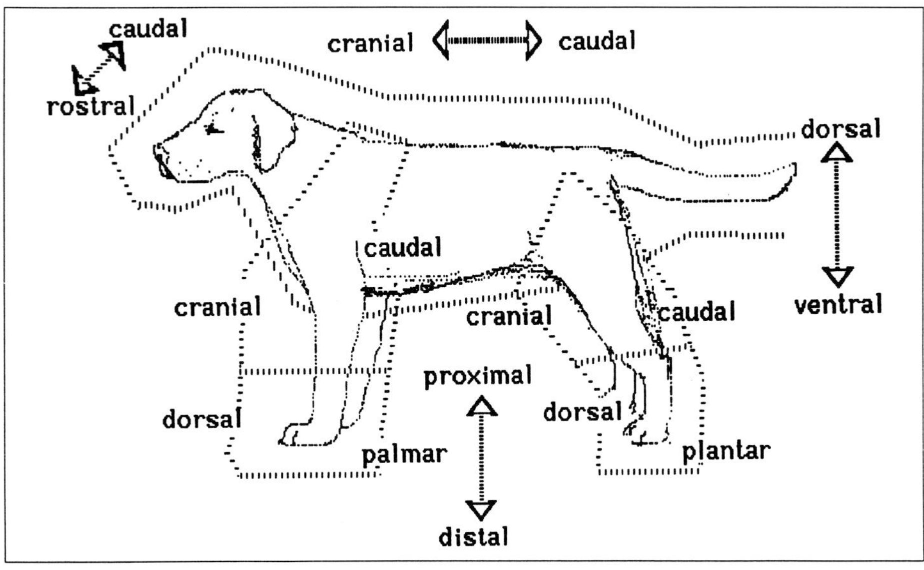

Positioning For Radiographs of the Skull

Correct positioning is extremely important when radiographing the skull. The symmetry of the skull is used when interpreting the films. Even a little deviation can cause misinterpretations.

General anesthesia is required for proper patient positioning. The number of radiographs made depends upon the clinical signs exhibited by the patient. Always begin with lateral and ventrodorsal (VD) radiographs. Because the animal is under anesthesia and motion is not a factor, the grid is used to increase the detail and contrast on the radiograph. Positioning aids, such as tape, sandbags and clean dry roll cotton or foam wedges, are used to minimize personnel exposure.

Lateral

Place the patient in lateral recumbency and position the head so the tympanic bullae and the rami of the mandibles are superimposed. This is accomplished by padding beneath the dependent mandible with roll cotton or a clean foam wedge. Roll the head so an imaginary line can be drawn superimposing one eye over the other, perpendicular to the table. Also pad under the nose so that an imaginary line can be drawn from the nose to between the eyes parallel to the table. Center the primary beam on the skull, making sure that the collimation light illuminates the tip of the nose, the top of the head, the base of the skull and off the mandible (Figs 2, 3).

Ventrodorsal (VD)

Place the patient in ventrodorsal position, with the front limbs extended caudally. The hard palate should be parallel to the table. This can be achieved by taping across the incisor teeth from one side of the table to the other, or by placing rolled cotton beneath the neck. Check the symmetry of the skull from the end of the table, making sure it is not obliqued. Center the primary beam on the skull, making sure the collimation light illuminates the tip of the nose, the base of the skull, and both right and left sides of the skull. Identify the left or right with labels on the cassette. Before the exposure is made, remove the endotracheal tube to avoid superimposition over the skull (Figs 4, 5).

Chapter 9, Figures 2-108 begin on page 100.

Ventrodorsal Open Mouth (Maxillary)
(Ventral 15- to 20-Degree Rostral-Dorsocaudal Oblique)

This view shows the nasal and ethmoid regions without superimposition of the mandible. Place the patient in ventrodorsal position, with the front limbs extended caudally. Place tape across the incisor teeth to bring the hard palate parallel to the table. Then place tape around the mandible, pulling it caudally, opening the mouth as wide as possible. Angle the x-ray tube rostral to caudal no more than 20 degrees. The degree of angle depends upon how wide the mouth can be opened. Identify the left or right side with labels on the cassette. The endotracheal tube need not be removed, but just included in the tape that is pulling the mandible caudal (Figs 6, 7).

90-Degree Frontal (Rostrocaudal)

This view shows the frontal sinuses. Place the patient in ventrodorsal position, with the front limbs extended caudally. Place tape around the nose so that it can be pulled caudally. Position the nose so that the hard palate is perpendicular to the table. Center the primary beam on the frontal sinuses and collimate the beam. Finally, measure the thickness for the kVp setting at the level of the sinuses, between the eyes. Identify the right or left side with labels on the cassette (Figs 8, 9).

15- to 20-Degree Frontal
(Rostral 15-20 Dorsal-Caudoventral)

This view shows the cranial vault, calvarium and sagittal crest. Place the patient in ventrodorsal position, with the front limbs extended caudally. Place tape around the nose so that it can be pulled caudally. Position the skull so that the hard palate is pulled caudally 15-20 degrees off of perpendicular. Measure thickness for the kVp setting at the level of the frontal sinuses. Identify the right or left side with labels on the cassette (Figs 10, 11).

Open-Mouth Tympanic Bulla
(Rostral 30-Degree Ventral-Caudodorsal)

This view shows the tympanic bulla with minimal superimposition of the petrous temporal bone. Place the patient in ventrodorsal

Chapter 9, Figures 2-108 begin on page 100.

position, with the front limbs extended caudally. Place tape around the mandible, including the tongue and endotracheal tube, to keep the tube near the mandible and on the midline of the tongue. With tape, pull the maxilla rostrally and the mandible caudally so that the primary beam is centered over the tympanic bulla perpendicular to the table. Measure for the kVp setting from the table to the commissure of the mouth. Collimate the beam and identify the right or left side with labels on the cassette (Figs 12, 13).

Intraoral

This view shows the rostral portion of the mandible or maxilla without superimposition of the opposite dental arcade. Use of direct-exposure film is recommended to maximize the detail of the image. With either image, the skull must be in strict ventrodorsal or dorsoventral position.

Maxilla: Place the patient in sternal recumbency, with the endotracheal tube tied to the mandible. Place a corner of the direct-exposure film into the mouth as far in as possible. Collimate and identify the right or left side with labels on the film (Figs 14, 15).

Mandible: Place the patient in ventrodorsal position, with the front limbs extended caudally. Place a corner of the direct-exposure film as far into the mouth as possible, with the tongue positioned in the center of the mandible. Collimate and identify the right or left side with labels on the film (Figs 16, 17).

Lateral Oblique Positioning for the Tympanic Bullae and Temporomandibular Joints
(Left 20-Degree Ventral, Right Dorsal Oblique) (Right 20-Degree Ventral, Left Dorsal Oblique)

This projection separates the bullae and temporomandibular joints. Place the patient in right lateral recumbency to image the right bulla and temporomandibular joint, and in left lateral recumbency for the left bulla and temporomandibular joint. Position the skull obliquely 15-20 degrees toward ventrodorsal and raise the nose slightly (Figs 18, 19).

Chapter 9, Figures 2-108 begin on page 100.

Positioning For Radiographs
of the Vertebral Column

General anesthesia is mandatory for obtaining quality radiographs of the vertebral column. If radiographs are made without anesthesia, false narrowing of the intervertebral disk spaces can occur from muscle spasm. Because the patient is anesthetized and motion is not a factor, a grid is always used to increase the detail and contrast of the radiograph.

With all radiographic procedures involving the vertebral column, place the longitudinal center of the primary beam on the vertebrae and collimate the width of the beam to increase the detail. Clean, dry padding should always be used. Use of tape or sandbags also aids in positioning the limbs.

Cervical Vertebrae

Lateral: Place the patient in lateral recumbency, with the front limbs extended caudally. Do not overextend the limbs, as this can cause rotation of the spine. Pad beneath the mandible to superimpose the wings of the atlas. Padding may also be needed under the neck so that the spine does not sag in the middle, causing false narrowing. However, too much padding can cause the spine to bulge, also producing false narrowing.

The cranial landmark is the base of the skull and the caudal landmark is the spine of the scapula. Place the wings of the atlas and the center of the spine of the scapula in the longitudinal center of the primary beam. Measure over the spine of the scapula for the kVp setting (Figs 20, 21).

Ventrodorsal (VD): Place the patient in ventrodorsal position, with the front limbs extended caudally. Place the head and spine in a natural position without padding, making sure they are not obliqued. The cranial landmark is the base of the skull and the caudal landmark is the spine of the scapula. Measure at the manubrium for the kVp setting. Remove the endotracheal tube before making the exposure (Figs 22, 23).

Dorsoventral (DV): Place the patient in sternal recumbency. Pad under the head, keeping the vertebrae parallel to the table and not

Chapter 9, Figures 2-108 begin on page 100.

in an oblique position. The cranial landmark is the base of the skull and the caudal landmark is the spine of the scapula. Measure at the level of the manubrium for the kVp setting. Remove the endotracheal tube before making the exposure (Fig 24).

Oblique Projections: The purpose of this view is to help localize a lesion observed on the lateral and ventrodorsal projections during myelography. Position the patient in lateral recumbency, with the front limbs extended slightly caudally. Place padding under the cranial thorax to give a 45-degree oblique projection. Pad the head so that it is also at a 45-degree angle. Both oblique projections should be made for comparison (Fig 25).

Flexed Lateral: This view is sometimes made during myelography to visualize spinal cord impingement by extradural changes that are associated with vertebral instability. Position the patient in lateral recumbency, with the front limbs extended slightly caudally. Flex the head and neck caudoventrally. It is important to flex C5-6 as much as C2-3 (Fig 26).

Extended Lateral: This view is sometimes made during myelography to visualize spinal cord impingement by extradural changes that are associated with vertebral instability. Position the patient in lateral recumbency, with the front limbs extended slightly caudally. With sandbags, hyperextend the head and neck caudodorsally. The cranial landmark is the base of the skull and the caudal landmark is the spine of the scapula (Fig 27).

Thoracic Vertebrae

Lateral: Place the patient in lateral recumbency, with the front limbs extended cranially. Pad under the sternum or the spine to position the sternum and the spinous processes in a plane parallel to the table. This superimposes the ribs over one another, providing better visualization of the intervertebral disk spaces. The cranial landmark is the base of the skull. The caudal landmark is the spine of the scapula. The caudal landmark is halfway between the xiphoid and the last rib, from that point dorsal to the vertebrae. Measure the thickest area of the thorax for the kVp setting (Figs 28, 29).

Ventrodorsal (VD): Place the patient in ventrodorsal position, with the front limbs extended cranially. Position the patient so the ster-

Chapter 9, Figures 2-108 begin on page 100.

num and vertebrae are superimposed in a plane perpendicular to the table. The cranial landmark is the spine of the scapula. The caudal landmark is halfway between the xiphoid and the last rib, from that point dorsal to the vertebrae. Measure the thickest area of the thorax for the kVp setting (Figs 30, 31).

Thoracolumbar Vertebrae (T-L)

Lateral: Place the patient in lateral recumbency. Center the primary beam on the T-L junction by finding the point halfway between the xiphoid and the last rib, from that point dorsal to the vertebrae. Pad under the sternum or the spine to position the sternum and spinous processes in a plane parallel to the table. This superimposes the ribs over one another, providing better visualization of the intervertebral disk spaces. Measure the thickest area for the kVp setting (Figs 32, 33).

Ventrodorsal (VD): Place the patient in ventrodorsal position, with the front limbs extended cranially. Position the patient so the sternum and vertebrae are superimposed in a plane perpendicular to the table. Center the primary beam on the T-L junction by finding the point midway between the xiphoid and the last rib, then dorsal to the vertebrae. Measure the thickest area for the kVp setting (Figs 34, 35).

Lumbar Vertebrae

Lateral: Place the patient in lateral recumbency, with the rear limbs extended caudally. Position it so the sternum and the spinous processes are in a plane parallel to the table and the wings of the ilium are superimposed. Padding may be required in the mid-lumbar area to prevent sagging of the vertebral column. The cranial landmark is halfway between the xiphoid and the last rib, from that point dorsal to the vertebrae. The caudal landmark is the wings of the ilium. Measure over the T-L junction for the kVp setting (Figs 36, 37).

Ventrodorsal (VD): Place the patient in ventrodorsal position, with the front limbs extended cranially. Position the patient so the sternum and vertebrae are superimposed in a plane perpendicular to the table. Also, the wings of the ilium should be in a plane parallel to the table. The cranial landmark is midway between the xiphoid and the last rib, from that point dorsal to the vertebrae. The caudal landmark

Chapter 9, Figures 2-108 begin on page 100.

is the wings of the ilium. Measure over the T-L junction for the kVp setting (Figs 38, 39).

Lumbosacral Vertebrae

Some patient preparation is necessary before making lumbosacral radiographs. Give cleansing enemas 1-2 hours before imaging to evacuate feces from the colon. On the ventrodorsal view the colon is superimposed over the vertebral column. Excessive amounts of feces can make visualization difficult.

Lateral: Place the patient in lateral recumbency, with the rear limbs extended caudally. Position the animal so the wings of the ilium are superimposed by padding under the nondependent limb. Place the center of the primary beam on the wings of the ilium. Measure the thickest area for the kVp setting. Sometimes the kVp must be increased because of the thick subject density (Figs 40, 41).

Ventrodorsal (VD): Place the patient in ventrodorsal position, with the front limbs extended cranially. Position the animal so the wings of the ilium are in a plane parallel to the table. Center the primary beam on the wings of the ilium and angle the beam 20 degrees caudal to cranial. This is necessary to open the lumbosacral joint space. Measure the thickest area for the kVp setting (Figs 42, 43).

Positioning For Radiographs
of the Metacarpus and Digits

Mediolateral (ML)

Place the patient in lateral recumbency, with the area of interest down (closer to the table). Extend the unaffected limb caudally and out of the way. Center the primary beam on the metacarpus and collimate to include the carpal joint and digits. Place a right or a left marker on the dorsal side of the limb. Sometimes the usefulness of a lateral projection is limited because of superimposition of the digits. To open a space between each metacarpal bone, position at a slight oblique angle. To image only the digits, tape each digit so it is not superimposed over the others (Figs 44, 45).

Chapter 9, Figures 2-108 begin on page 100.

Dorsopalmar (DPa)

Position the patient in sternal recumbency, with the affected limb extended cranially. Move the patient's body to the right and left to get the limb in an accurate position. Center the primary beam on the metacarpus and collimate to include the carpal joint and digits. Place a right or a left marker on the lateral side of the limb (Figs 46, 47).

Positioning For Radiographs of the Carpus

Mediolateral (ML)

Place the patient in lateral recumbency, with the limb of interest down (closer to the table). Extend the unaffected limb caudally, out of the way. Place tape on the metacarpus and extend it cranially. Center the primary beam on the carpus and collimate. Place a right or a left marker on the dorsal side of the limb (Figs 48, 49).

Dorsopalmar (DPa)

Place the patient in sternal recumbency, with the affected limb extended cranially. Move the patient's body to the right and left to get the carpus in DPa position. Center the primary beam on the carpus and collimate. Place a right or a left marker on the lateral side of the limb (Figs 50, 51).

Positioning For Radiographs of the Radius and Ulna

Mediolateral (ML)

Place the patient in lateral recumbency, with the limb to be imaged down (closer to the table). Extend the unaffected limb caudally, out of the way. With tape, extend the metacarpus cranially. Center the primary beam on the center of the radius and collimate to include carpal and elbow joints. Place a right or a left marker on the cranial side of the limb (Figs 52, 53).

Craniocaudal (CrCd)

Place the patient in sternal recumbency, with the affected limb extended cranially. Move the patient's body to the right or left so the

Chapter 9, Figures 2-108 begin on page 100.

olecranon of the ulna can be palpated in the center of the joint. Center the primary beam on the center of the radius and collimate to include the carpal and elbow joints. Place a right or a left marker on the lateral side of the limb (Figs 54, 55).

Positioning For Radiographs of the Elbow Joint

Mediolateral (ML)

Place the patient in lateral recumbency, with the limb of interest closer to the table. Extend the unaffected limb caudally. Place tape around the metacarpus and extend the limb cranially. Center the primary beam on the elbow and collimate to include only the region of the joint. A flexed mediolateral may be necessary to better evaluate the joint. Position the flexed elbow the same as for the standard mediolateral, except flex the joint as much as possible. Place a right or a left marker on the cranial side of the limb (Figs 56, 57).

Craniocaudal (CrCd)

Place the patient in sternal recumbency, with the limb of interest extended cranially. Move the head dorsally and slightly caudally to get the soft tissues of the chest and neck away from the elbow area. Move the patient's body to the right or left so the olecranon of the ulna can be palpated in the center of the joint. Center the primary beam on the elbow and collimate to include only the region of the joint. Place a right or a left marker on the lateral side of the limb (Figs 58, 59).

Positioning For Radiographs of the Humerus

Mediolateral (ML)

Place the patient in lateral recumbency, with the limb of interest down (closer to the table). Extend the unaffected limb caudally. Extend the metacarpus cranially, securing it with tape. Center the primary beam on the humeral shaft and collimate, making sure the shoulder and elbow joints are included. Place a right or a left marker on the cranial side of the limb (Figs 60, 61).

Chapter 9, Figures 2-108 begin on page 100.

Caudocranial (CdCr)

Because of the structure of the humerus, it is difficult to extend it cranially enough to be parallel to the cassette. This causes foreshortening of the limb, altering the imaged length and shape of the bone.

There are 2 methods for positioning a CdCr projection of the humerus. The first is a *cross-table projection* (Fig 62). Position the patient in lateral recumbency, with the limb to be imaged up (farther from the table). Place the cassette cranial to the limb and perpendicular to the table. Keep the cassette close to the limb and parallel to the humerus. Abduct the limb by rotating the elbow. Move the x-ray tube head down toward the table and angle the primary beam perpendicular to the humerus. Center the primary beam on the center of the humeral shaft, making sure the elbow and shoulder joints are included.

A second method, the *ventrodorsal extended projection,* involves placing the patient in ventrodorsal position (Fig 63). Sedation may be necessary to achieve adequate muscle relaxation. Pull the limb of interest cranially to get the humerus parallel to the table. With this method, the increase in OFD causes magnification and a decrease in detail. Place a right or a left marker on the lateral side of the limb (Fig 64).

Positioning For Radiographs
of the Shoulder Joint

Mediolateral (ML)

Place the patient in lateral recumbency, with the joint of interest down (closer to the table). Pull the unaffected limb caudally to prevent superimposition of the manubrium over the joint. Extend the head caudodorsally to prevent superimposing the trachea over the joint. Extend the affected limb cranially. Center the primary beam on the shoulder joint and collimate to include only it. Place a right or left marker on the cranial side (Figs 65, 66).

Caudocranial (CdCr)

Place the patient in ventrodorsal position and extend the limb of interest cranially. Slightly roll the sternum away from the limb being

Chapter 9, Figures 2-108 begin on page 100.

imaged to prevent superimposition over the body wall. Center the primary beam on the shoulder joint and collimate to include only it. Place a right or left marker on the lateral side (Figs 67, 68).

Positioning For Radiographs of the Scapula

Mediolateral (ML)

Place the patient in lateral recumbency, with the limb to be imaged down (closer to the table). Pull the unaffected limb caudally and extend the head caudodorsally. Extend the affected limb cranially. Center the primary beam on the scapula, making sure the shoulder joint and the dorsal border of the scapula are included on the image. Place a right or left marker on the cranial side (Figs 69, 70).

Caudocranial (CdCr)

Place the patient in ventrodorsal position, with the limb of interest extended cranially. Slightly roll the sternum away from the limb being imaged to prevent superimposition over the body wall. Center the primary beam on the scapula, making sure the shoulder joint and the dorsal border of the scapula are included on the image. Place a right or a left marker on the lateral side (Figs 71, 72).

Positioning For Radiographs of the Thorax

Lateral

Place the patient in right lateral recumbency, with the front limbs extended cranially to avoid superimposing the triceps muscles on the cranial part of the lung field. Place the neck in a neutral position to prevent misinterpretation of the tracheal position. The cranial landmark is the manubrium and the caudal landmark is halfway between the xiphoid and the last rib. Use padding to keep the sternum and the dorsal spinous processes in a plane parallel to the table. Measure the thickest area for the kVp setting. Make the exposure during peak

Chapter 9, Figures 2-108 begin on page 100.

inspiration. If the thorax is being examined for tumor metastasis, imaging the right and left lateral thorax is helpful (Figs 73, 74).

Ventrodorsal (VD)

Place the patient in ventrodorsal position, with the front limbs extended cranially. The cranial landmark is the manubrium and the caudal is halfway between the xiphoid and the last rib. Position the thorax so the sternum and vertebrae are superimposed in a plane perpendicular to the table. Measure the thickest area for the kVp setting. Make the exposure during peak inspiration (Figs 75, 76).

Dorsoventral (DV)

This view is helpful for evaluating pneumothorax. Place the patient in dorsoventral position, with the front limbs extended cranially. The cranial landmark is the manubrium and the caudal landmark is halfway between the xiphoid and the last rib. Position the thorax so the sternum and vertebrae are superimposed in a plane perpendicular to the table. Measure the thickest area for the kVp setting. Make the exposure during peak inspiration (Fig 77).

Positioning For Radiographs
of the Abdomen

Lateral

Place the patient in right lateral recumbency, with the hind limbs extended caudally. The cranial landmark is 3 intercostal spaces cranial to the xiphoid and the caudal landmark is the greater trochanter of the femur. Use padding to keep the sternum and the dorsal spinous processes in a plane parallel to the table. Measure at the thickest point for the kVp setting. Make the exposure during peak expiration (Figs 78, 79).

Ventrodorsal (VD)

Place the patient in ventrodorsal position, with the hind limbs extended caudally. The cranial landmark is 3 intercostal spaces cranial to the xiphoid and the caudal landmark is the greater trochanter of the femur. Position the patient so the sternum and verte-

Chapter 9, Figures 2-108 begin on page 100.

brae are superimposed in a plane perpendicular to the table. Measure the thickest area for the kVp setting. Make the exposure during peak expiration (Figs 80, 81).

Positioning For Radiographs of the Pelvis

Lateral

Place the patient in lateral recumbency, with the wings of the ilium superimposed on each other, perpendicular to the table. Position the right limb slightly cranially and the left limb slightly caudally to separate the femoral heads. The cranial landmark is the wings of the ilium and the caudal landmark is the caudal border of the ischium. Measure the thickest area for the kVp setting. Sometimes the kVp must be increased because of the thick subject density (Figs 82, 83).

Ventrodorsal (VD) Flexed

Place the patient in ventrodorsal position, with the front limbs extended cranially. Position the patient so the wings of the ilium are in a plane parallel to the table and the stifles are pushed cranially. The cranial landmark is the wings of the ilium and the caudal landmark is the caudal border of the ischium. Measure the thickest area for the kVp setting. Identify the right or left side with labels on the cassette (Figs 84, 85).

Ventrodorsal (VD) Extended

General anesthesia may be necessary to achieve complete muscle relaxation and accurate positioning. Place the patient in ventrodorsal position, with the front limbs extended cranially. Position the patient so the wings of the ilium are in a plane parallel to the table. The cranial landmark is the wings of the ilium and the caudal landmark is the stifle joint. Holding the tarsi, pull both hind limbs caudally, rotating the stifle joints medially (inward). The femora should be parallel to the table and to each other. Measure the thickest area for the kVp setting. Identify the right or left side with labels (Figs 86, 87).

Chapter 9, Figures 2-108 begin on page 100.

Positioning For Radiographs
of the Femur

Mediolateral (ML)

Place the patient in lateral recumbency, with the limb of interest down (closer to the table). Abduct the unaffected limb out of the way. Center the primary beam on the femoral shaft and collimate to include the coxofemoral and stifle joints. Measure the thickest area for the kVp setting. Place a right or a left marker on the cranial side of the limb (Figs 88, 89).

Craniocaudal (CrCd)

Because of the structure of the femur, it is sometimes difficult to position it parallel to the table. This causes foreshortening of the limb, altering the imaged length and shape of the bone.

There are 2 methods for positioning a CrCd projection of the femur. The first is a *cross-table projection* (Fig 90). Position the patient in lateral recumbency, with the limb to be imaged farther from the table. Place the cassette caudal to the limb and perpendicular to the table. Keep the cassette as close to the limb as possible and parallel to the femur. Slightly abduct the limb by rotating the stifle joint. Bring the tube head down toward the table and angle the primary beam perpendicular to the femur. Center the primary beam on the femoral shaft and collimate to include the coxofemoral and stifle joints.

The second method is the *ventrodorsal extended projection.* This may require some sedation to achieve proper extension of the femur (Fig 91). Place the patient in ventrodorsal position. Extend the limb caudally so that the femur is parallel to the table. With this method, the increase in OFD causes magnification and a decrease in detail. For both methods, measure the thickest area for the kVp setting. Place a right or a left marker on the lateral side of the limb (Fig 92).

Chapter 9, Figures 2-108 begin on page 100.

Figure 14. Positioning for an intraoral image of the maxilla.

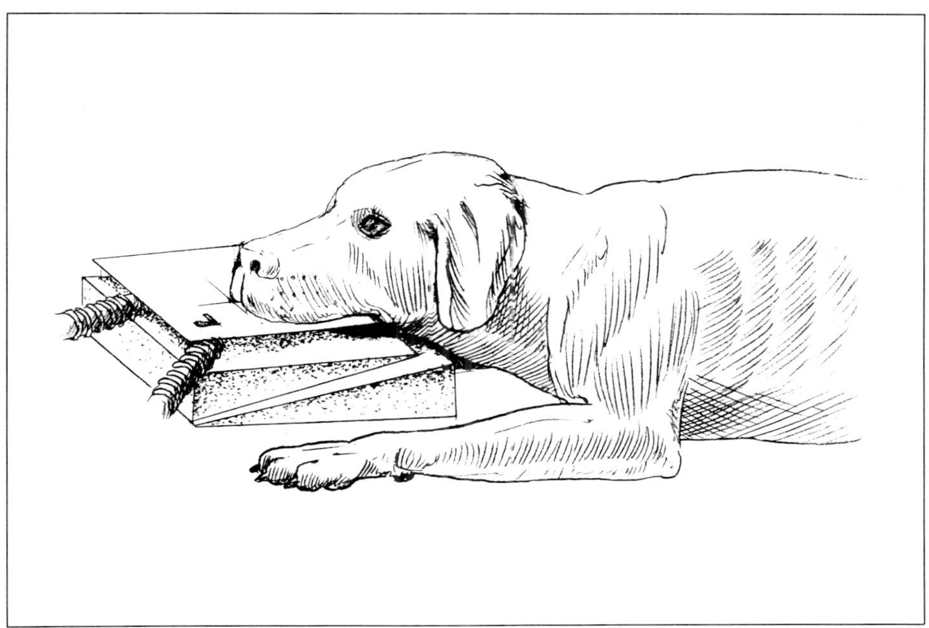

Figure 15. Intraoral image of the maxilla.

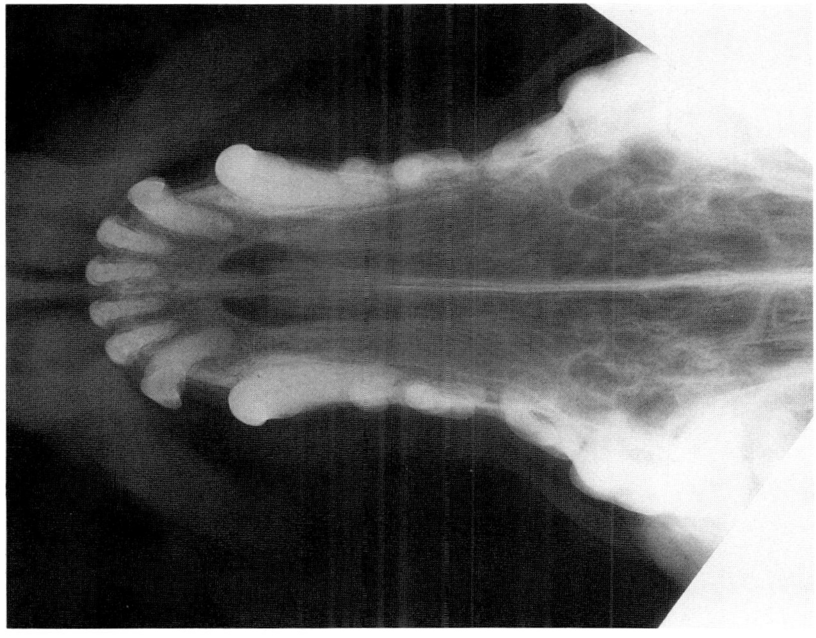

Figure 16. Positioning for an intraoral image of the mandible.

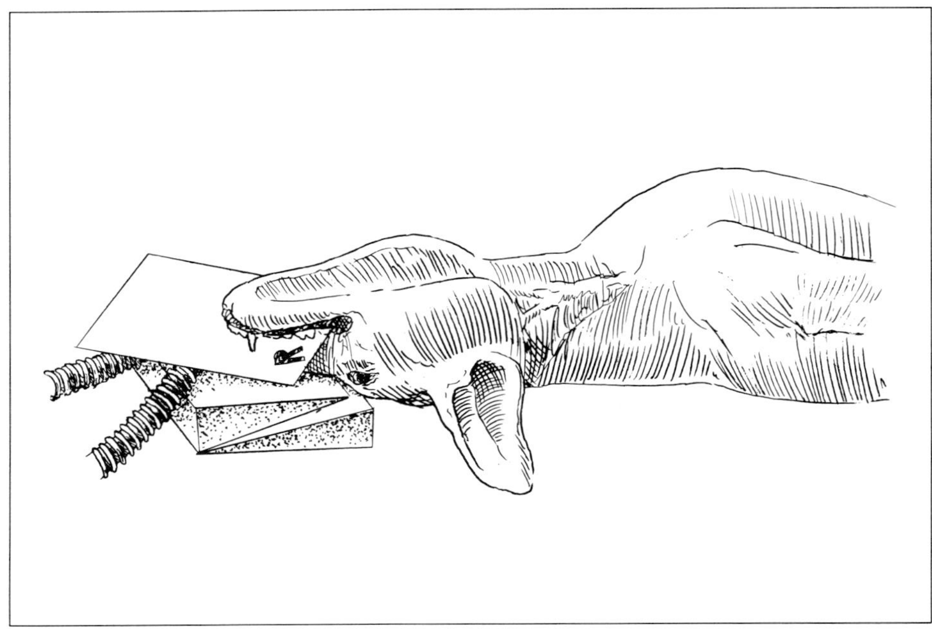

Figure 17. Intraoral image of the mandible.

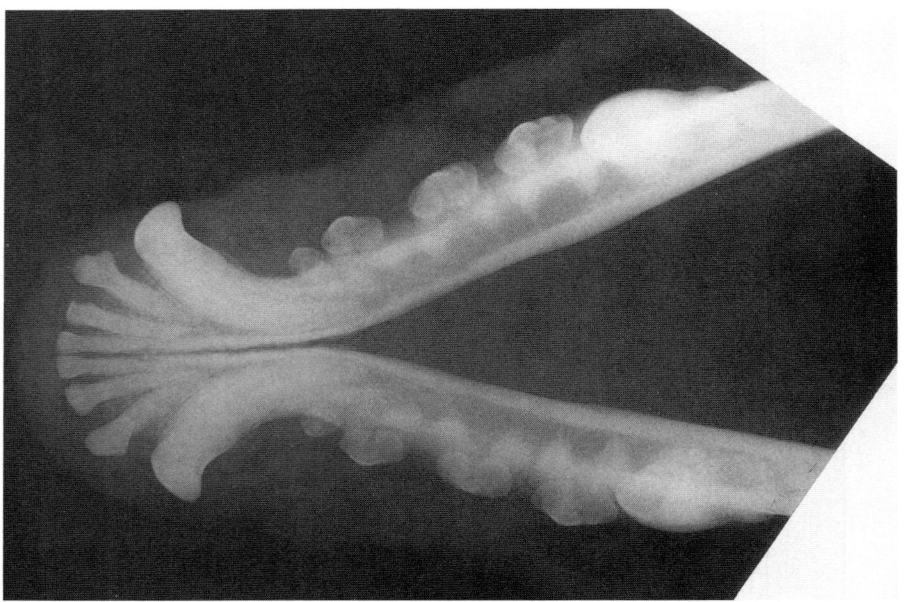

Figure 18. Positioning for a lateral oblique projection of the skull to image the tympanic bulla and temporomandibular joint.

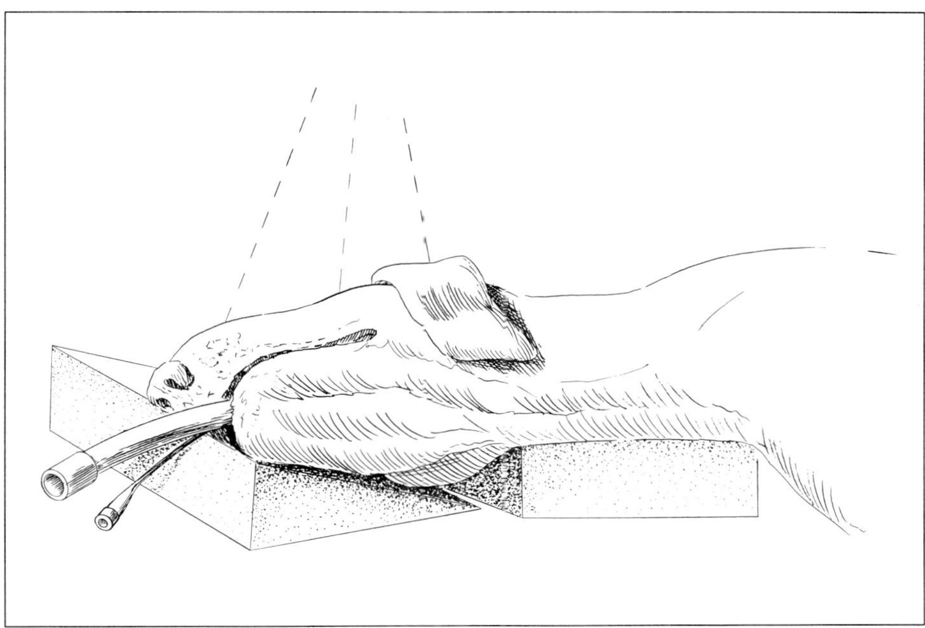

Figure 19. Lateral oblique projection of the skull to image the tympanic bulla and temporomandibular joint.

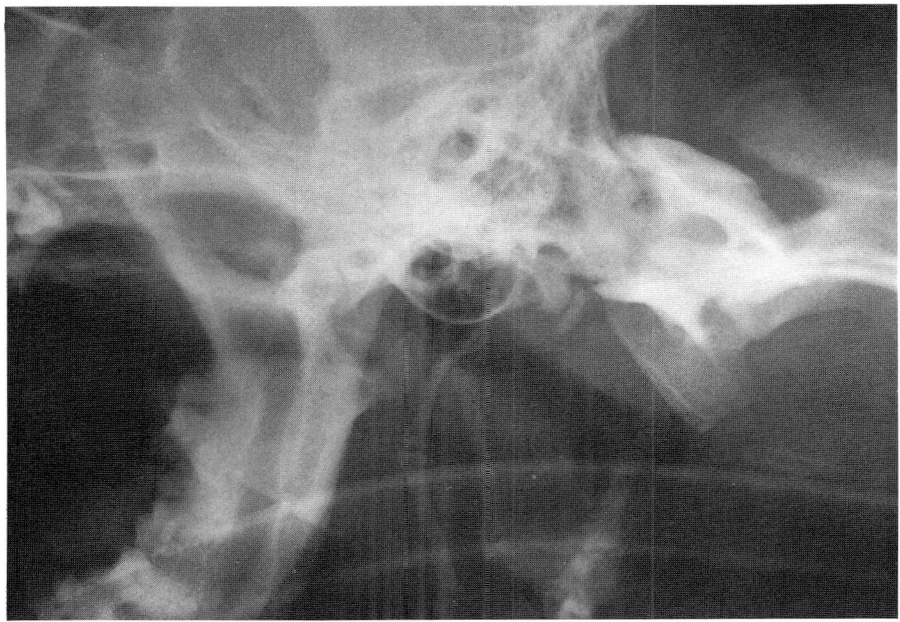

Figure 20. Positioning for a lateral projection of the cervical vertebrae.

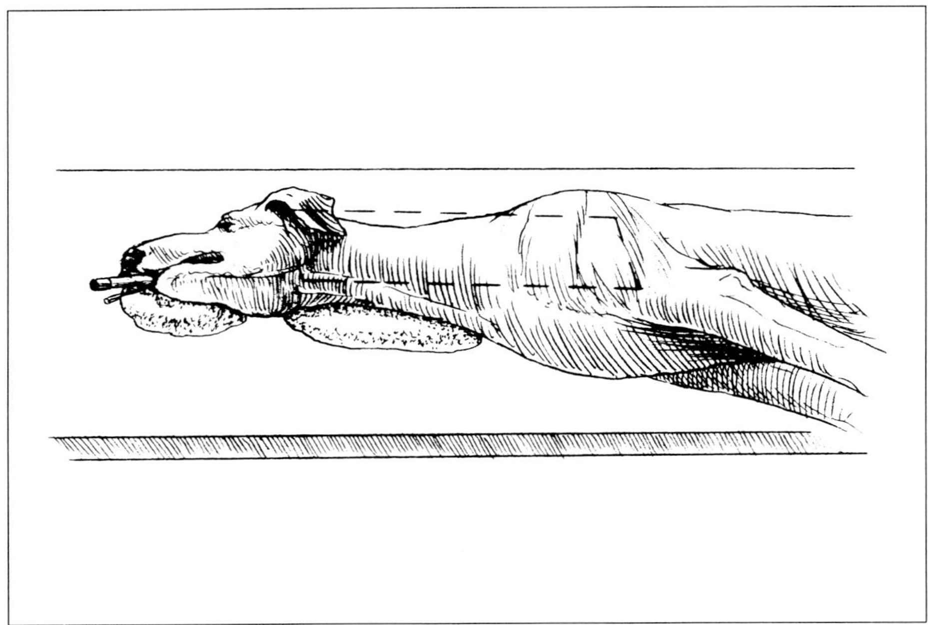

Figure 21. Lateral projection of the cervical vertebrae.

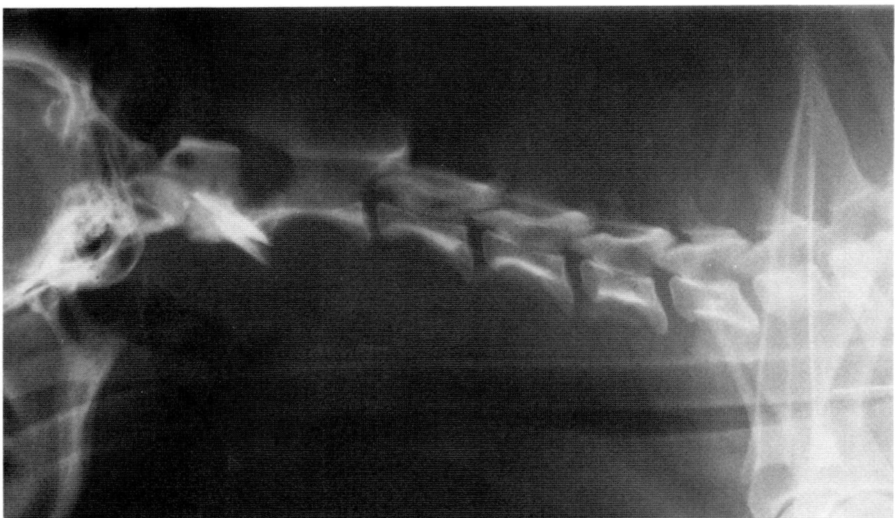

Figure 22. Positioning for a ventrodorsal projection of the cervical vertebrae.

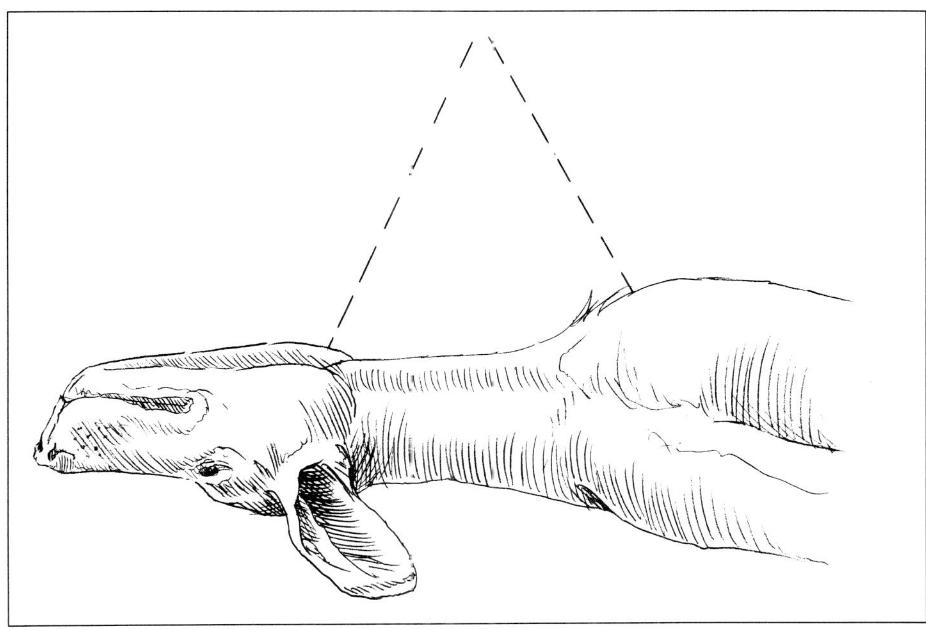

Figure 23. Ventrodorsal projection of the cervical vertebrae.

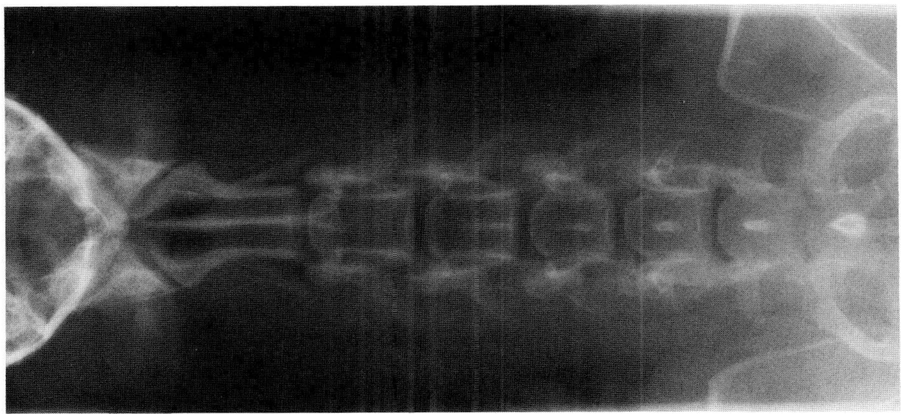

Figure 24. Positioning for a dorsoventral projection of the cervical vertebrae.

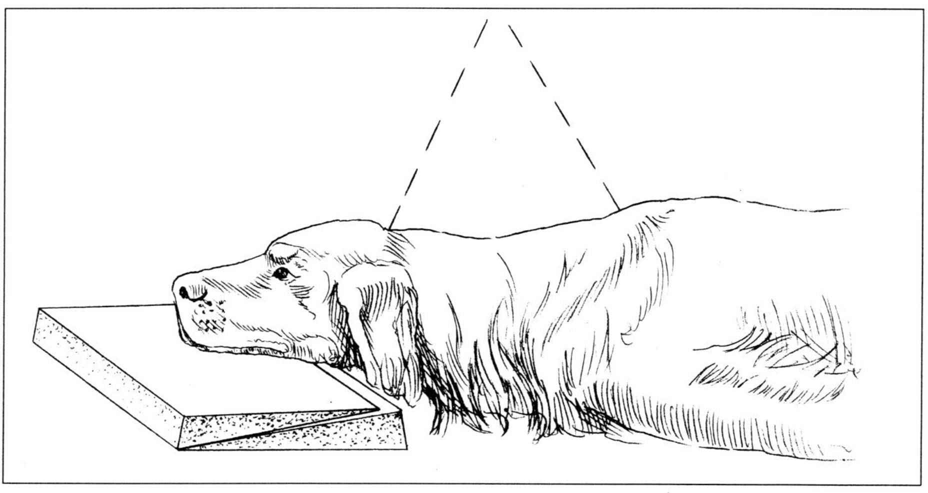

Figure 25. Positioning for a 45-degree oblique projection of the cervical vertebrae.

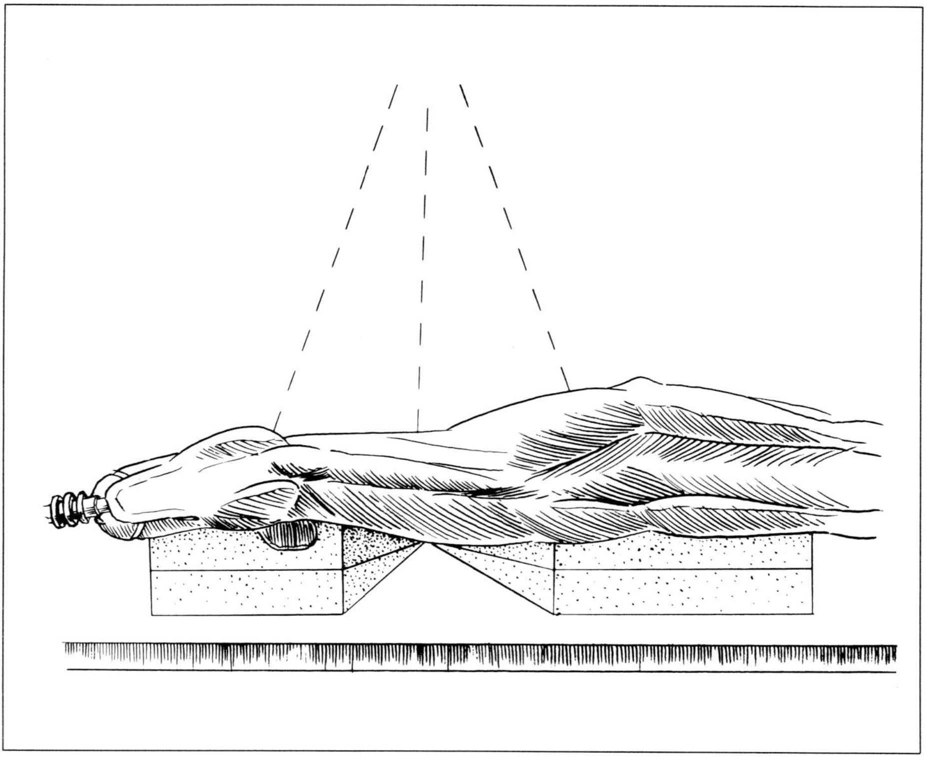

Figure 26. Positioning for a flexed lateral projection of the cervical vertebrae.

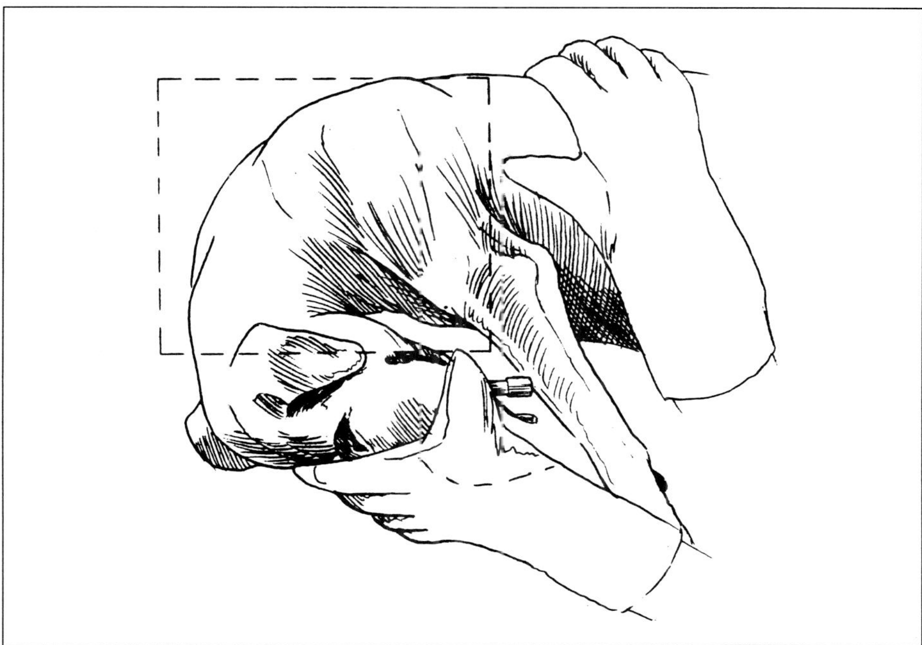

Figure 27. Positioning for an extended lateral projection of the cervical vertebrae.

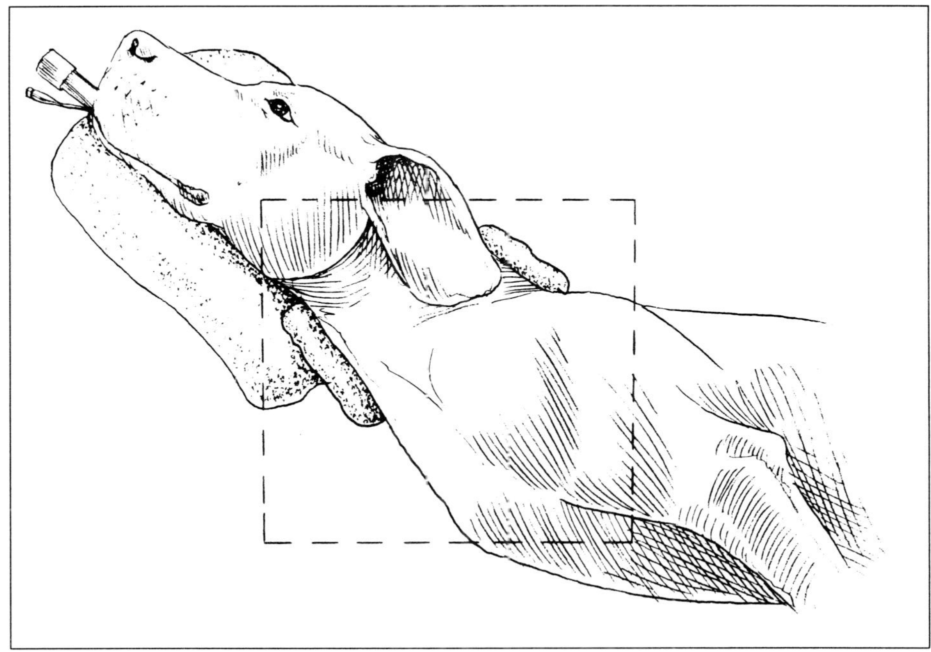

Figure 28. Positioning for a lateral projection of the thoracic vertebrae.

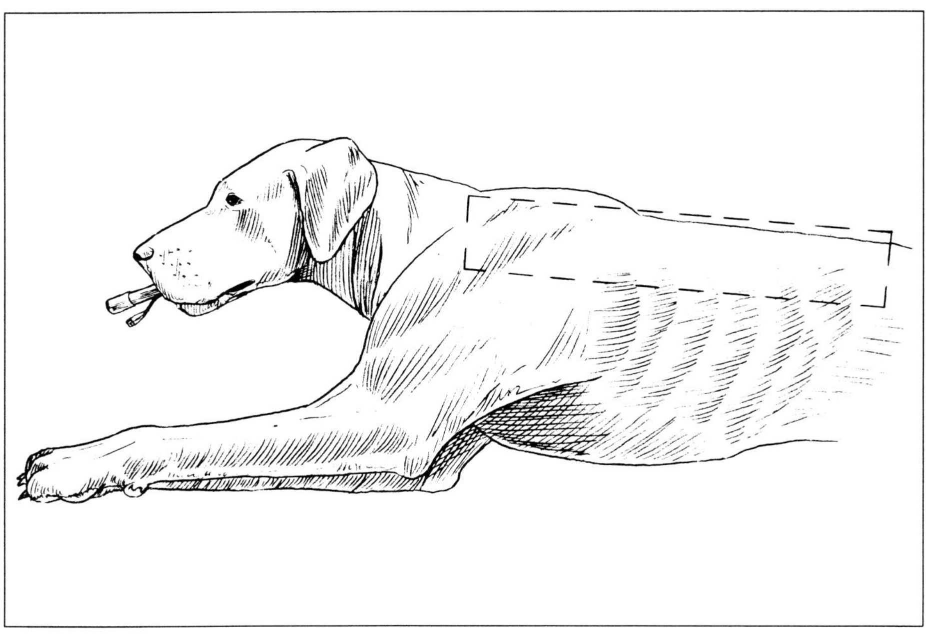

Figure 29. Lateral projection of the thoracic vertebrae.

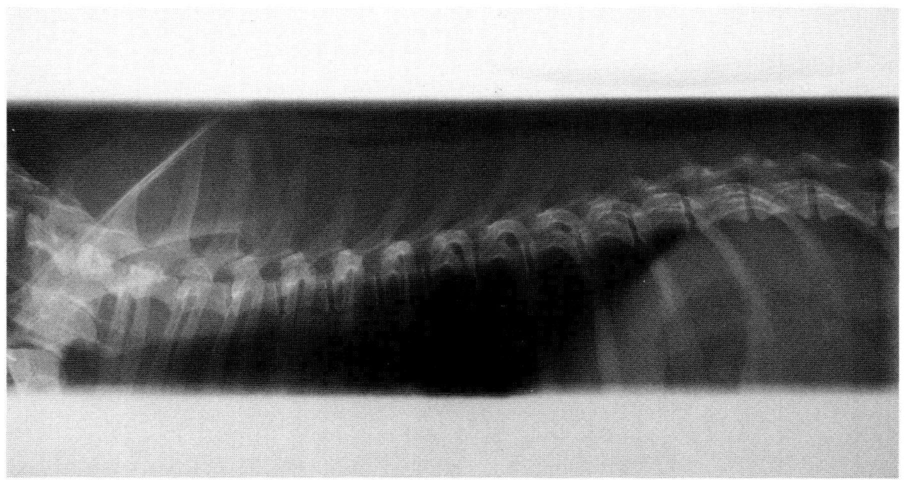

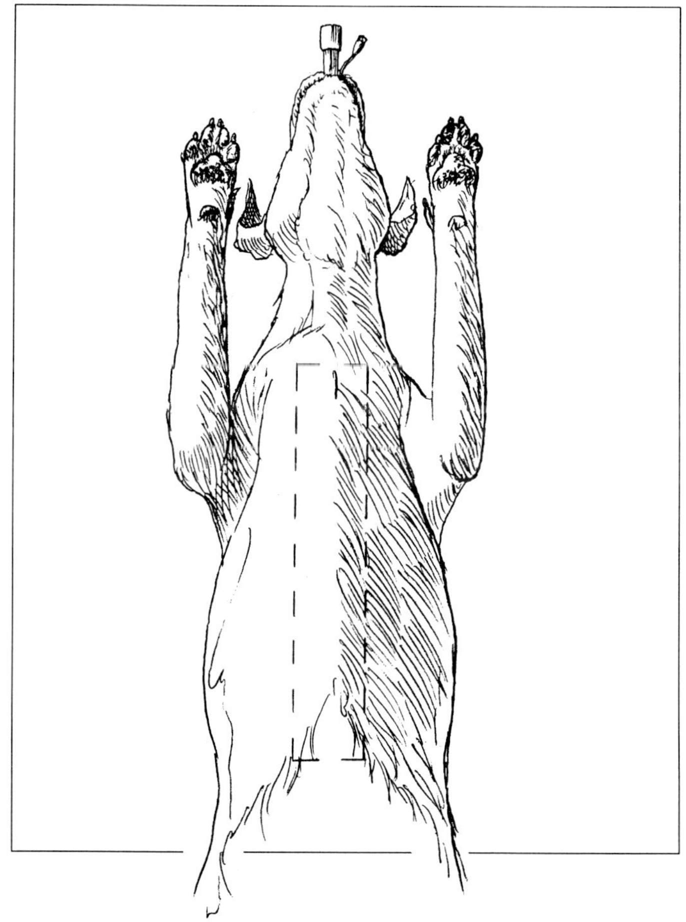

Figure 30. Positioning for a ventrodorsal projection of the thoracic vertebrae.

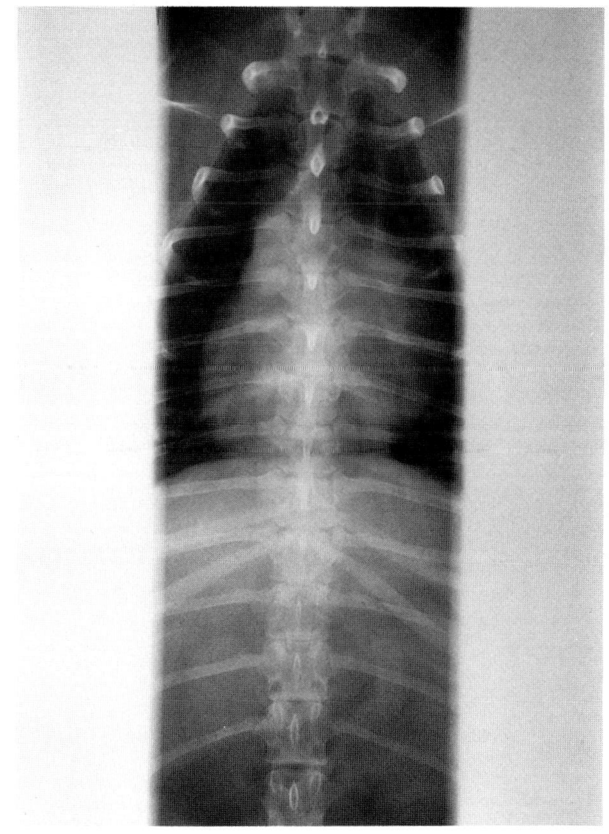

Figure 31. Ventrodorsal projection of the thoracic vertebrae.

Figure 32. Positioning for a lateral projection of the thoracolumbar vertebrae.

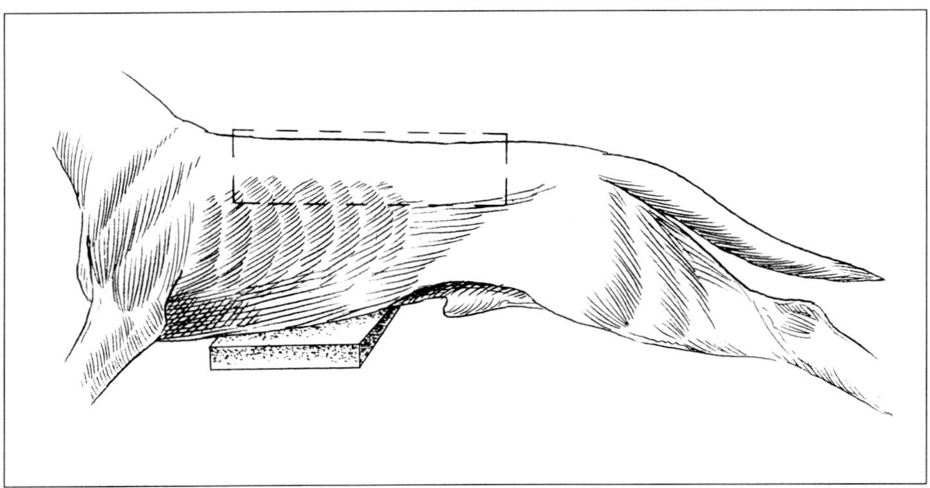

Figure 33. Lateral projection of the thoracolumbar vertebrae.

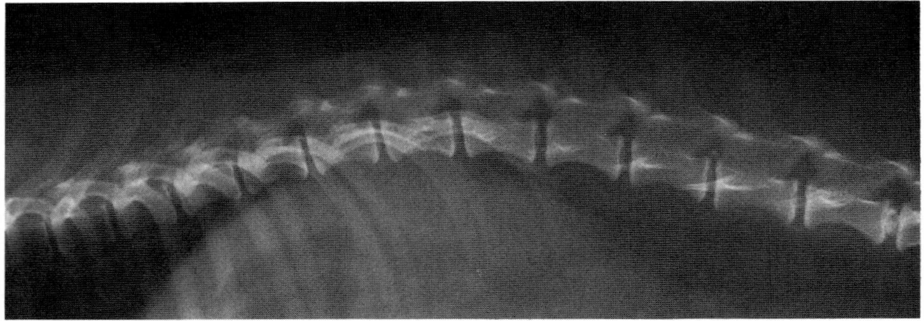

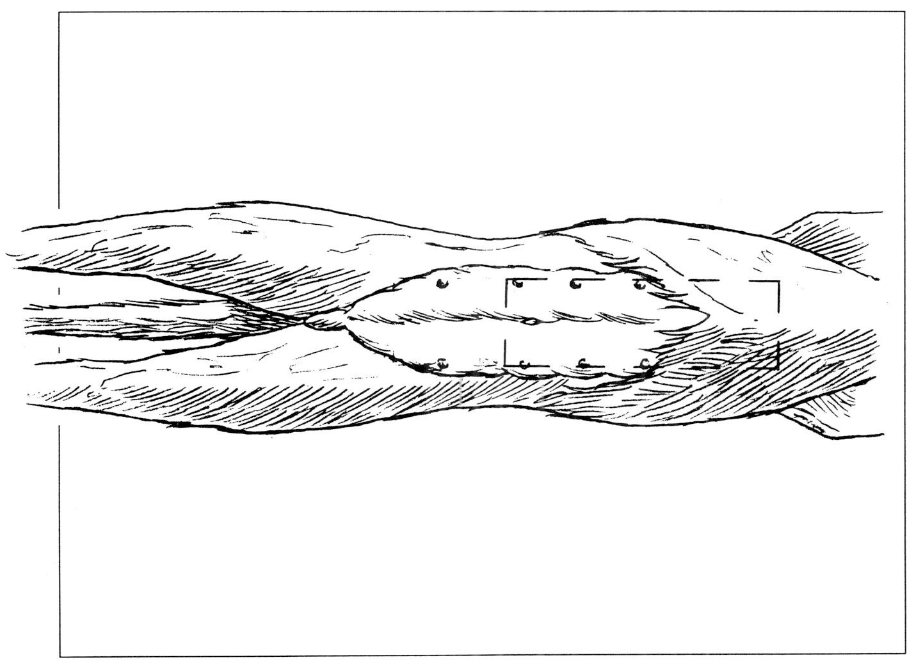

Figure 34. Positioning for a ventrodorsal projection of the thoracolumbar vertebrae.

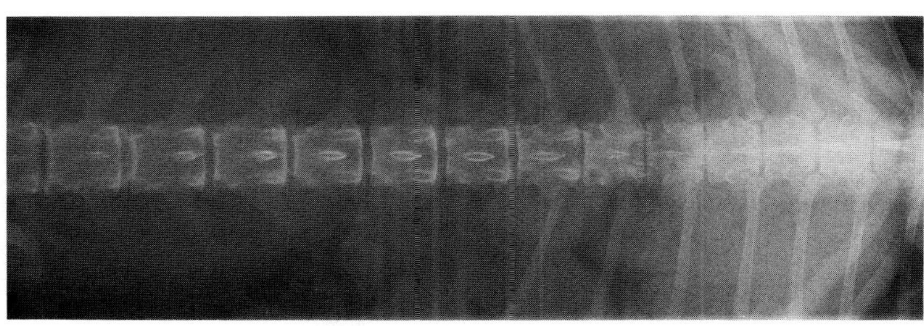

Figure 35. Ventrodorsal projection of the thoracolumbar vertebrae.

Figure 36. Positioning for a lateral projection of the lumbar vertebrae.

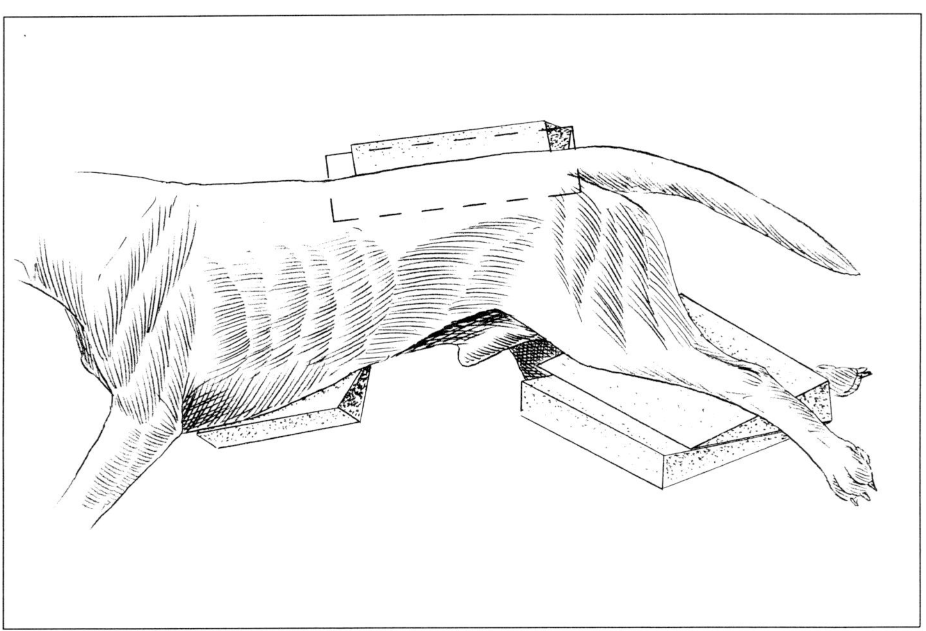

Figure 37. Lateral projection of the lumbar vertebrae.

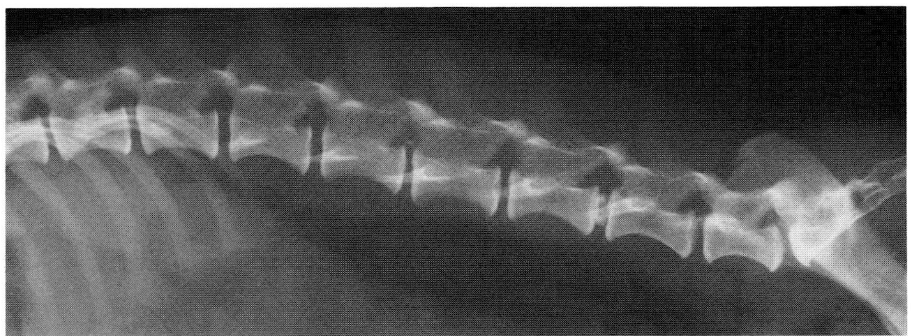

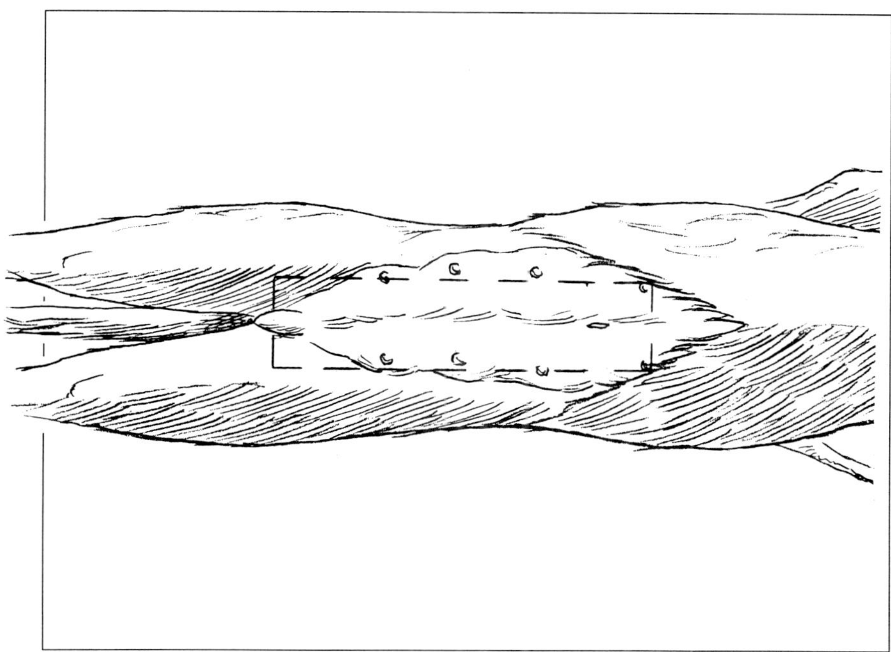

Figure 38. Positioning for a ventrodorsal projection of the lumbar vertebrae.

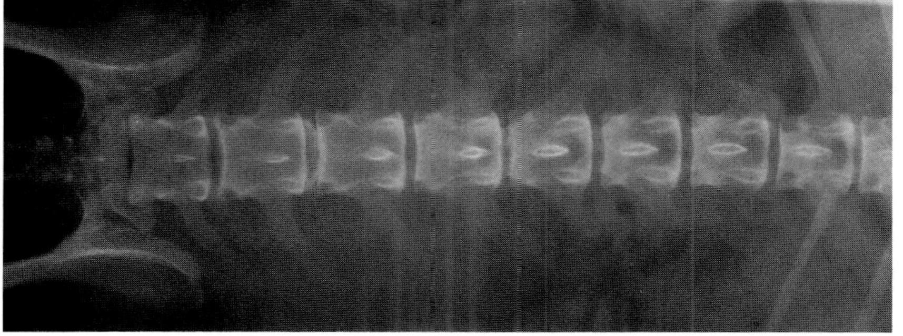

Figure 39. Ventrodorsal projection of the lumbar vertebrae.

Figure 40. Positioning for a lateral projection of the lumbosacral vertebrae.

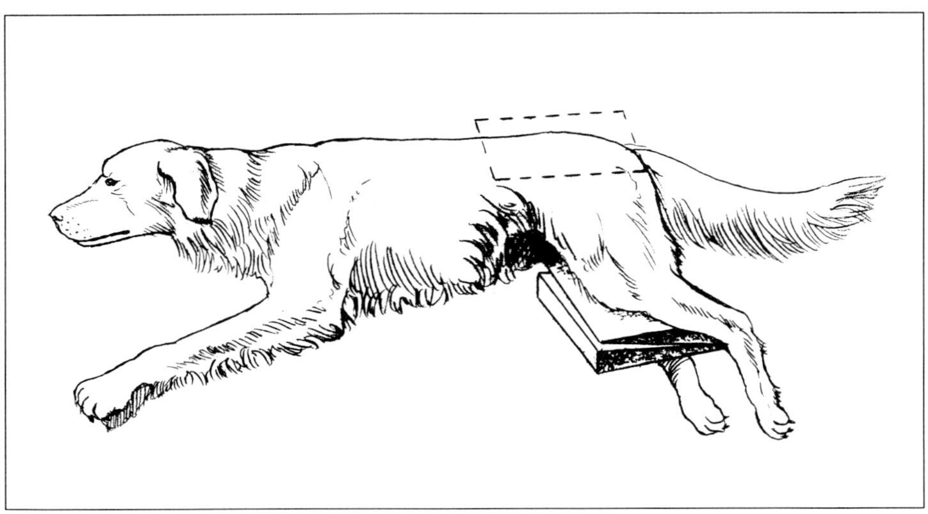

Figure 41. Lateral projection of the lumbosacral vertebrae.

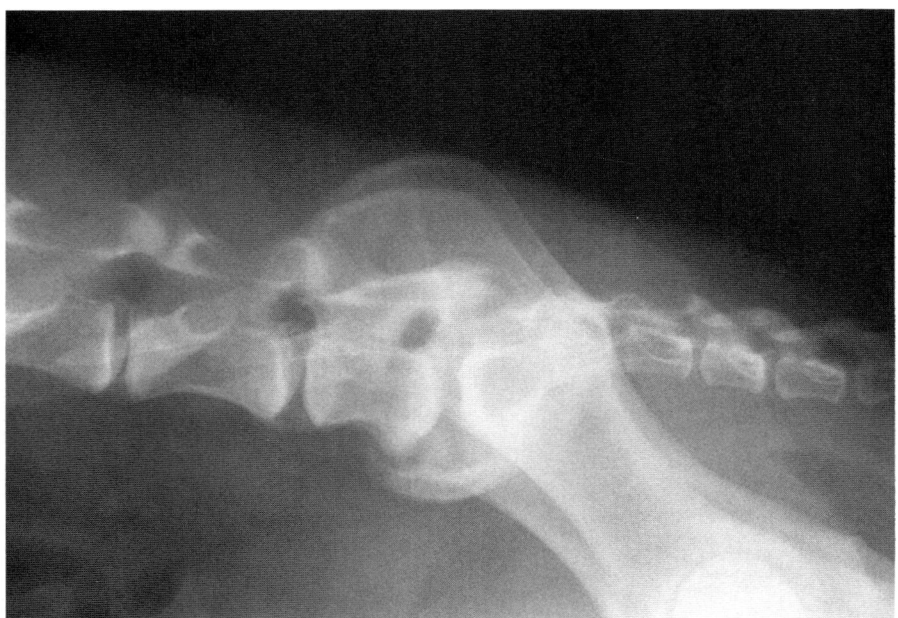

Figure 42. Positioning for a ventrodorsal projection of the lumbosacral vertebrae.

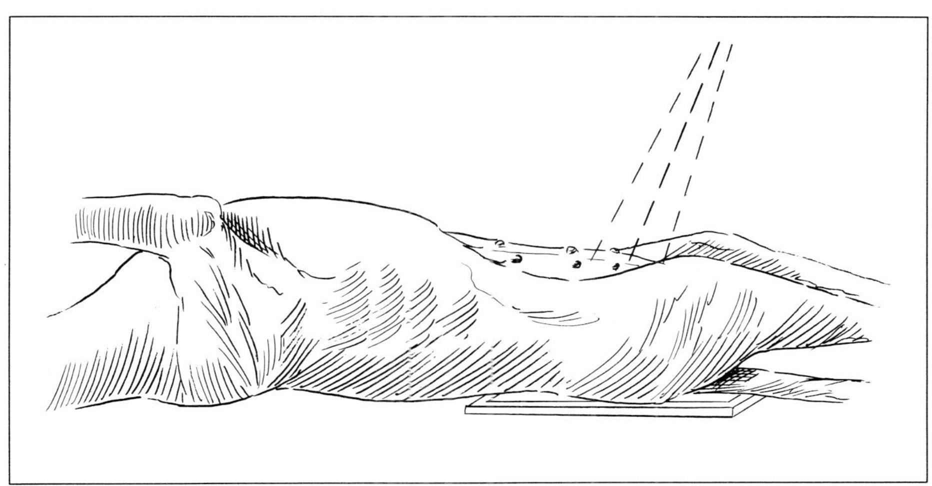

Figure 43. Ventrodorsal projection of the lumbosacral vertebrae.

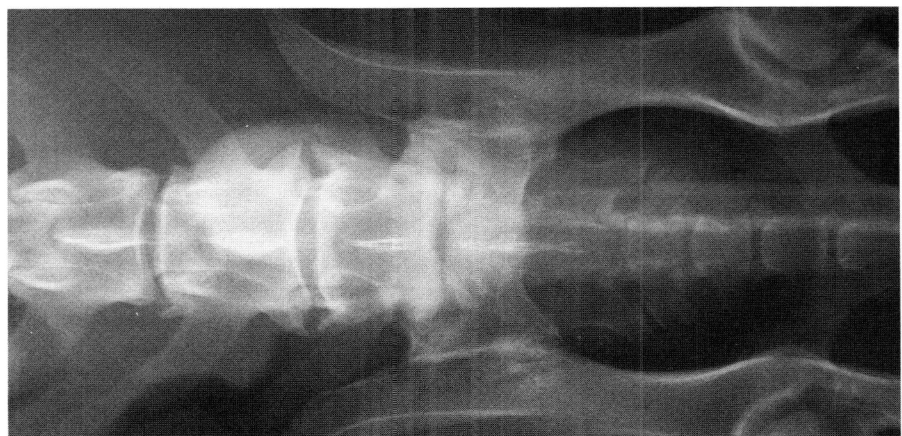

Figure 44. A. Positioning for a mediolateral projection of the metacarpus and digits. B. Positioning for a lateral oblique of the metacarpus. This sets off each metacarpus without the others being superimposed. C. Positioning for a lateral projection of the digits.

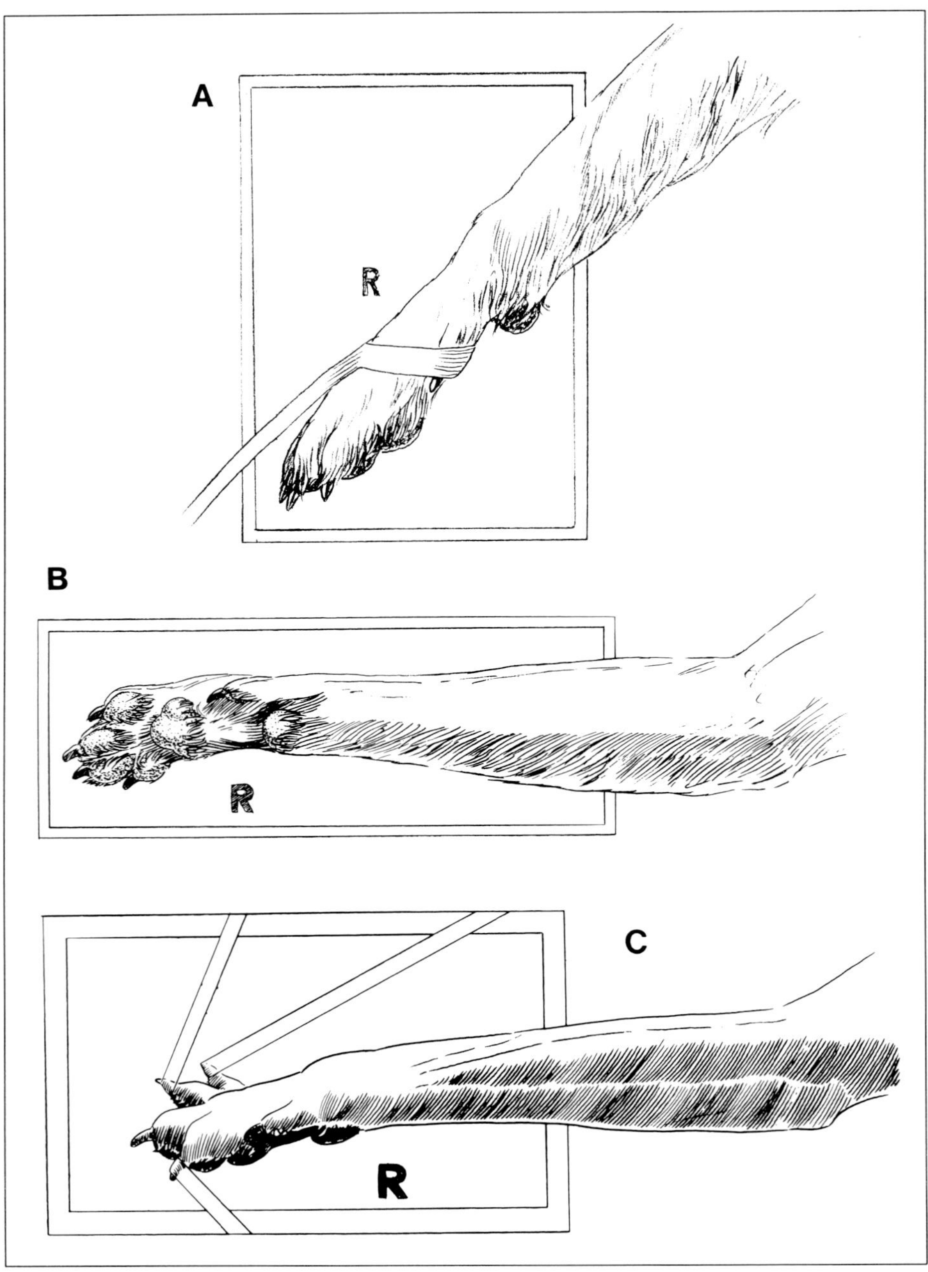

Figure 45. Image A is a lateral projection of the metacarpus and digits. Image B is a lateral oblique projection of the metacarpus. Image C is a lateral projection of the digits, using tape to separate the digits.

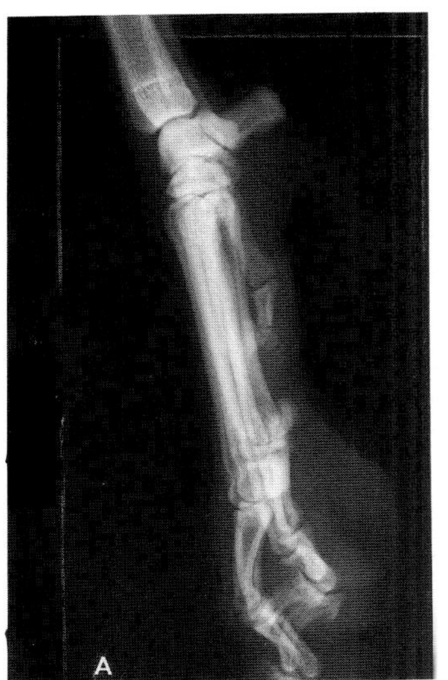
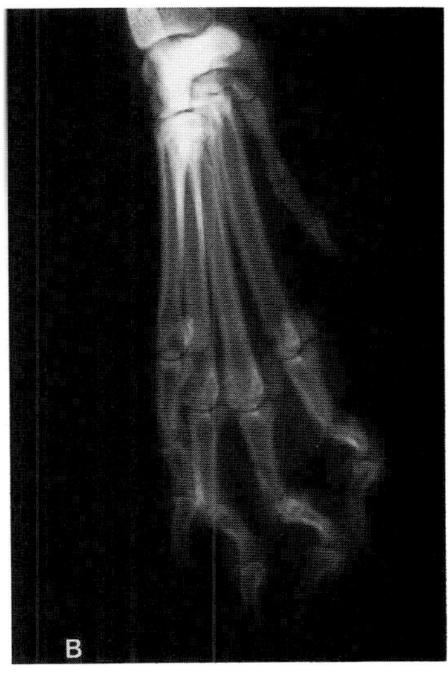
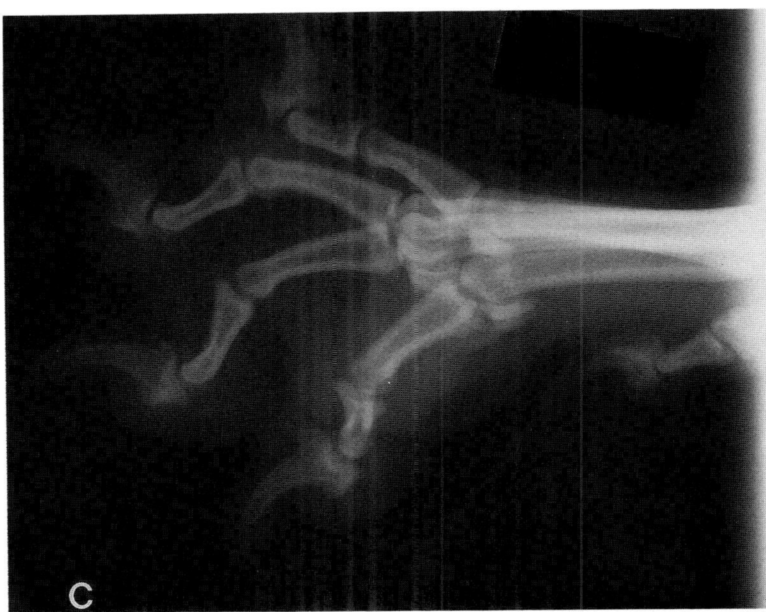

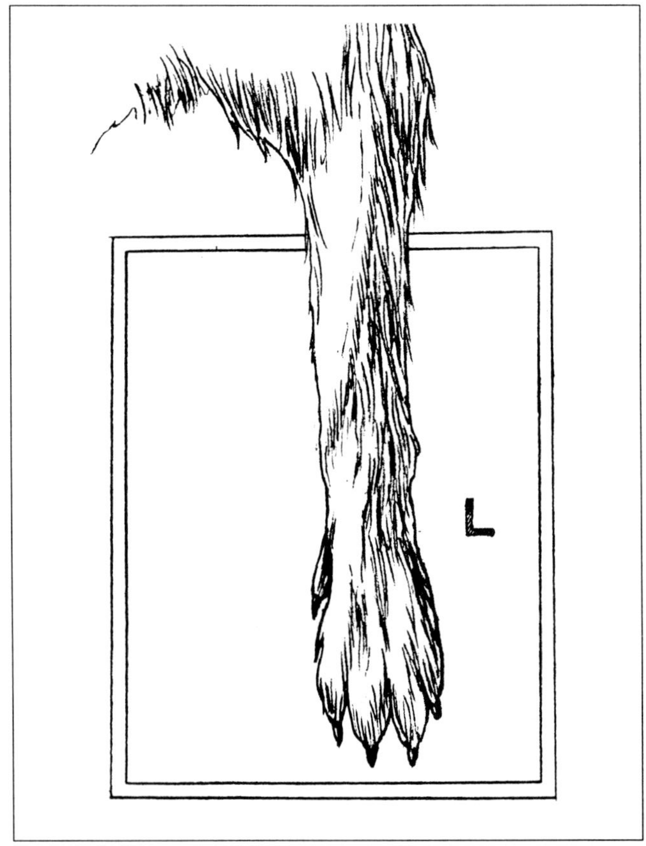

Figure 46. Positioning for a dorsopalmar projection of the metacarpus and digits.

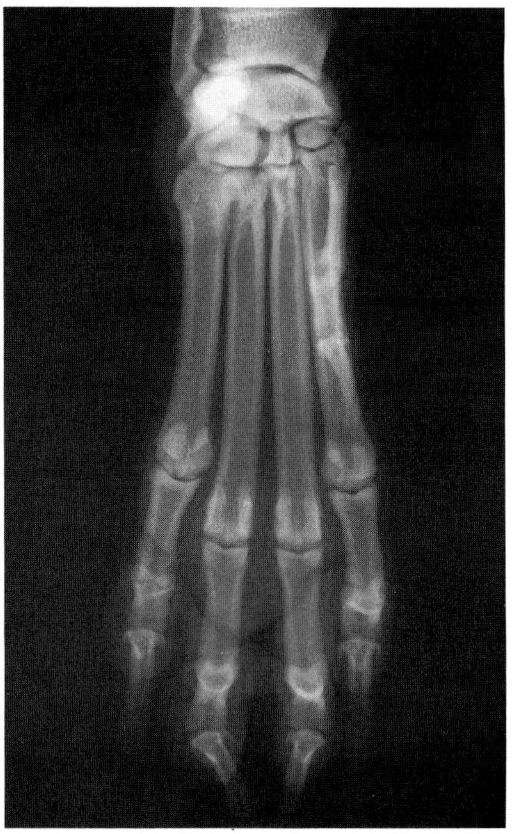

Figure 47. Dorsopalmar projection of the metacarpus and digits.

Figure 48. Positioning for a mediolateral projection of the carpus.

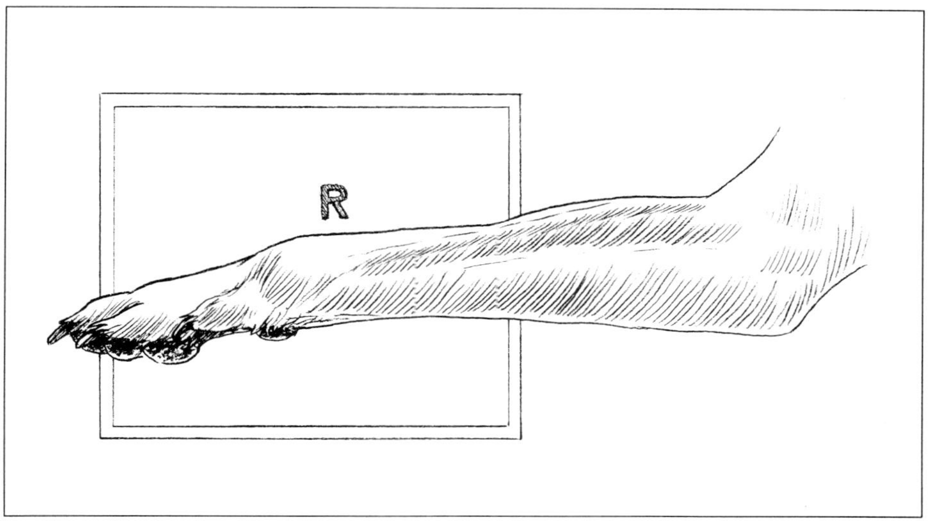

Figure 49. Mediolateral projection of the carpus.

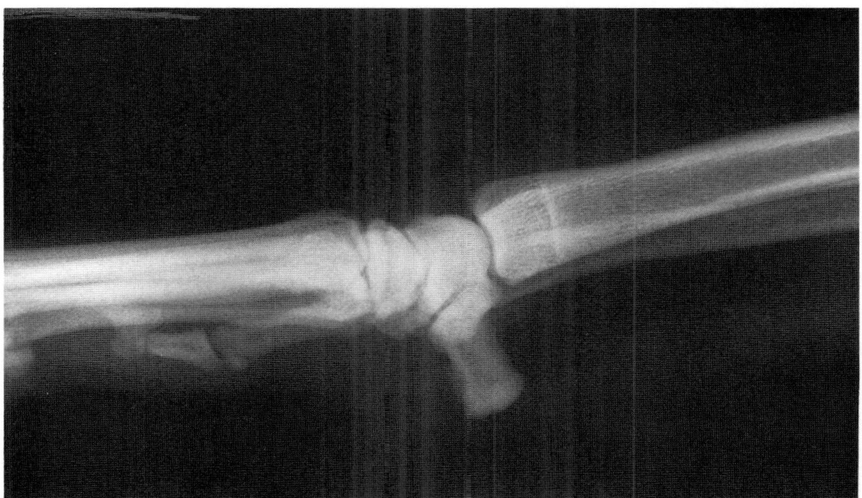

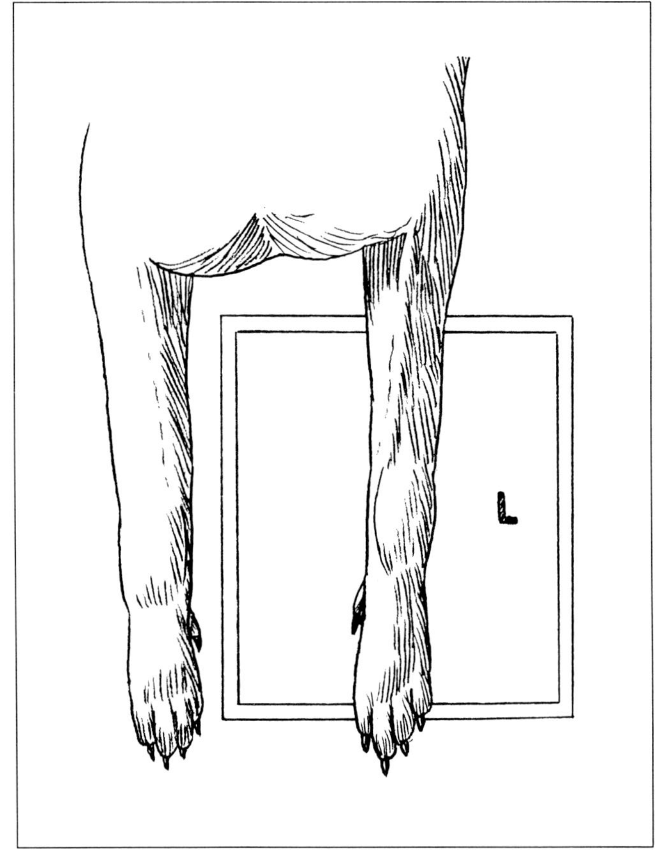

Figure 50. Positioning for a dorsopalmar projection of the carpus.

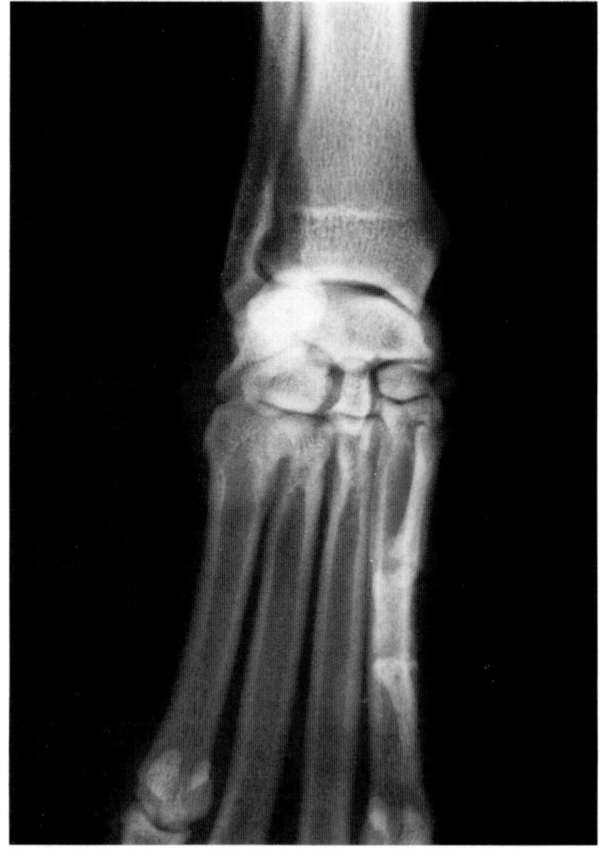

Figure 51. Dorsopalmar projection of the carpus.

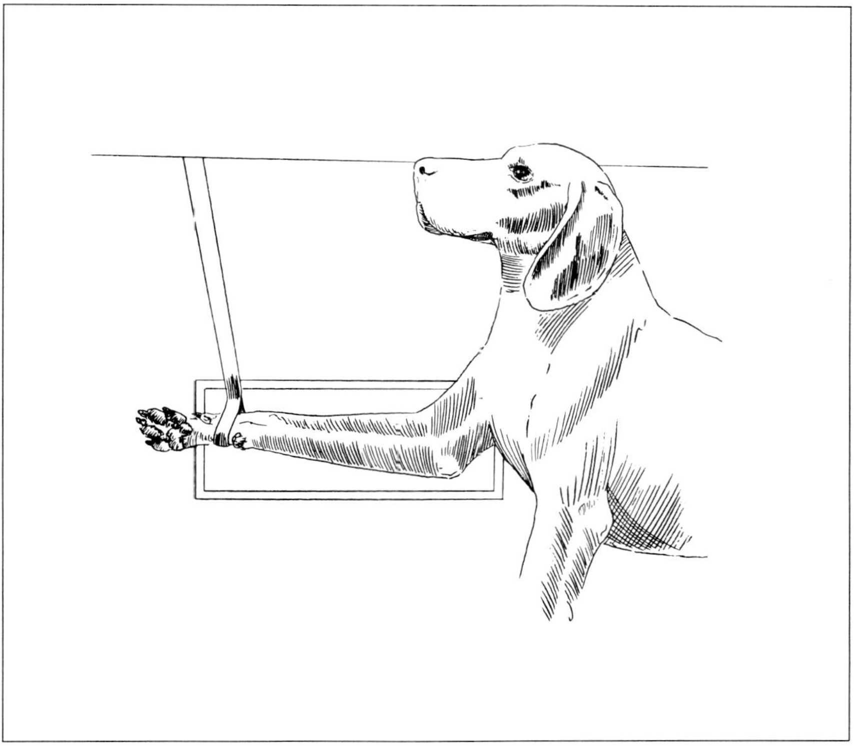

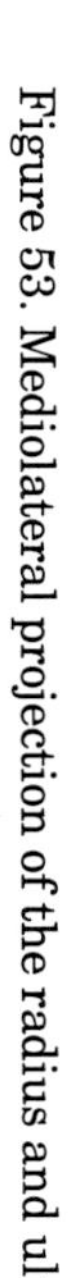

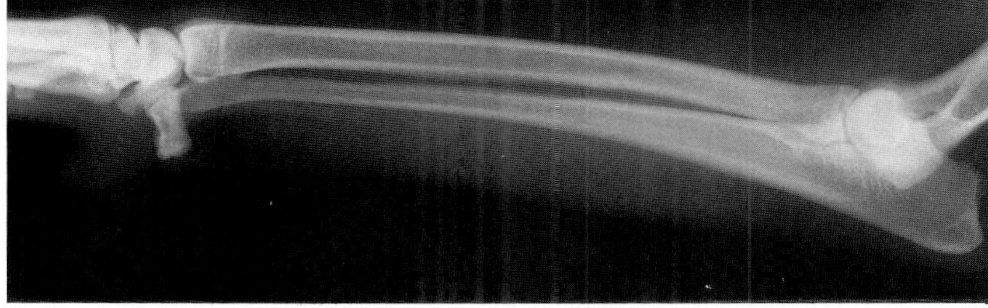

Figure 52. Positioning for a mediolateral projection of the radius and ulna.

Figure 53. Mediolateral projection of the radius and ulna.

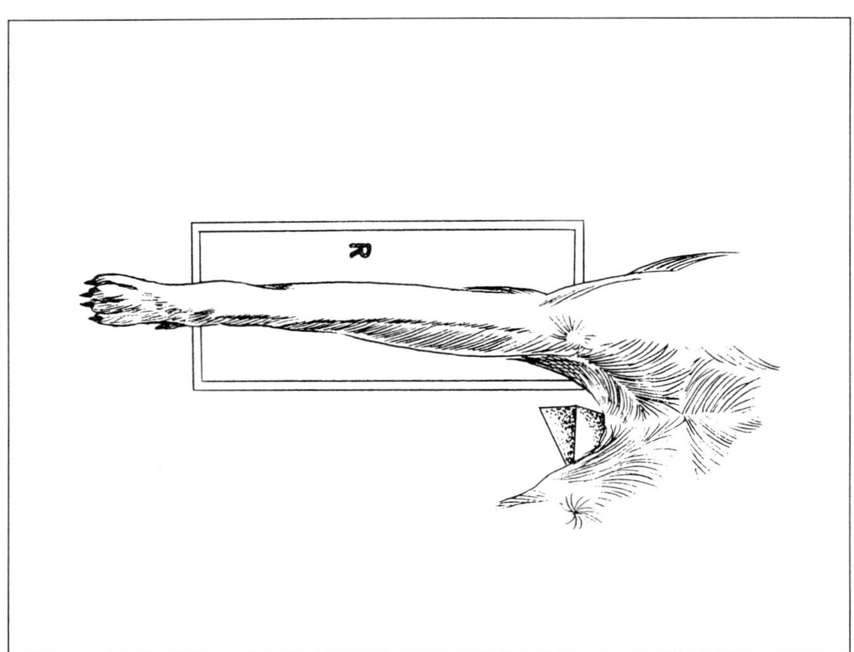

Figure 54. Positioning for a craniocaudal projection of the radius and ulna.

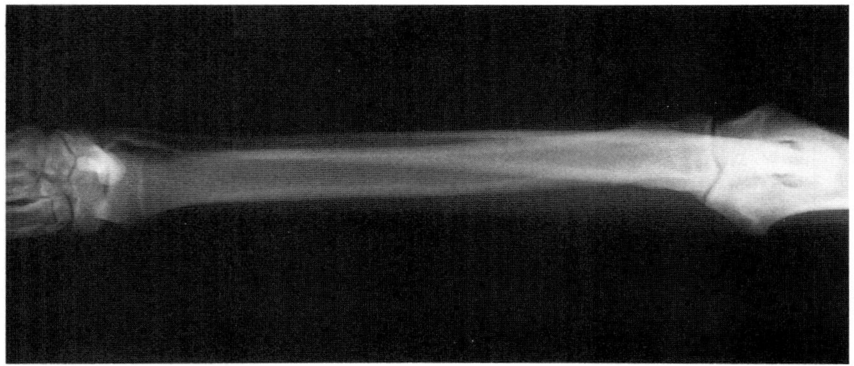

Figure 55. Craniocaudal projection of the radius and ulna.

Figure 56. Positioning for a mediolateral projection of the elbow (left). Positioning for a mediolateral projection of the elbow in the flexed position (right).

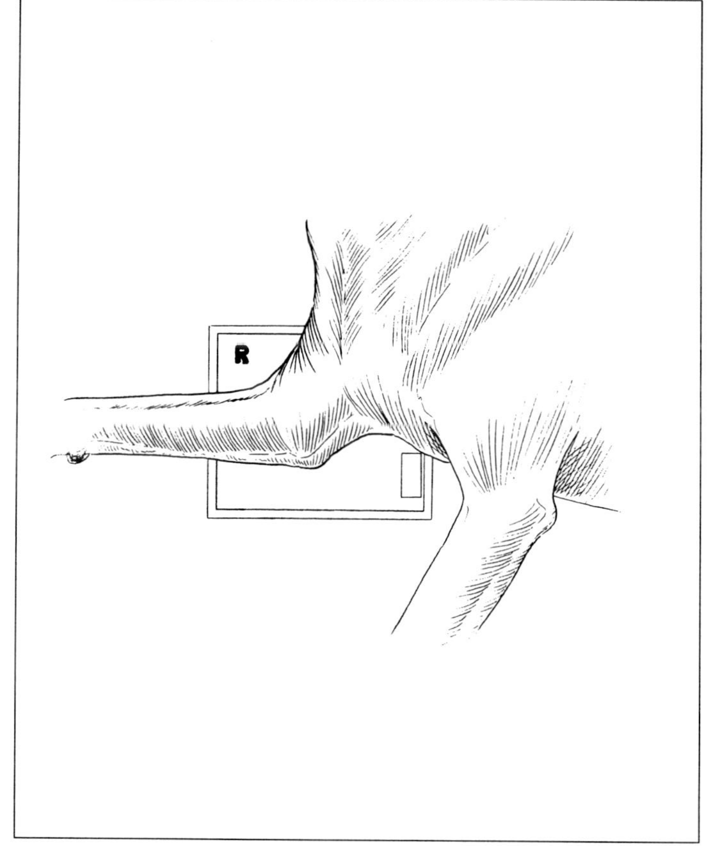
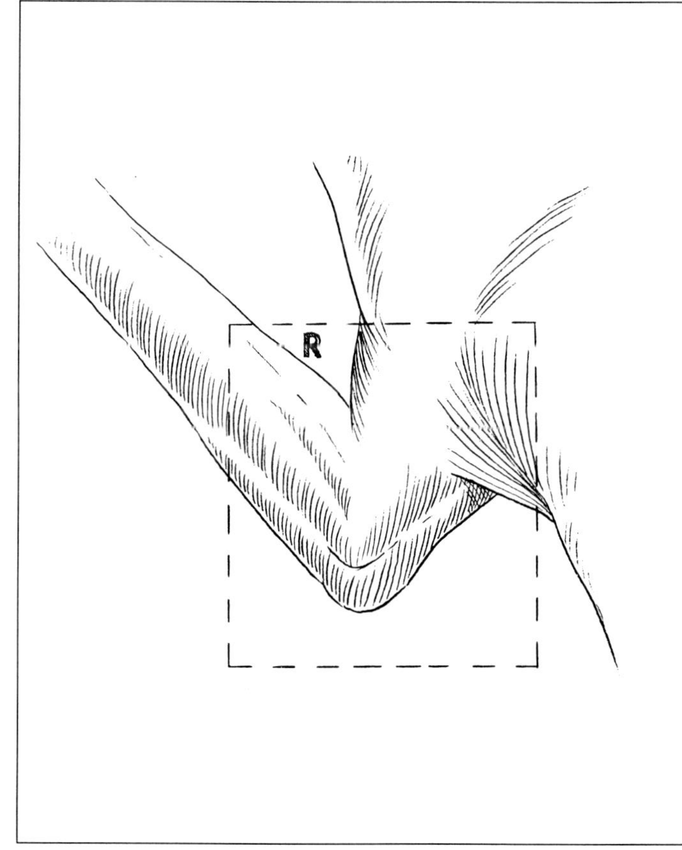

Figure 57. Mediolateral projection of the elbow (top). Mediolateral projection of the elbow in the flexed position (bottom).

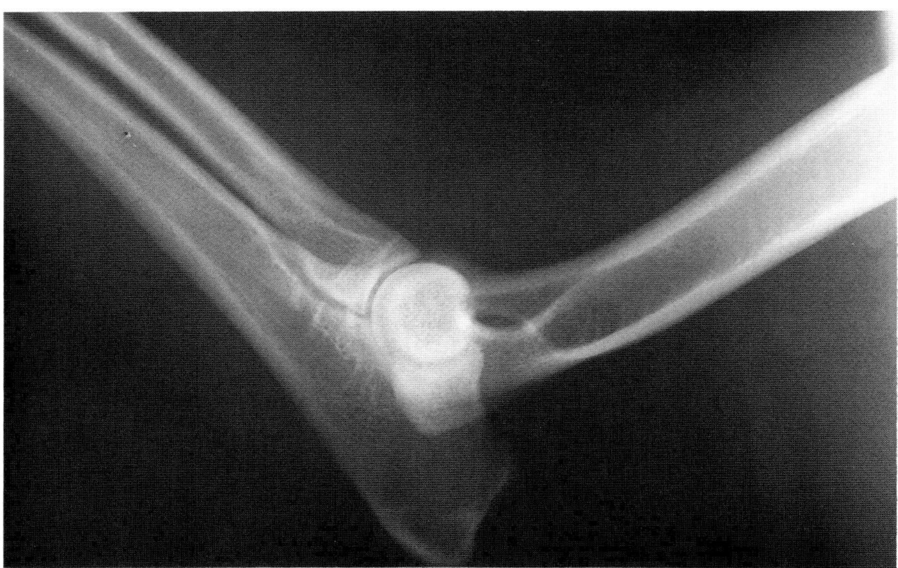

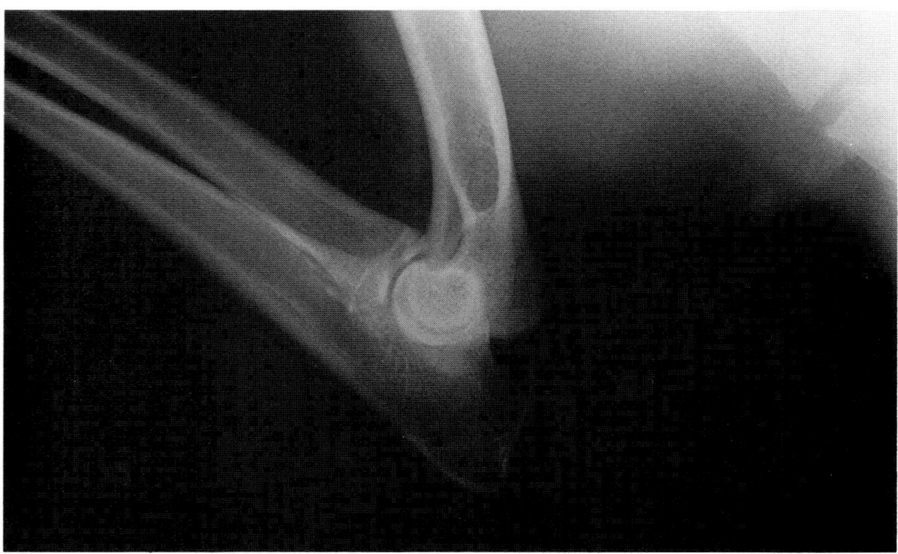

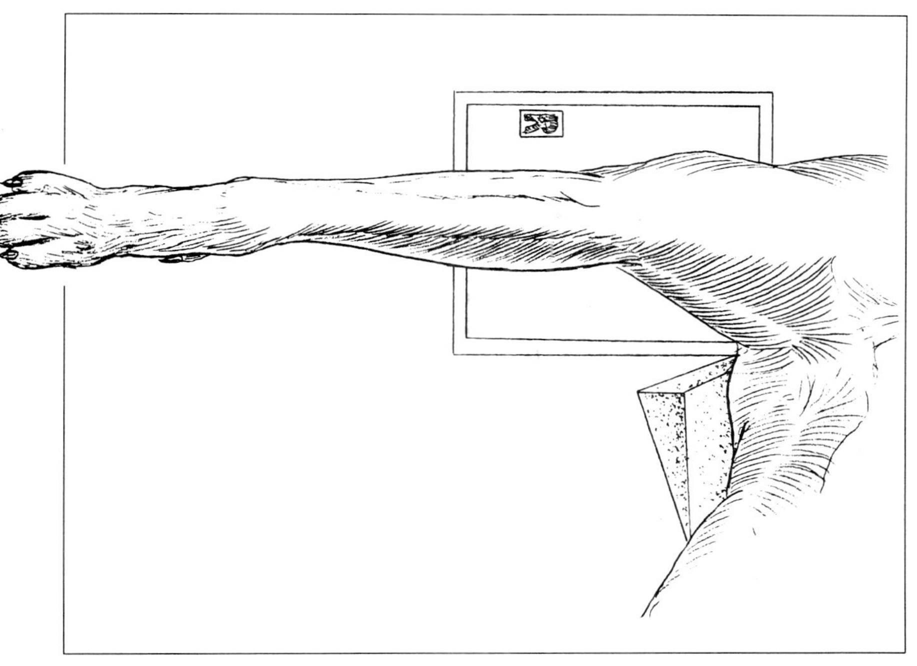

Figure 58. Positioning for a craniocaudal projection of the elbow.

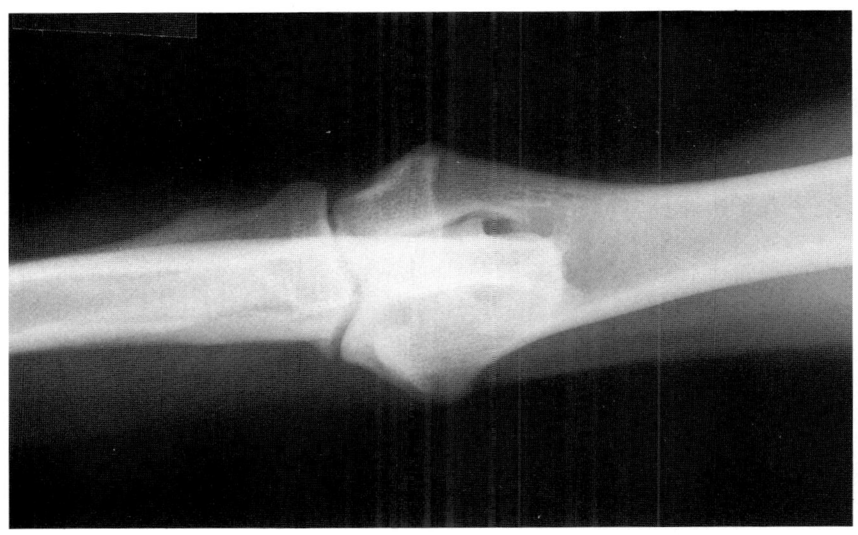

Figure 59. Craniocaudal projection of the elbow.

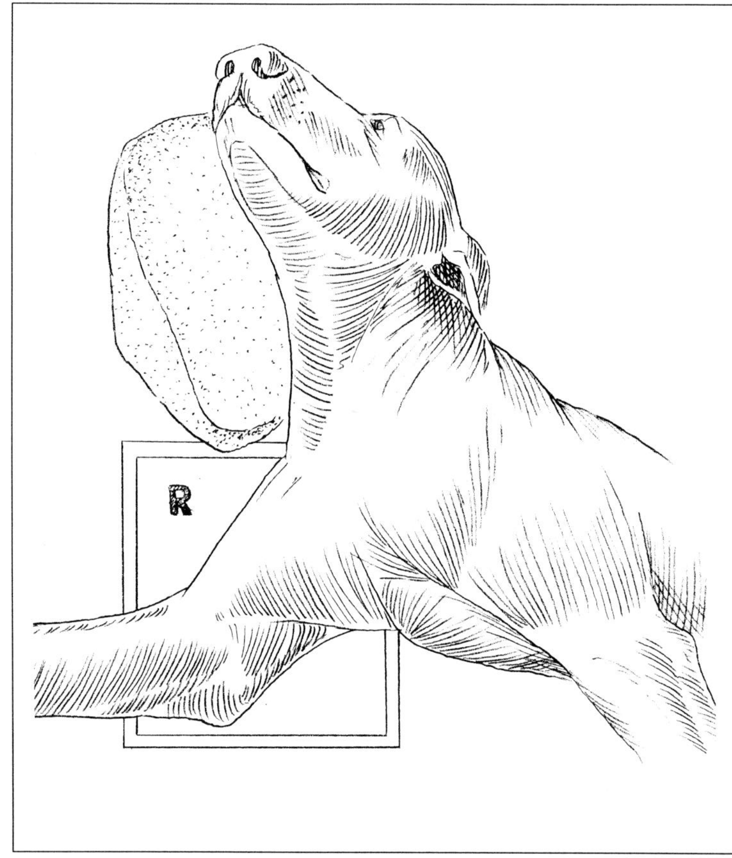

Figure 60. Positioning for a mediolateral projection of the humerus.

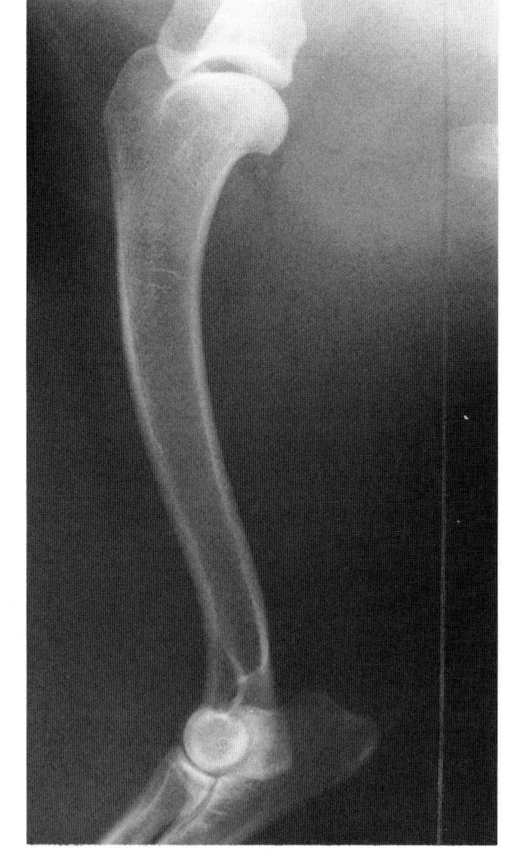

Figure 61. Mediolateral projection of the humerus.

Figure 62. Positioning for a cross-table caudocranial projection of the humerus (top). Figure 63. Positioning for a ventrodorsal extended caudocranial projection of the humerus (bottom right).

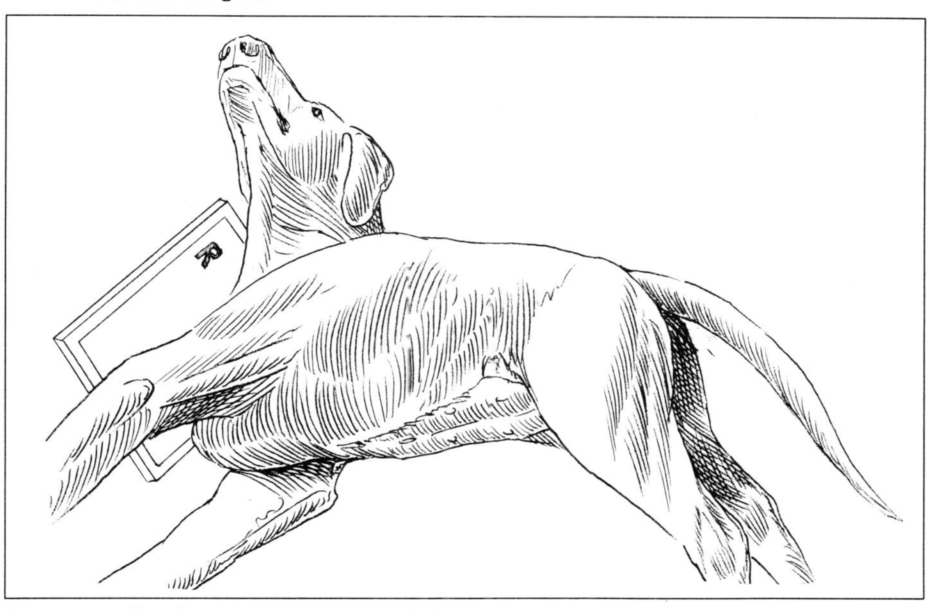

Figure 64. Caudocranial projection of the humerus.

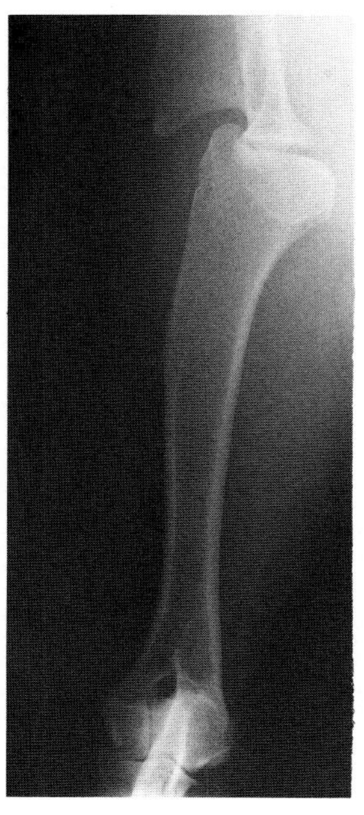

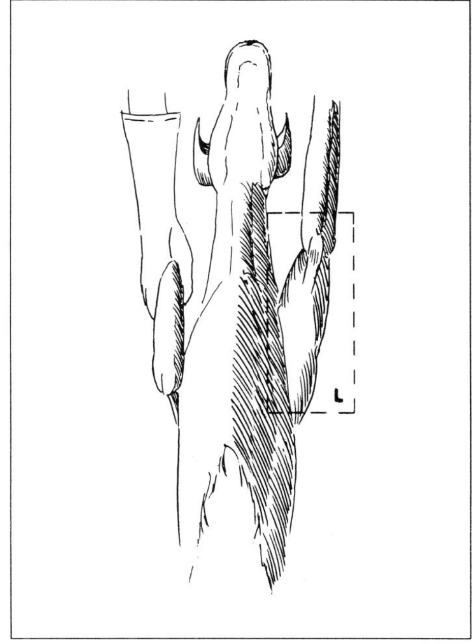

Figure 65. Positioning for a mediolateral projection of the shoulder joint.

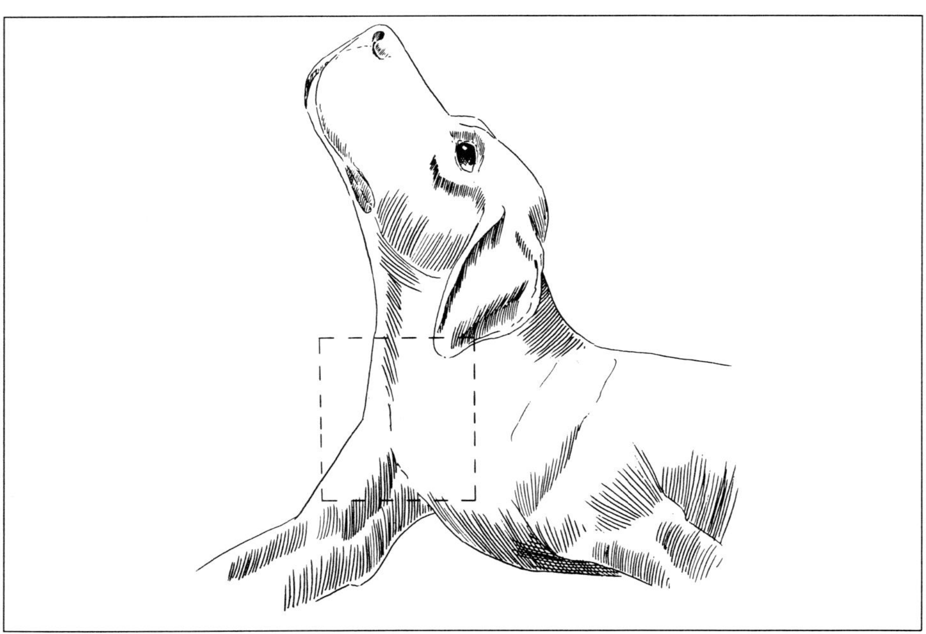

Figure 66. Mediolateral projection of the shoulder joint.

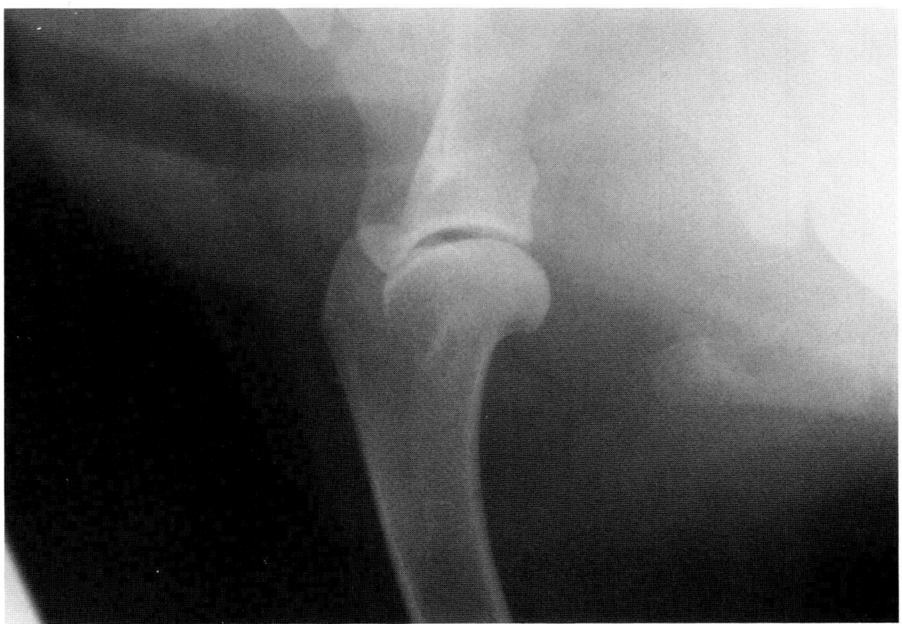

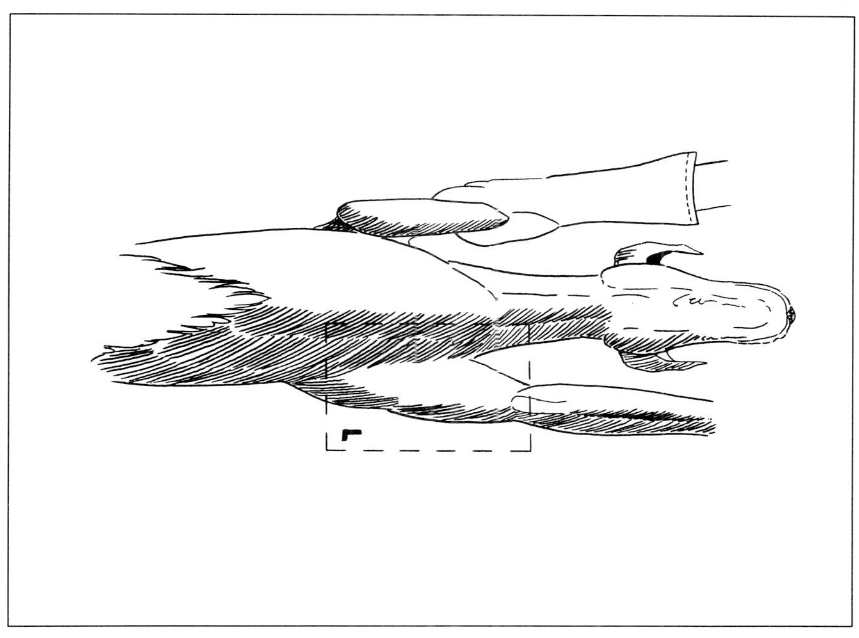

Figure 67. Positioning for a caudocranial projection of the shoulder joint.

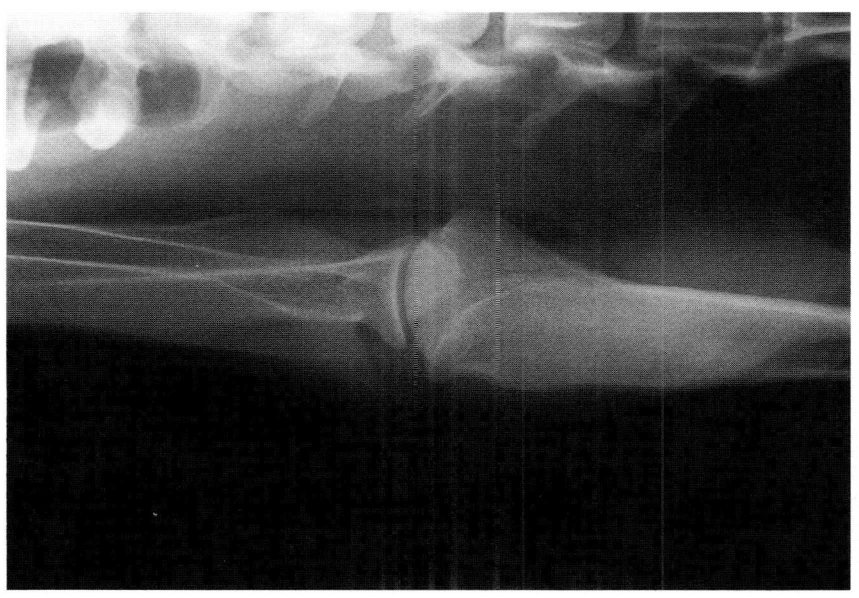

Figure 68. Caudocranial projection of the shoulder joint.

Figure 69. Positioning for a mediolateral projection of the scapula.

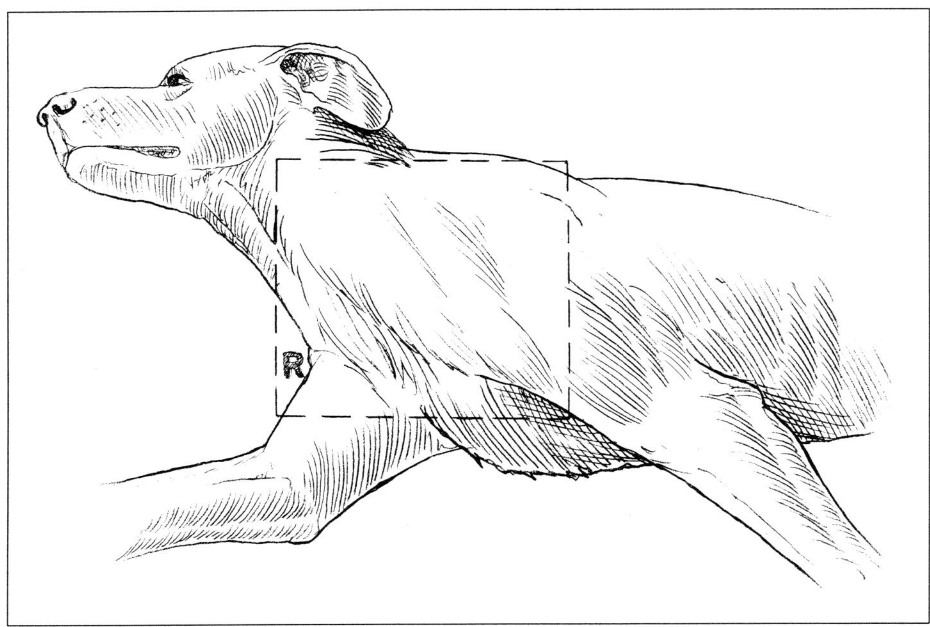

Figure 70. Mediolateral projection of the scapula.

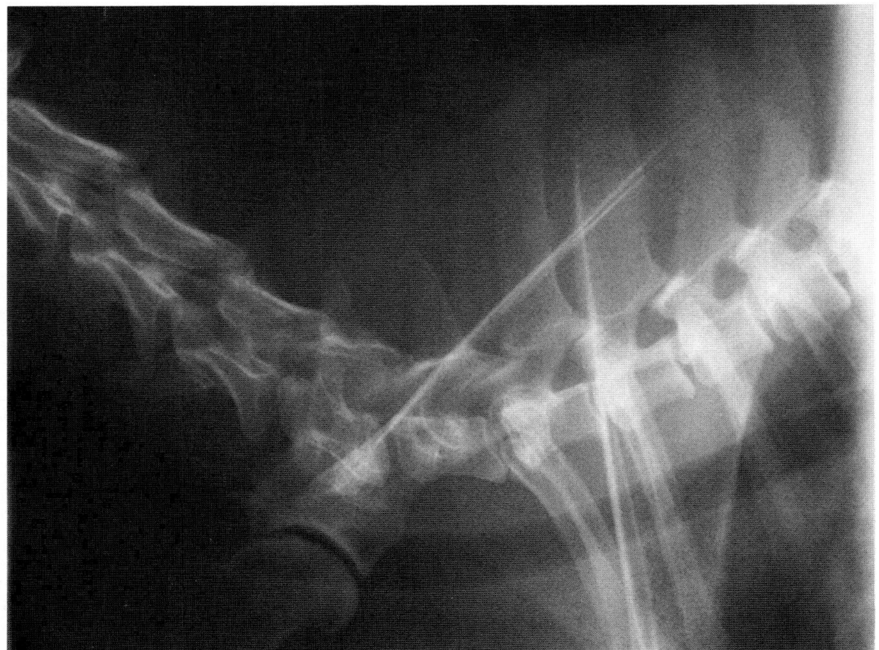

Figure 71. Positioning for a caudocranial projection of the scapula.

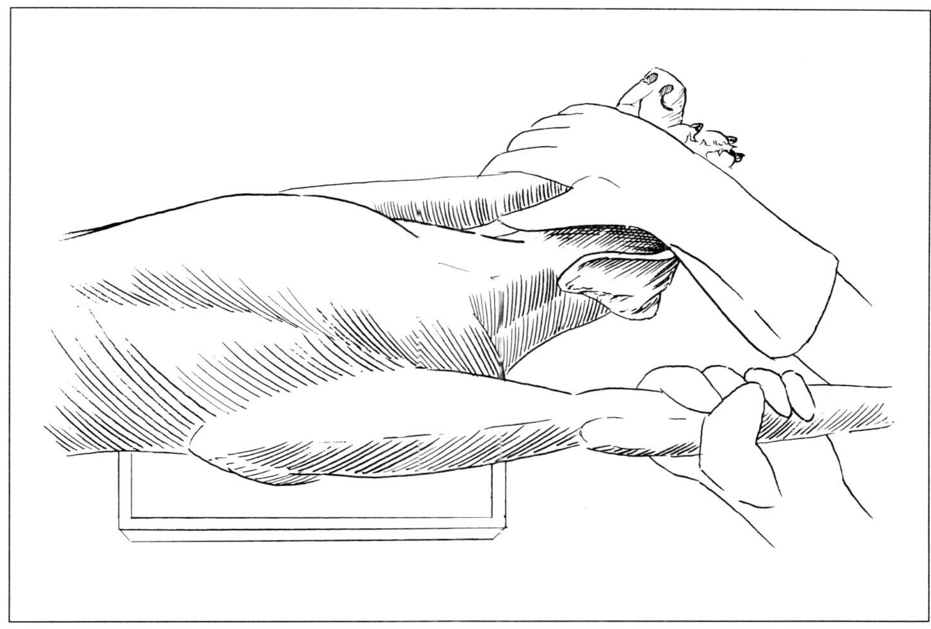

Figure 72. Caudocranial projection of the scapula.

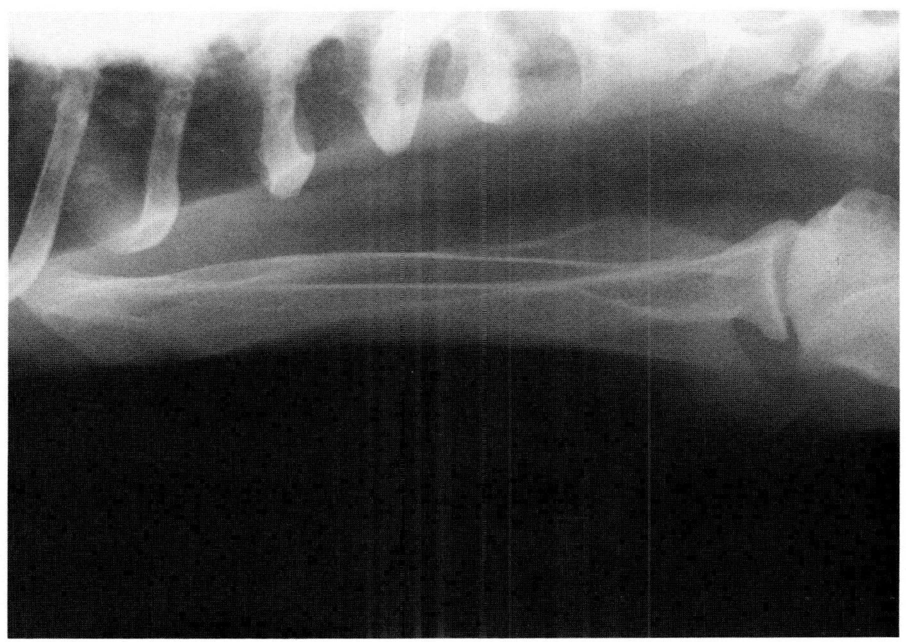

Figure 73. Positioning for a lateral projection of the thorax.

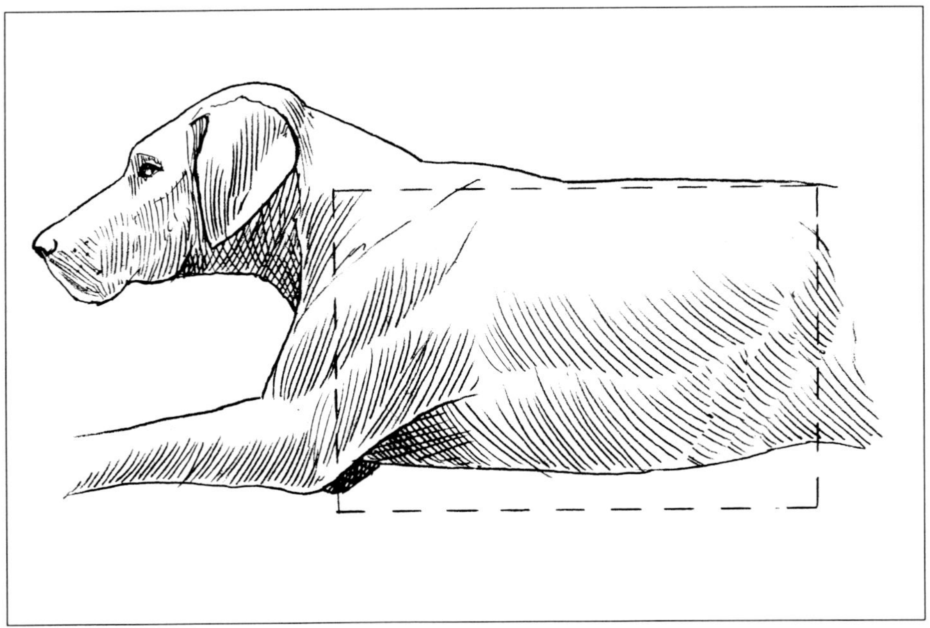

Figure 74. Lateral projection of the thorax.

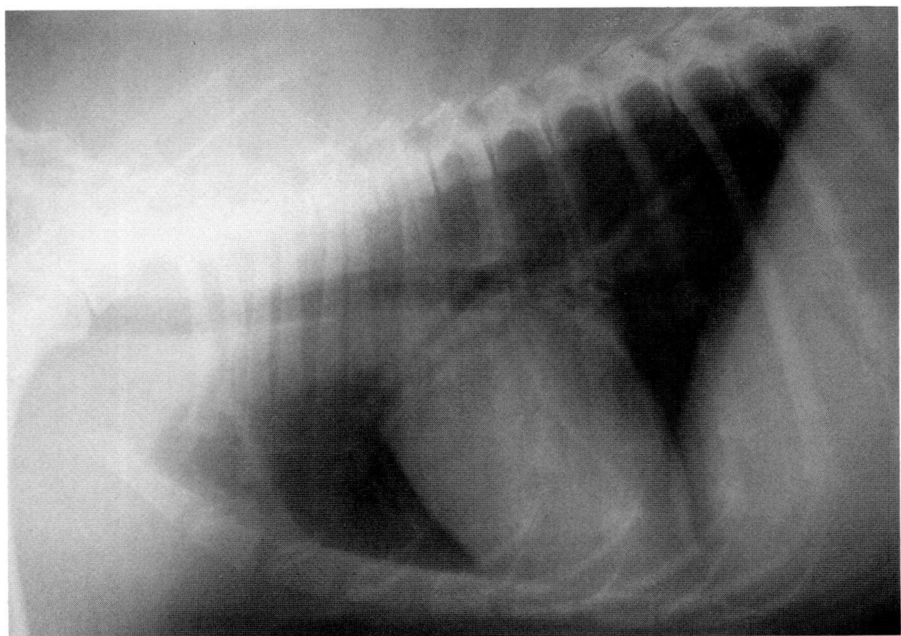

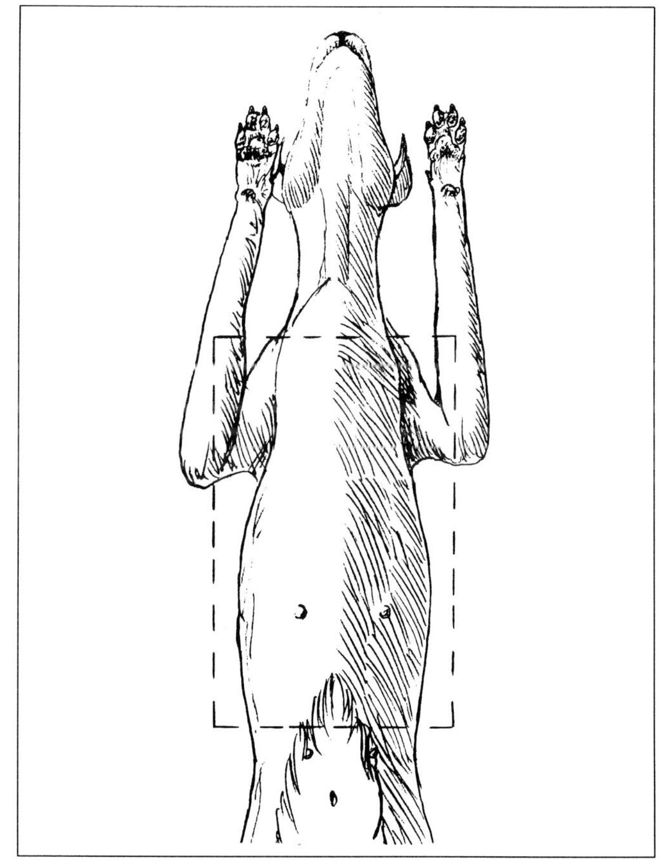

Figure 75. Positioning for a ventrodorsal projection of the thorax.

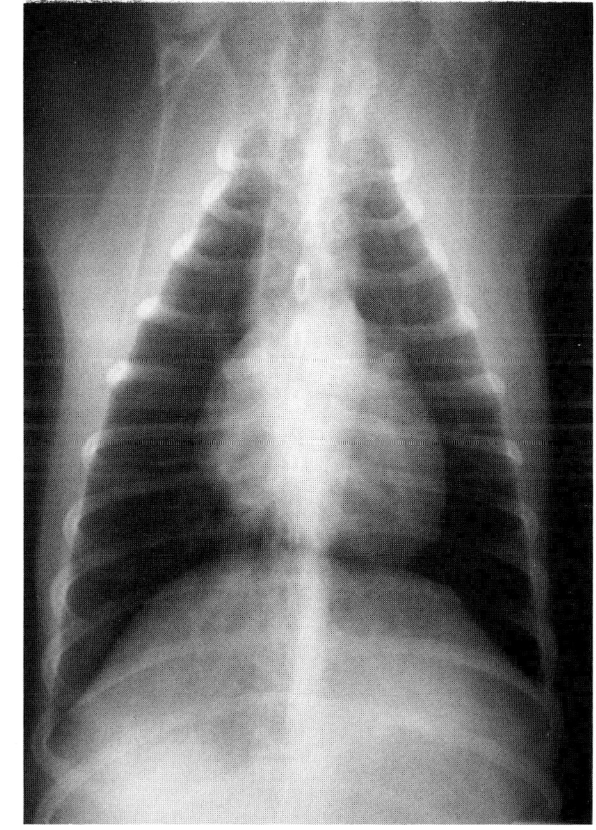

Figure 76. Ventrodorsal projection of the thorax.

Figure 77. Positioning for a dorsoventral projection of the thorax.

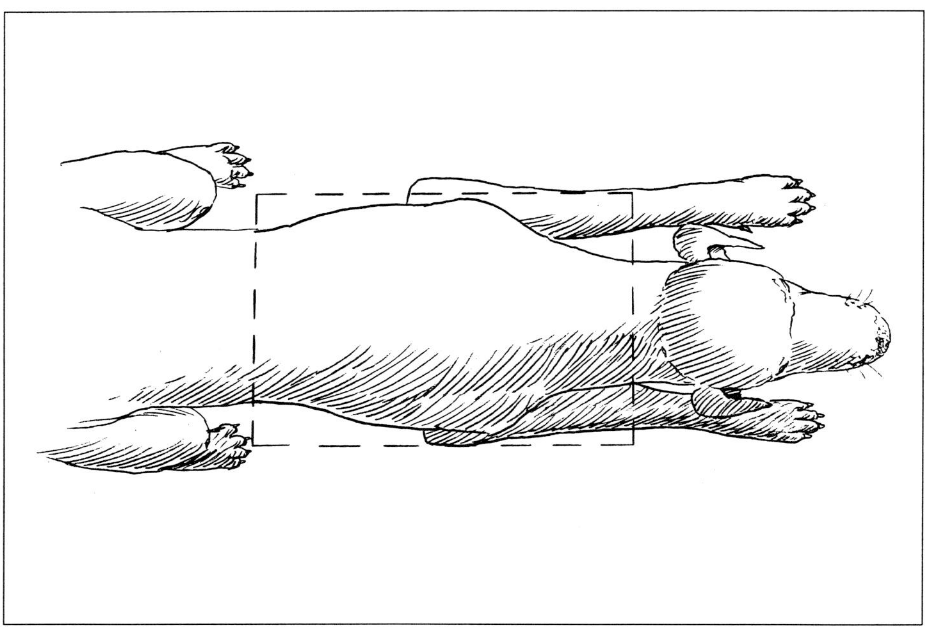

Figure 78. Positioning for a lateral projection of the abdomen.

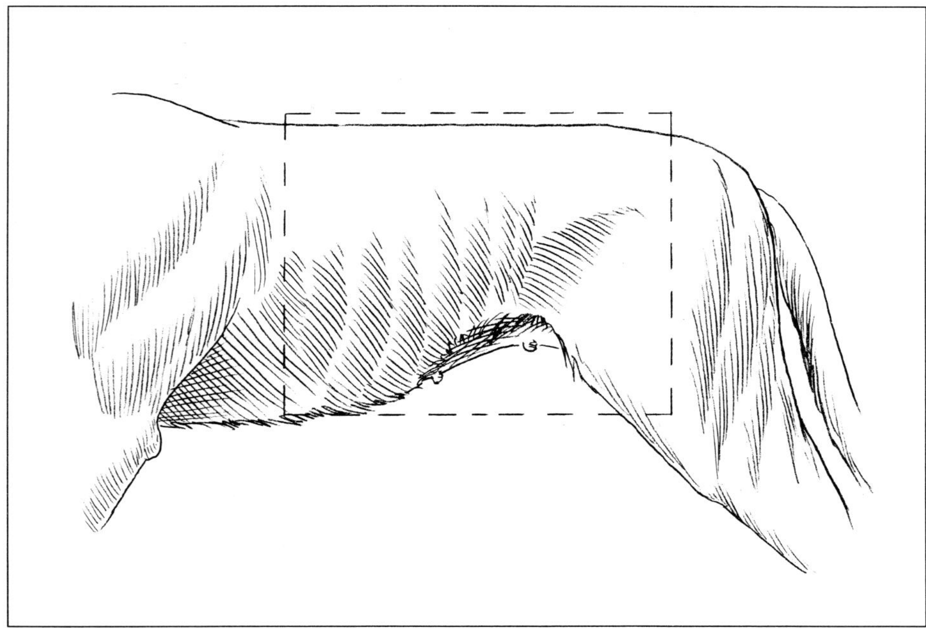

Figure 79. Lateral projection of the abdomen.

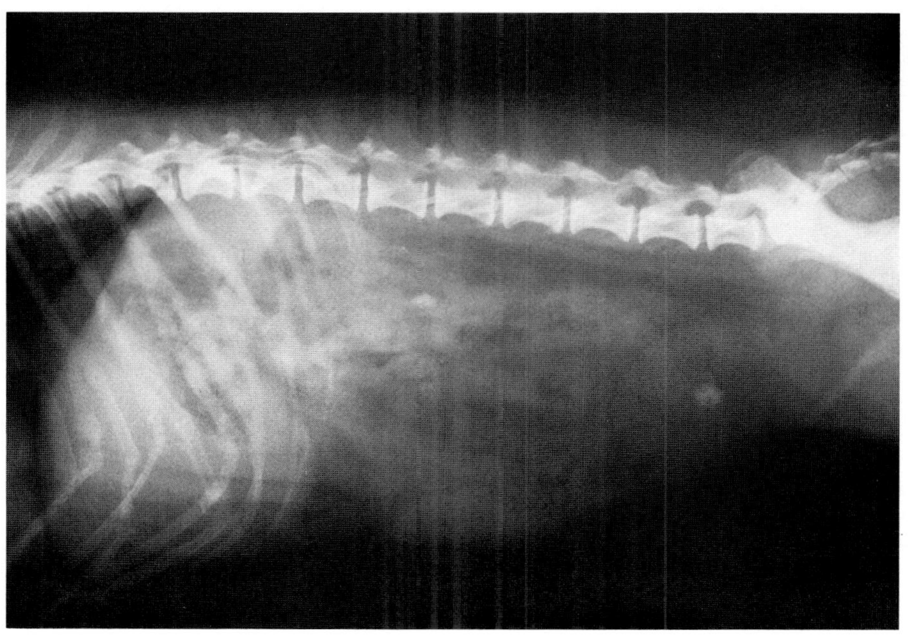

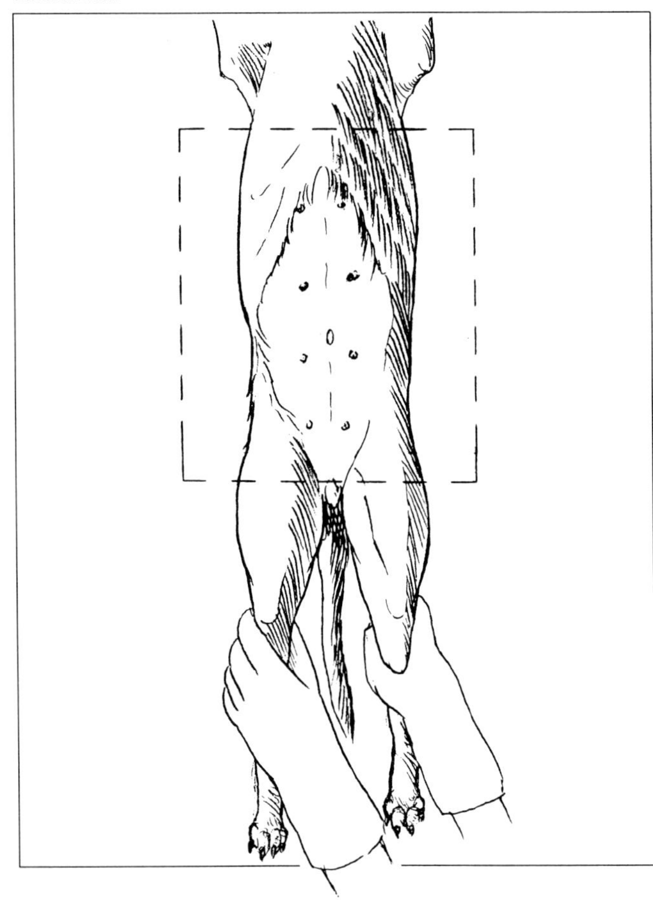

Figure 80. Positioning for a ventrodorsal projection of the abdomen.

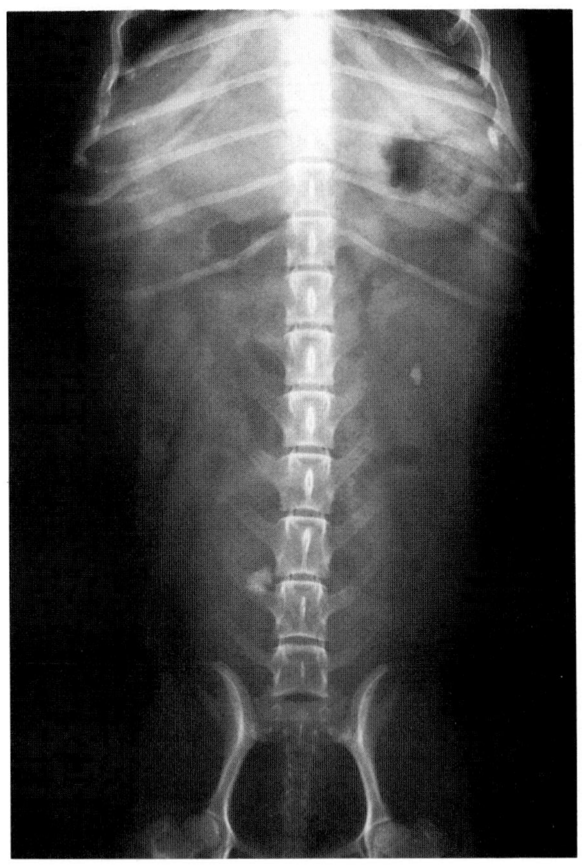

Figure 81. Ventrodorsal projection of the abdomen.

Figure 82. Positioning for a lateral projection of the pelvis.

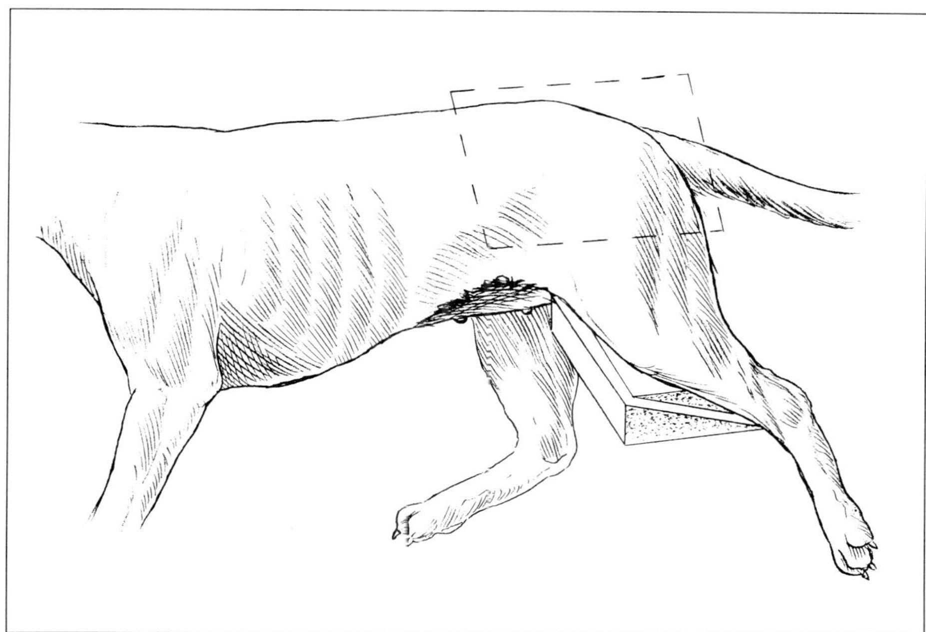

Figure 83. Lateral projection of the pelvis.

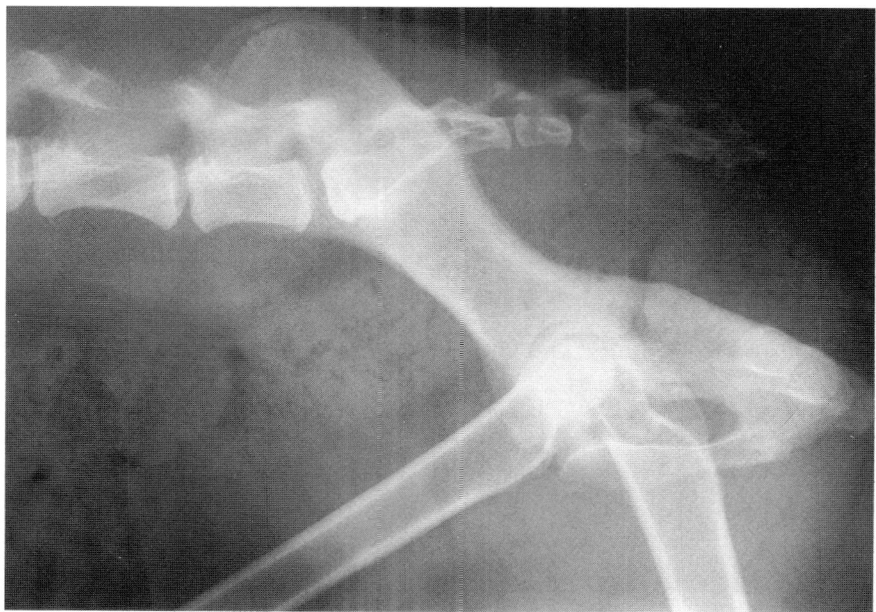

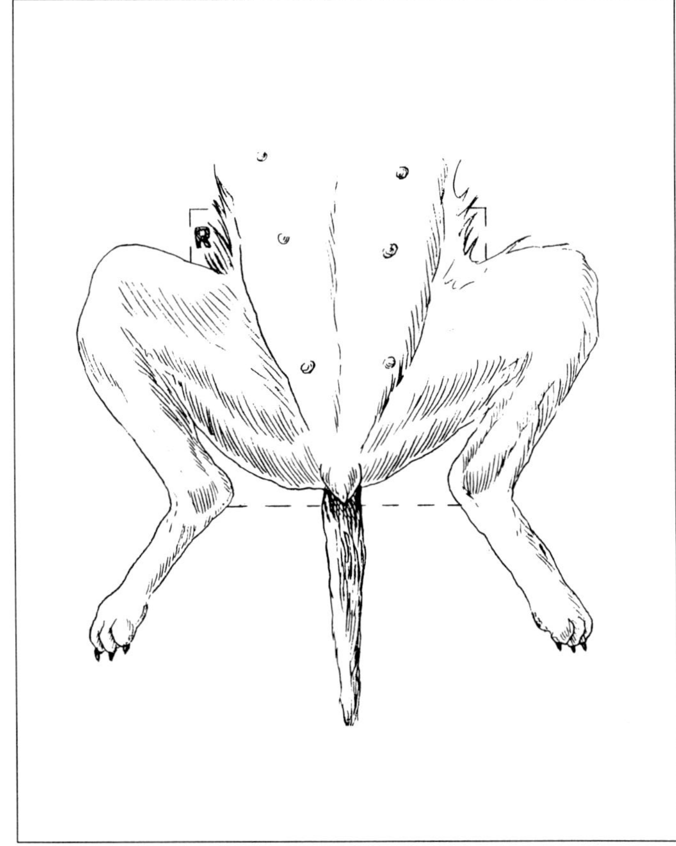

Figure 84. Positioning for a ventrodorsal projection of the pelvis in the flexed position.

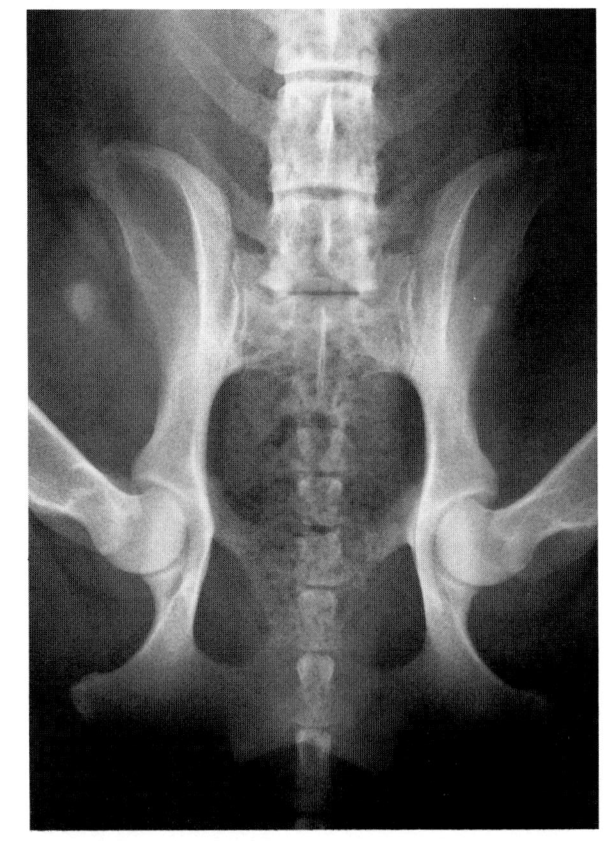

Figure 85. Ventrodorsal projection of the pelvis in the flexed position.

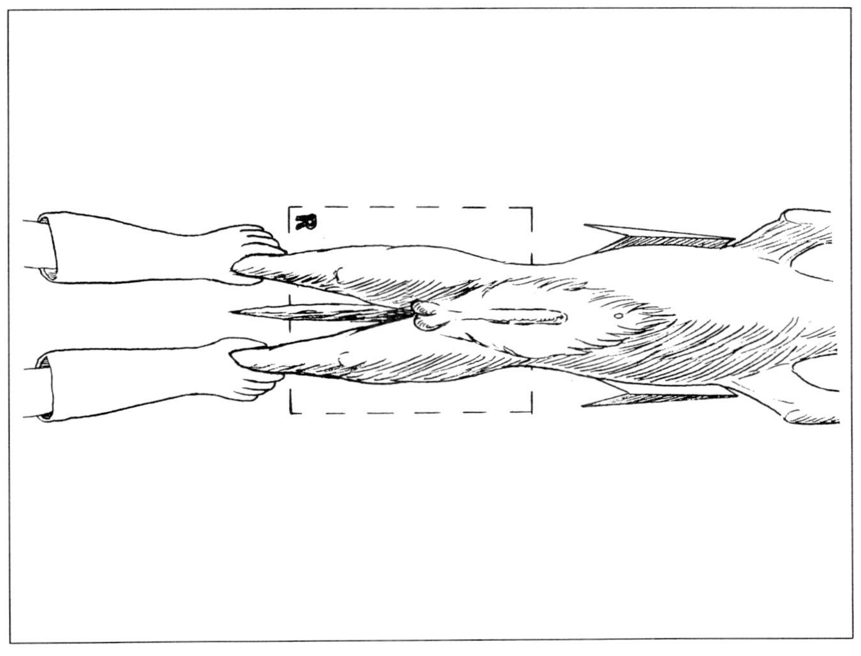

Figure 86. Positioning for a ventrodorsal projection of the pelvis in the extended position.

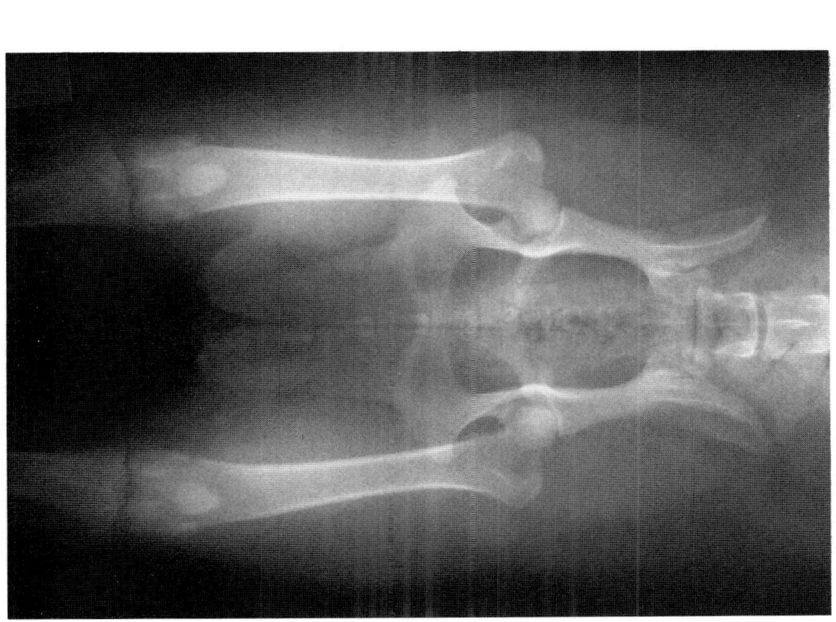

Figure 87. Ventrodorsal projection of the pelvis in the extended position.

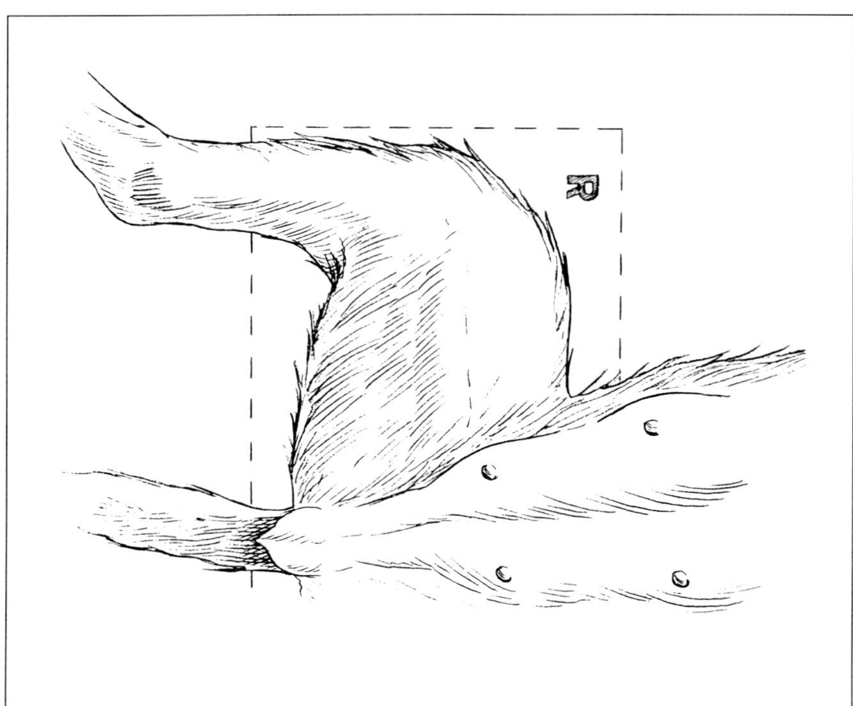

Figure 88. Positioning for a mediolateral projection of the femur.

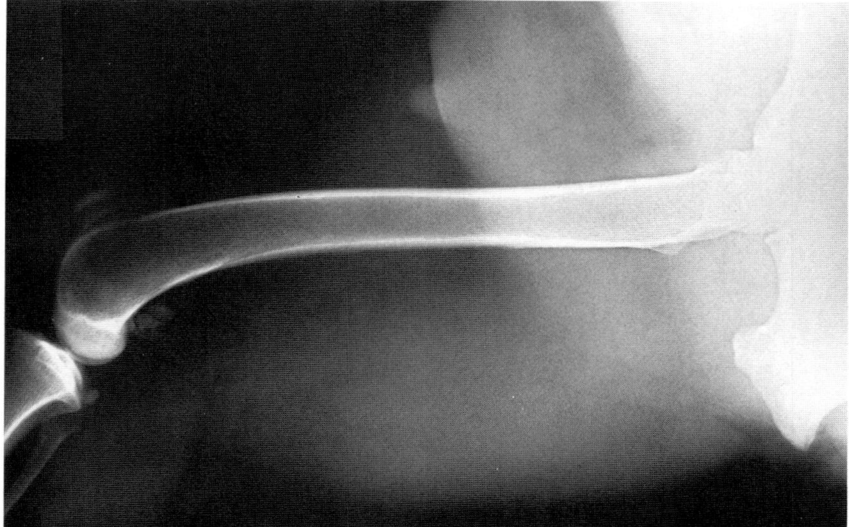

Figure 89. Mediolateral projection of the femur.

Figure 90. Positioning for a cross-table craniocaudal projection of the femur.

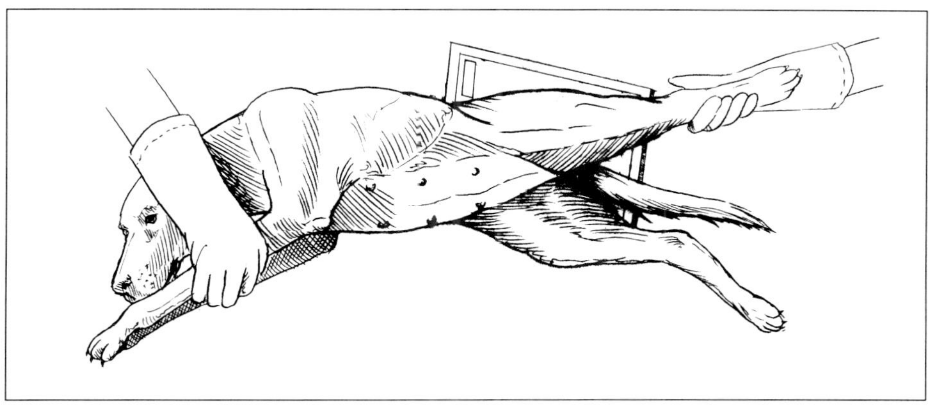

Figure 91. Positioning for a ventrodorsal extended craniocaudal projection of the femur.

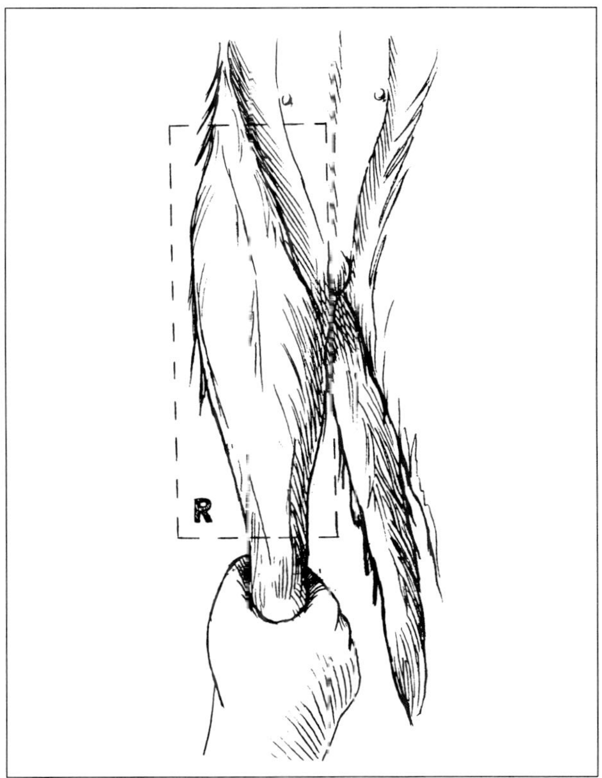

Figure 92. Craniocaudal projection of the femur.

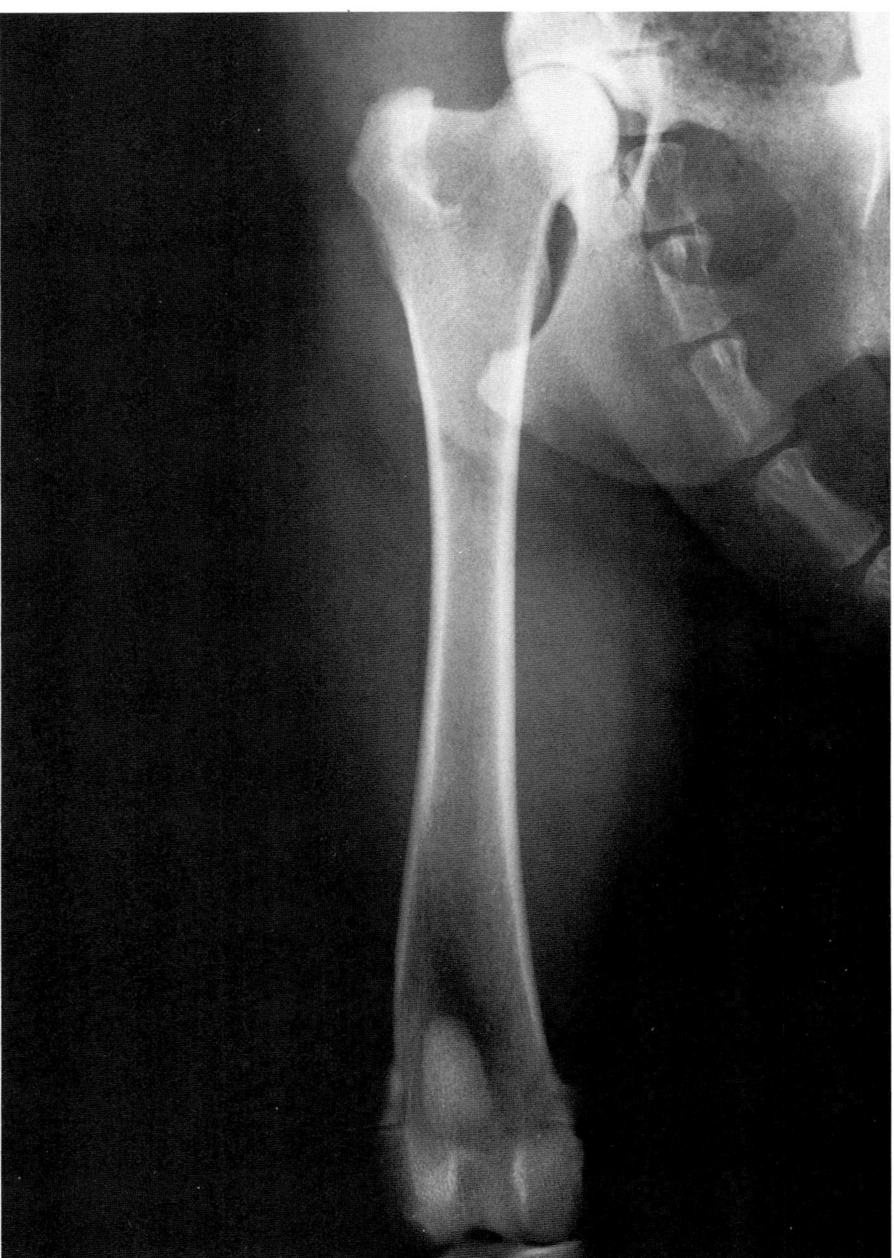

Figure 93. Positioning for a mediolateral projection of the stifle joint.

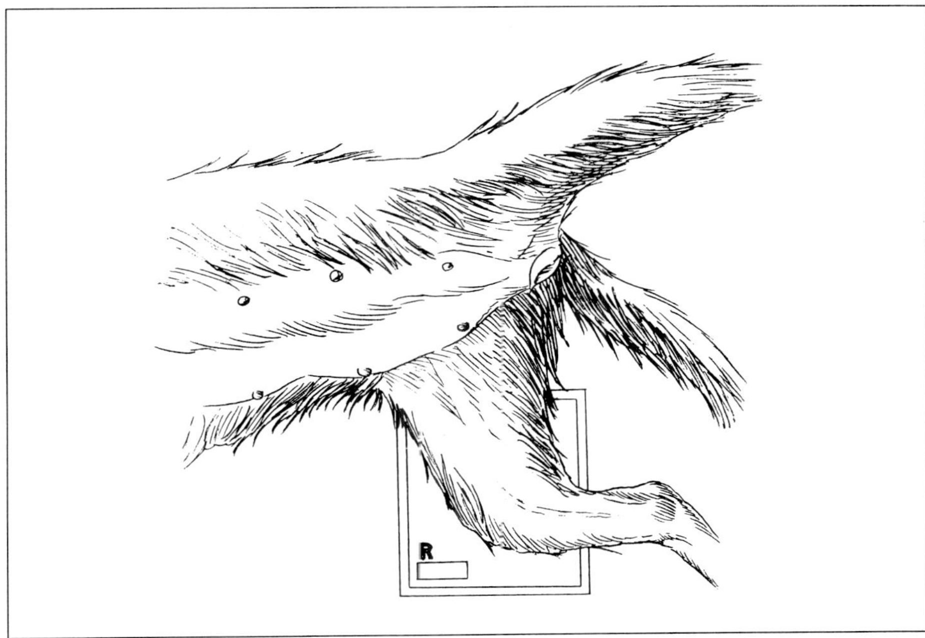

Figure 94. Mediolateral projection of the stifle joint.

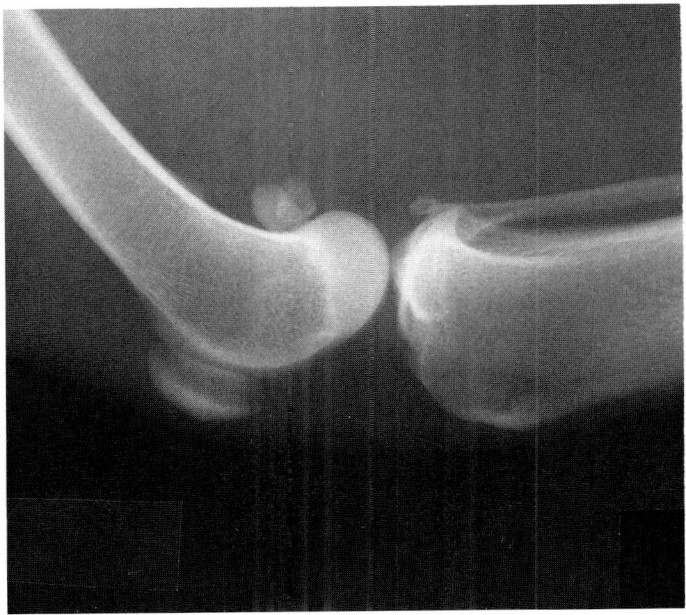

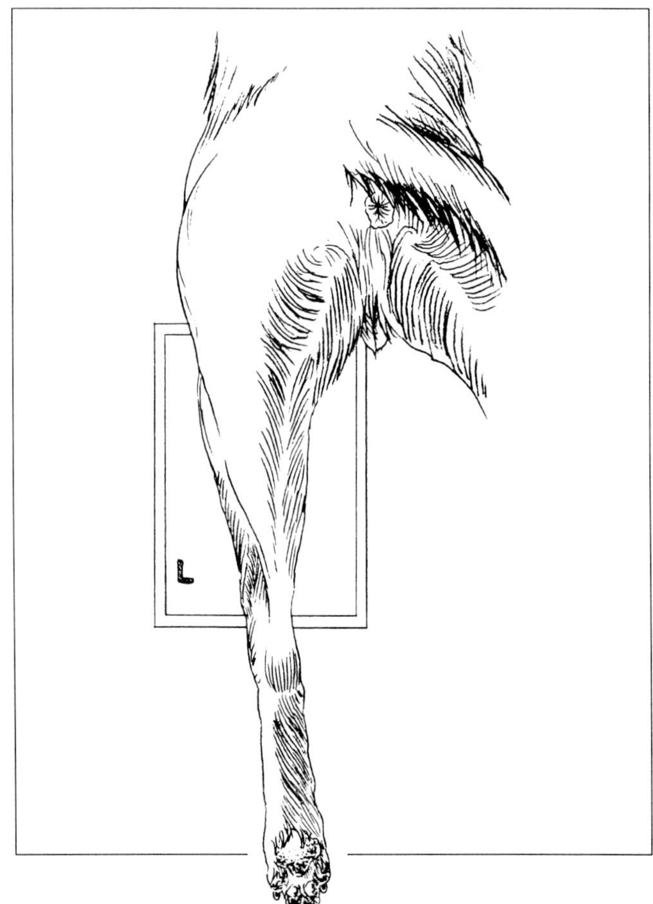

Figure 95. Positioning for a caudocranial projection of the stifle joint.

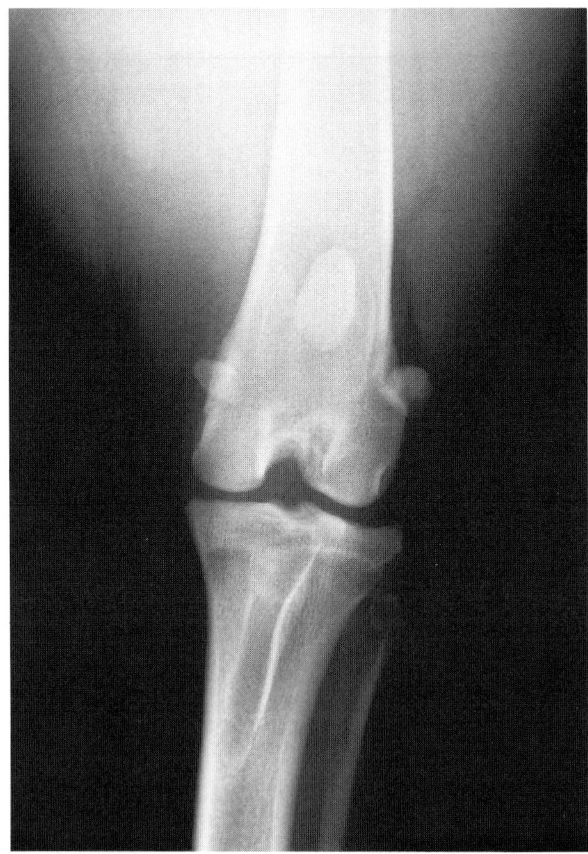

Figure 96. Caudocranial projection of the stifle joint.

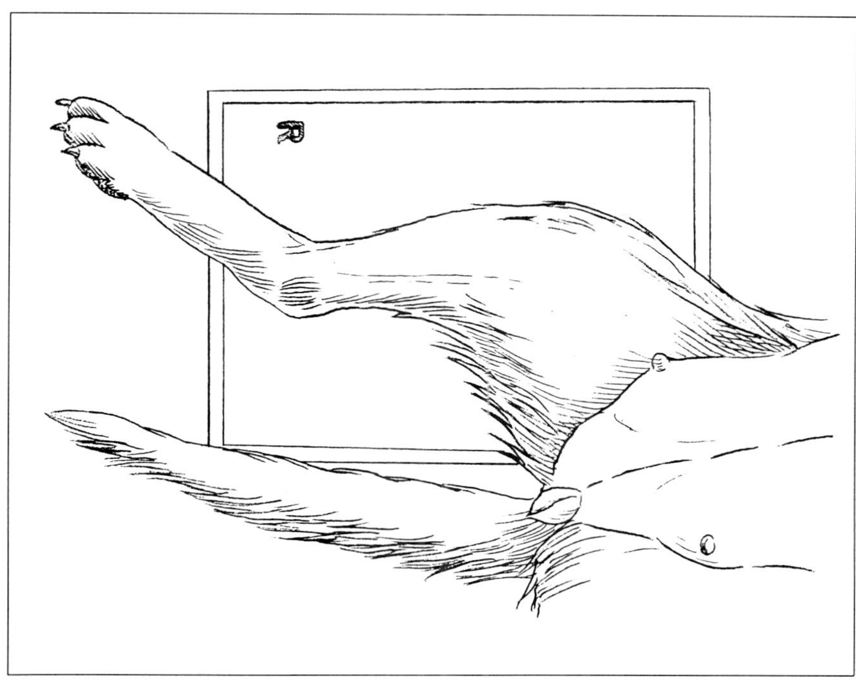

Figure 97. Positioning for a mediolateral projection of the tibia.

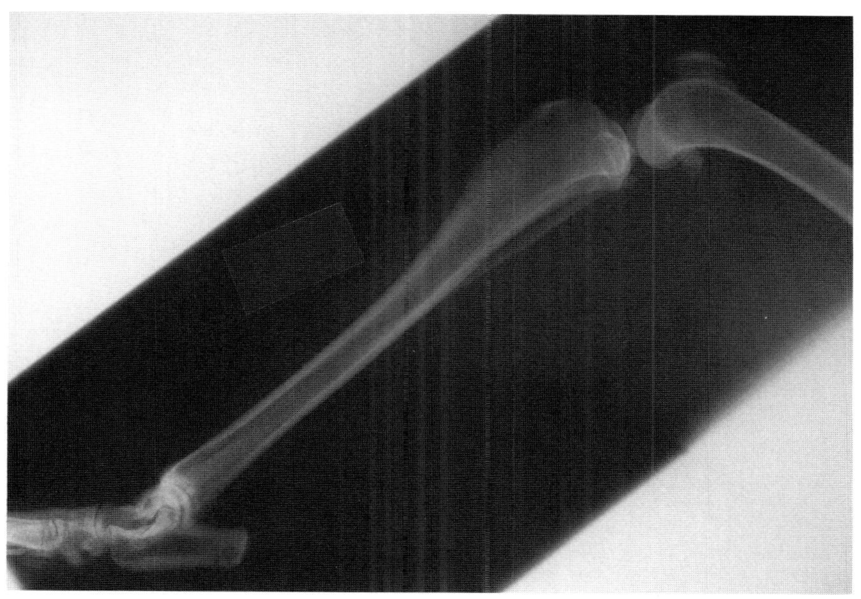

Figure 98. Mediolateral projection of the tibia.

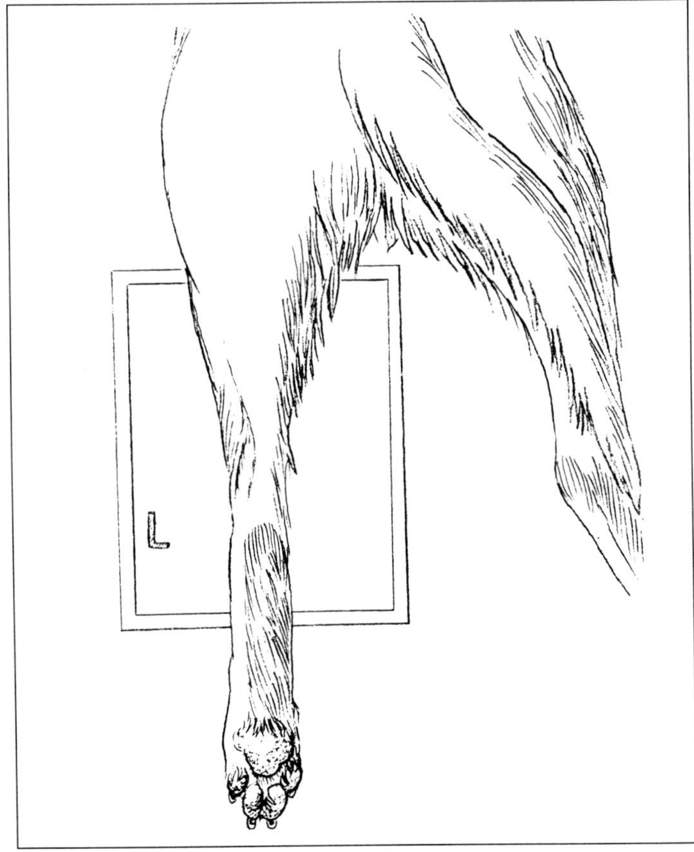

Figure 99. Positioning for a caudocranial projection of the tibia.

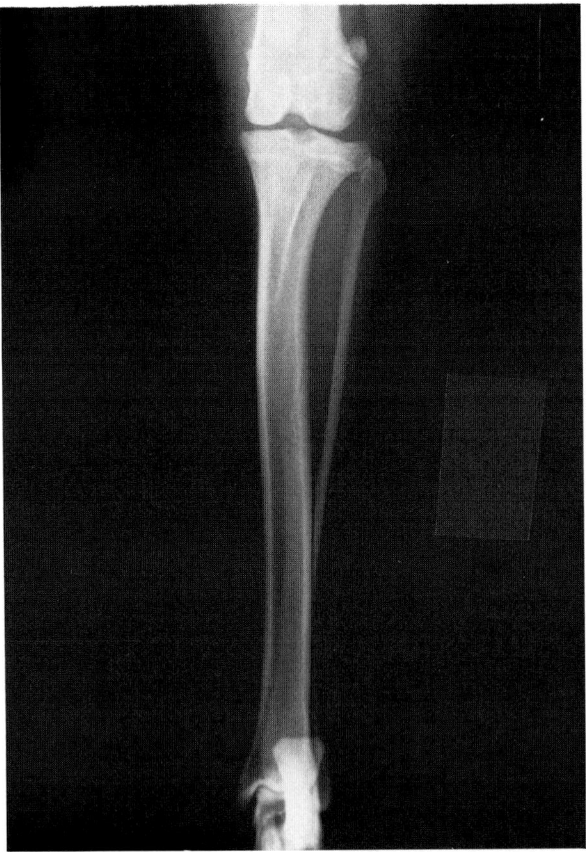

Figure 100. Caudocranial projection of the tibia.

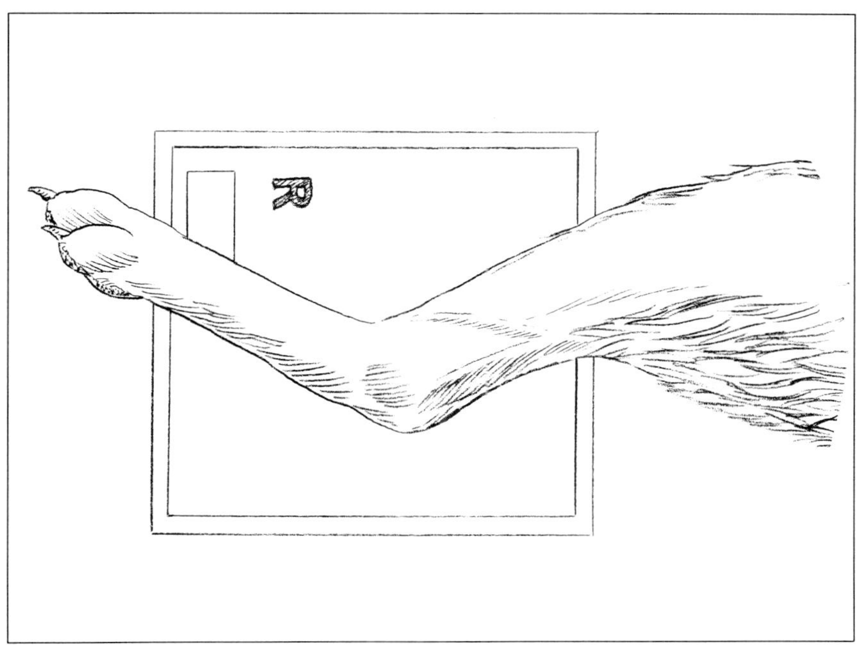

Figure 101. Positioning for a mediolateral projection of the tarsal joint.

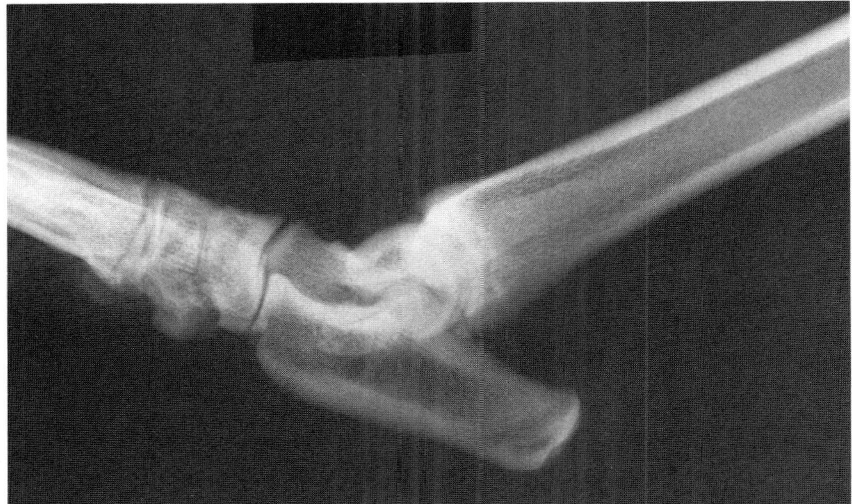

Figure 102. Mediolateral projection of the tarsal joint.

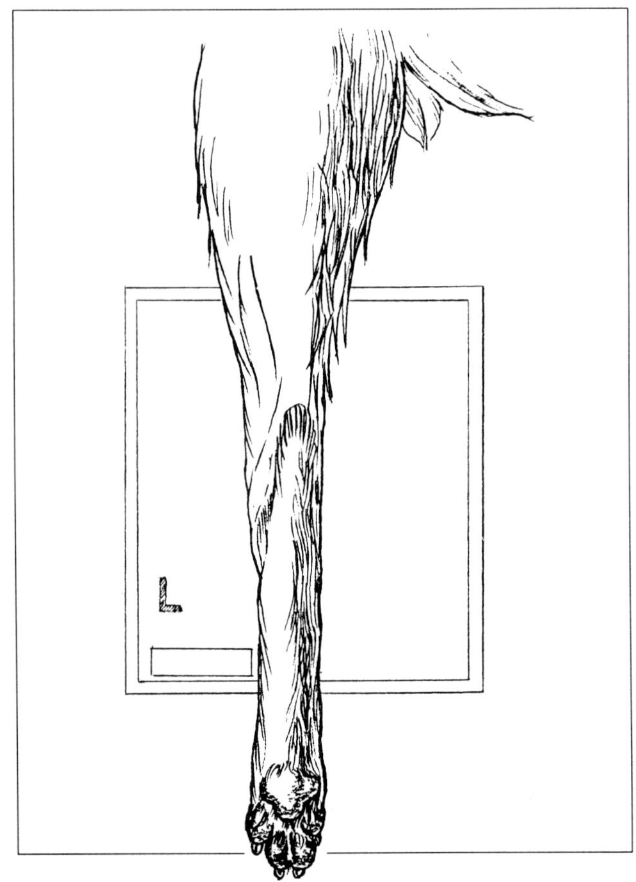

Figure 103. Positioning of the plantarodorsal projection of the tarsal joint.

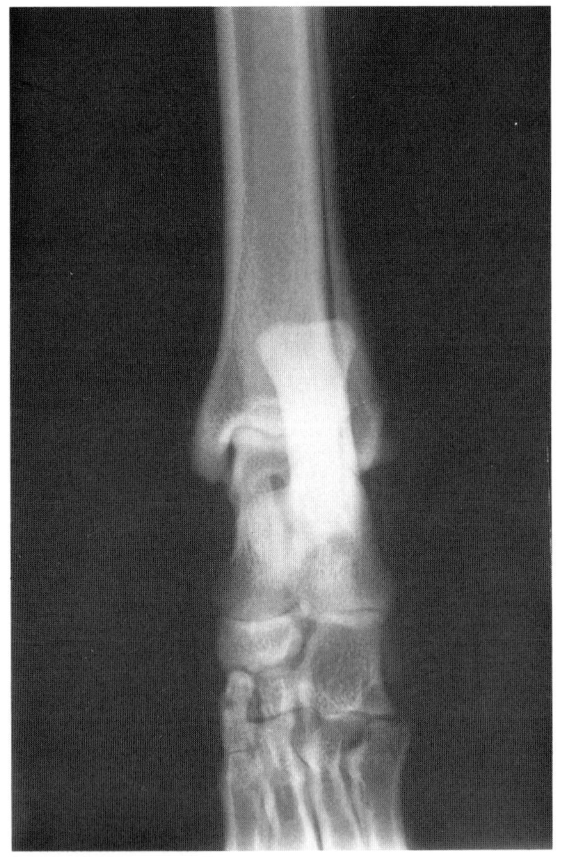

Figure 104. Plantarodorsal projection of the tarsal joint.

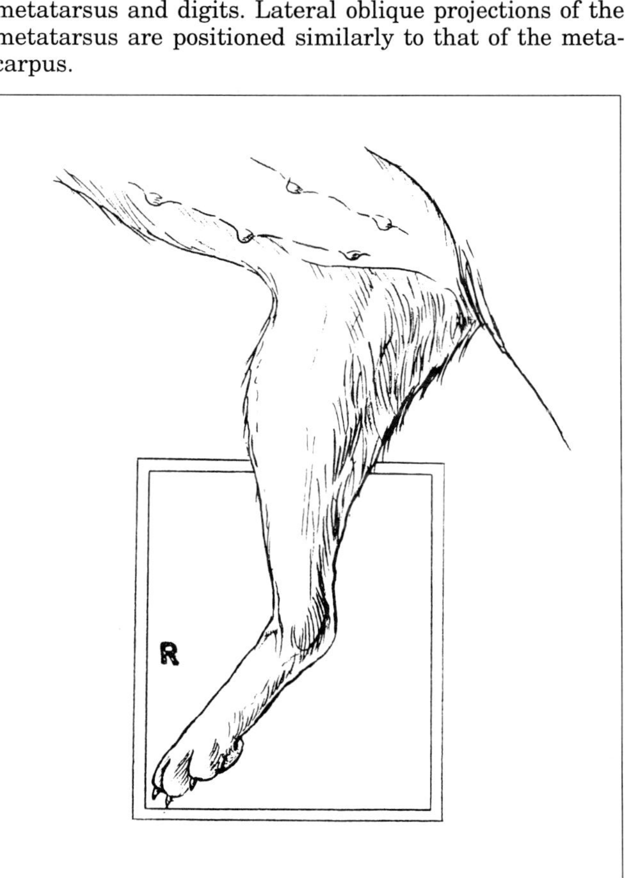

Figure 105. Positioning for a mediolateral projection of the metatarsus and digits. Lateral oblique projections of the metatarsus are positioned similarly to that of the metacarpus.

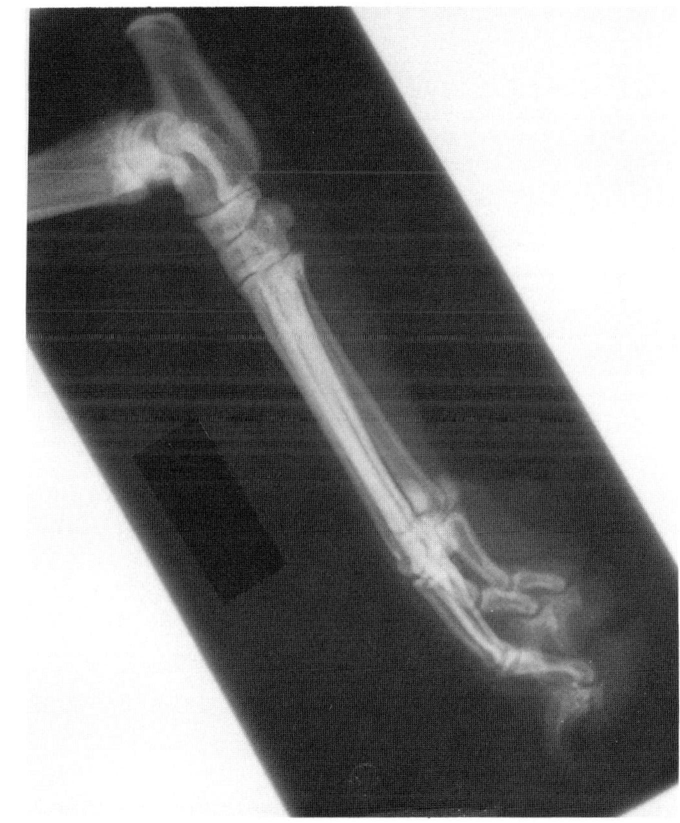

Figure 106. Mediolateral projection of the metatarsus and digits.

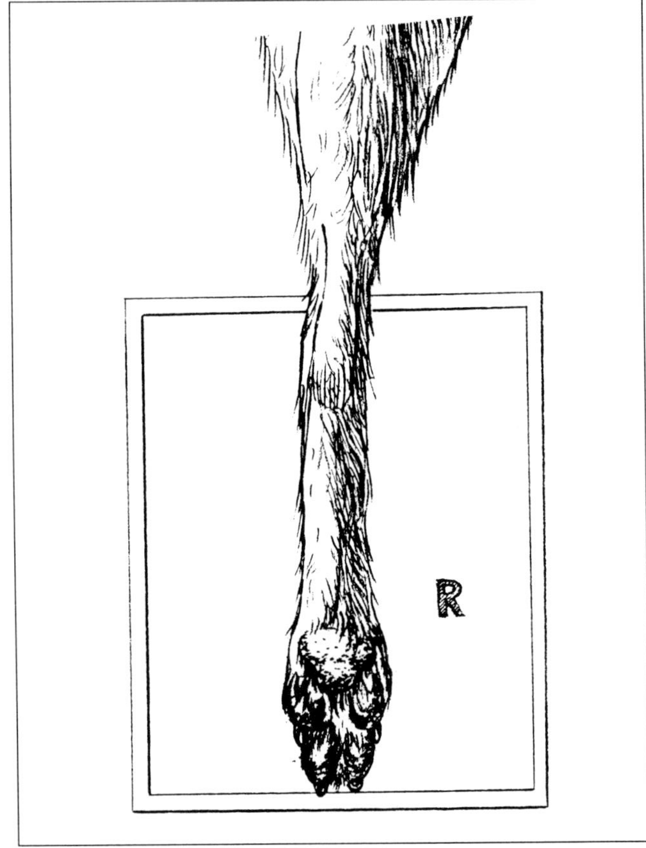

Figure 107. Positioning for a plantarodorsal projection of the metatarsus and digits.

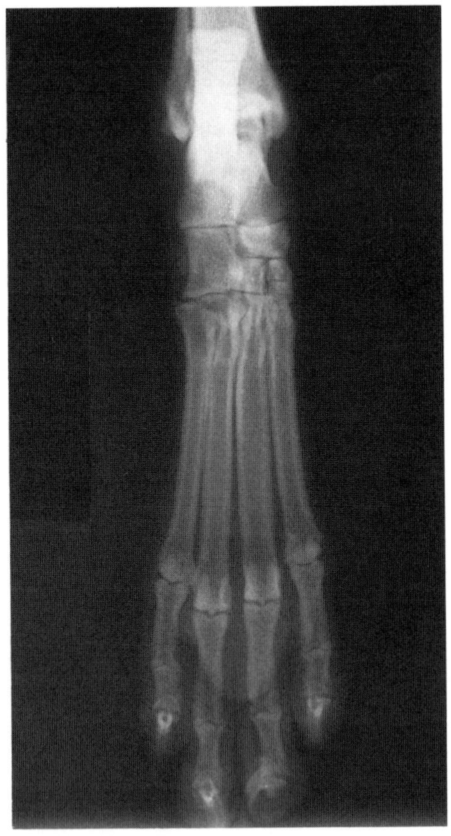

Figure 108. Plantarodorsal projection of the metatarsus and digits.

10

Contrast Radiographic Studies

The purpose of a contrast radiographic study is to delineate an organ or organ system against surrounding soft tissues. They are useful in determining the size, shape, position, location and function of an organ. The information obtained from a contrast study complements or confirms the information from survey (plain) radiographs. A contrast study should never be used in place of survey radiographs.

In contrast studies, areas of interest appear either radiopaque or radiolucent on the finished radiograph. Areas that are radiopaque appear white. Positive-contrast agents appear radiopaque (white) on a radiograph. Radiolucent areas on the finished radiograph appear black. Negative-contrast agents produce radiolucencies (black areas) on a radiograph.

Survey radiographs made before a contrast study establish proper exposure technique and patient preparation. In addition, a diagnosis may be achieved from the survey radiographs, eliminating the need for the contrast study. Because most contrast studies require multiple images, it is very important to label each film with the time and sequence. Always record the amount, type and route of administration of the contrast medium.

Illustrations for Chapter 10 begin on page 178.

Positive-Contrast Media

Positive-contrast media contain elements with a high atomic number (very dense). Elements with a high atomic number absorb more x-rays. Thus, fewer x-rays penetrate the patient and expose the film, making a white area on the radiograph. Two common types of positive-contrast agents are barium sulfate and water-soluble organic iodides.

Barium Sulfate

Barium sulfate is commonly used for positive-contrast studies of the gastrointestinal tract. It is insoluble and is not affected by gastric secretions. Therefore, it provides good mucosal detail on the radiograph. Barium sulfate preparations are relatively inexpensive and are manufactured in the form of powders, colloid suspensions or pastes.

One disadvantage of using barium sulfate is that it can take 3 or more hours to travel from the stomach to the colon. Also, it can be harmful to the peritoneum, so it should never be used when gastrointestinal perforations are suspected. Barium sulfate is insoluble and the body cannot eliminate it, resulting in granulomatous reactions. While administering barium sulfate per os, care must be taken to prevent the patient from aspirating. Aspiration of large amounts into the lungs could be fatal. Barium sulfate may also aggravate an already obstructed bowel by causing further impactions.

Organic Iodides

Water-soluble organic iodides in ionic or nonionic forms are also used for positive-contrast procedures. Different forms of the water-soluble organic iodides can be administered intravenously, orally, into a hollow viscus or into the subarachnoid space. Being water soluble, they are absorbed into the bloodstream and excreted by the kidneys.

Ionic Iodides: A commonly used oral form of ionic water-soluble organic iodide is a solution of meglumine and sodium diatrizoate. It is used for contrast studies of the gastrointestinal tract when perforation is suspected. When this iodide is administered orally, transit through the gastrointestinal system is rapid, usually within 45-60

Illustrations for Chapter 10 begin on page 178.

minutes. However, it is a hypertonic solution that draws fluid into the bowel lumen. Thus, the contrast medium is diluted, decreasing the quality of the resultant films. Fluid loss may further complicate hypovolemia in a dehydrated animal. Water-soluble organic iodides should never be used in place of barium sulfate, only when perforations are suspected.

Ionic water-soluble organic iodides for intravenous use are prepared in various combinations of meglumine and sodium diatrizoate. Diatrizoate can also be infused into hollow organs, such as the urinary bladder, or into fistulous tracts. Sodium diatrizoate is commonly used for excretory urography because it provides better opacification of the kidneys. Nausea, vomiting or decreased blood pressure can occur after rapid administration of a large intravenous bolus of contrast medium. Ionic water-soluble organic iodides cannot be used for myelography because they are irritating to the brain and spinal cord.

Nonionic Iodides: Nonionic water-soluble organic iodides are used for myelography. Because of their low osmolarity and chemical nature, there are fewer adverse effects when they are placed in the subarachnoid space. Three commonly used media are metrizamide, iopamidol and iohexol.

Nonionic water-soluble organic iodides are suitable for myelography and also can be given intravenously. However, they are approximately 10 times more expensive than ionic iodides. Metrizamide is available as a powder because it cannot be heat sterilized and is unstable in solution. Before use, it must be reconstituted and filtered through a 0.22-μ bacteriostatic filter.

Negative-Contrast Media

Negative-contrast agents include air, oxygen and carbon dioxide. They all have a low atomic number (low density), and appear radiolucent on the finished radiograph. Oxygen and carbon dioxide are more soluble than water. Care must be taken not to overinflate organs, such as the bladder, with these gases. Air embolism can occur when ulcerative lesions cause organ rupture, leading to cardiac arrest.

Illustrations for Chapter 10 begin on page 178.

Double-Contrast Procedures

Double-contrast procedures use both positive- and negative-contrast media to image an organ or organ system. The most common organs imaged with double-contrast studies are the urinary bladder, stomach and colon. In most cases the negative-contrast medium is added first, then the positive-contrast medium. Adding negative-contrast medium to the positive-contrast medium can cause air bubbles to form, which might be misinterpreted as lesions.

Table 1 lists commonly used contrast agents.

Table 1. Commonly used contrast agents.

Trade Name	Generic Name	Iodine Content	Manufacturer
Barium			
Liquid E-Z Paque	Barium sulfate suspension 60%	—	E-Z-EM
Novopaque	Barium sulfate suspension 60%	—	Lafayette
Gastrografin	Sodium diatrizoate and meglumine diatrizoate	367 mg/ml	Solvay
Ionic Water-Soluble Organic Iodides			
Hypaque sodium 50%	Sodium diatrizoate 50%	300 mg/ml	Sanofi Winthrop
Hypaque meglumine 60%	Meglumine diatrizoate 60%	282 mg/ml	Sanofi Winthrop
Renografin 60	Sodium diatrizoate 8% and meglumine diatrizoate 52%	292 mg/ml	Squibb
Renografin 76	Sodium diatrizoate 10% and meglumine diatrizoate 66%	370 mg/ml	Squibb

Illustrations for Chapter 10 begin on page 178.

(Table 1, continued)

| Conray 60 | Meglumine iothalamate 60% | 282 mg/ml | Mallinckrodt |
| Conray 325 | Sodium iothalamate 66.8% | 325 mg/ml | Mallinckrodt |

Nonionic Water-Soluble Organic Iodides

Metrizamide	Metrizamide analytical grade	—	Nycomed
Isovue-M200	Iopamidol	200 mg/ml	Squibb Diagnostic
Omnipaque 240	Iohexol	240 mg/ml	Sanofi Winthrop
Omnipaque 180	Iohexol	180 mg/ml	Sanofi Winthrop

Gastrointestinal Tract Studies

Esophagography

Esophagography is used to evaluate functional and structural alterations of the esophagus. Esophagography is a dynamic study and should be ideally performed with fluoroscopy. If fluoroscopic equipment is not available, conventional radiography may also be successful (Fig 1).

Indications: Dysphagia, regurgitation, foreign body, mass, suspected rupture, stricture, megaesophagus, tracheo-esophageal fistula, esophageal dysfunction.

Precautions: Water-soluble organic iodides should be used in cases of suspected perforation or rupture.

Contrast Agents	**Dosage**
Barium sulfate paste 60%	1 ml/lb
Barium sulfate liquid 60%	3 ml/lb
Barium sulfate mixed with canned food	1/2-1 can of food
(add enough liquid barium to thoroughly coat food)	
Water-soluble organic iodide	1 ml/lb

Illustrations for Chapter 10 begin on page 178.

Equipment: Large dosing syringe and canned food.

Survey: Lateral and VD views of thoracic and cervical areas, including the total length of the esophagus.

Patient Preparation: If ingesta is seen in the esophagus on survey radiographs, fast the animal for 12 hours and repeat the survey radiographs.

Procedure: Administer the contrast medium via the buccal pouch using a large dosing syringe. Make lateral and VD views of the cervical and thoracic esophagus immediately after administration. If the contrast medium alone passes, repeat the procedure with the barium sulfate mixed with canned food.

Comments: Administer the contrast medium slowly to avoid aspiration. Use a slightly oblique VD projection to avoid superimposition of the spine on the esophagus.

Upper Gastrointestinal Series

Upper gastrointestinal studies are dynamic and can be imaged with fluoroscopy, though studies are usually recorded with multiple radiographs. Contrast medium is administered orally and films are made during transit of contrast through the stomach and small bowel into the colon (Fig 2).

Indications: Vomiting, small bowel diarrhea, melena, obstruction, wall distortions (dilatation, stenosis), wall lesions (ulcers, neoplasia), abdominal organ displacement, and to observe GI function.

Precautions: In cases of suspected perforation or rupture, water-soluble organic iodides should be used rather than barium. Water-soluble organic iodides should be avoided in dehydrated patients.

Contrast Agents	Dosage
Barium sulfate liquid 60%	3-5 ml/lb
Water-soluble organic iodide	1 ml/lb

Equipment: Large dosing syringe, stomach tubes and towels.

Survey: VD and lateral views of abdomen before enemas.

Illustrations for Chapter 10 begin on page 178.

Patient Preparation: Animal should be free of ingesta. Fast the animal 24 hours before the study. Give enemas the previous night, and 3 hours and 1 hour before the study.

Procedure: Make lateral and VD views of the abdomen before administering the contrast medium. Administer the medium into the buccal pouch or by a stomach tube. Immediately after administration, make lateral and VD views of the abdomen. Repeat abdominal views 15, 30 and 60 minutes postadministration. Repeat abdominal views hourly until the contrast medium has reached the colon.

Comments: If tranquilization is necessary, acepromazine in the dog and ketamine in the cat are the drugs of choice. Give enough contrast medium to fully distend the stomach. If stomach or bowel perforation is suspected, use a water-soluble organic iodide. All films should be marked with the time after administration.

Gastrography

Pneumogastrograms are helpful in determining the position of the stomach. Double-contrast gastrograms best demonstrate the gastric mucosa for ulcerations and mass lesions (Fig 3).

Indications: Suspected gastric masses, radiolucent foreign bodies, outflow obstructions.

Precautions: Contraindicated if fluid, ingesta or diarrhea is present. Double-contrast gastrography preceded by glucagon is contraindicated in patients with diabetes mellitus or pheochromocytoma.

Contrast Agents	**Dosage**
Negative-contrast gastrography or in conjunction with an upper gastrointestinal series:	
Air	6-12 ml/kg
Carbonated beverages	30-60 ml
Effervescent granules or tablets	Enough to produce 6-12 ml of gas/kg
Positive-contrast gastrography:	
Barium sulfate suspension 60%	6-12 ml/kg

Illustrations for Chapter 10 begin on page 178.

Water-soluble organic iodide solution (cannot be used with double-contrast gastrography)	6-12 ml/kg

Double-contrast gastrography without upper gastrointestinal series:

Glucagon hydrochloride (Lilly)

<8 kg body weight	0.10 ml/kg IV
8-20 kg body weight	0.20 ml/kg IV
20-40 kg body weight	0.30 ml/kg IV
>40 kg body weight	0.35 ml/kg IV

Barium sulfate suspension

<8 kg body weight	3 ml/kg
8-40 kg body weight	2 ml/kg
>40 kg body weight	1.5 ml/kg
Air	20 ml/kg

Equipment: Stomach tube, 3-way valve, mouth gag, large syringe.

Survey: VD and lateral views of the abdomen.

Patient Preparation: Fast the animal for 12-24 hours.

Negative-contrast Gastrography, Pneumogastrography: Place the stomach tube to administer air. If using effervescent granules, administer them in the buccal pouch via a dose syringe. This prevents loss of foam before it reaches the stomach. After the introduction of negative-contrast medium into the stomach, remove the tube. Make right lateral, left lateral, ventrodorsal and dorsoventral views of the cranial abdomen.

Positive-Contrast Gastrography: Place a stomach tube and administer either barium sulfate suspension or water-soluble organic iodide solution. Withdraw the stomach tube. Make right lateral, left lateral, ventrodorsal and dorsoventral views of the cranial abdomen.

Double-Contrast Gastrography With an Upper Gastrointestinal Series: When most of the barium sulfate has emptied from the

Illustrations for Chapter 10 begin on page 178.

stomach, place a stomach tube and administer the negative-contrast medium. Remove the tube and roll the patient from side to side to adequately coat the gastric mucosa. Make right lateral, left lateral, ventrodorsal and dorsoventral views of the cranial abdomen.

Double-Contrast Gastrography Without an Upper Gastrointestinal Series: Paralyze the stomach with glucagon. Place the stomach tube and administer positive-contrast medium. With the tube still in place, administer the negative-contrast medium. Remove the tube and roll the patient from side to side to adequately coat the gastric mucosa. Make right lateral, left lateral, ventrodorsal and dorsoventral views of the cranial abdomen.

Barium Enema

This procedure is used to study the position and contour of the colon. Do not attempt to study the colon using an upper gastrointestinal series (Fig 4).

Indications: Large bowel diarrhea, tenesmus, fresh blood in the feces, colonic/rectal neoplasia, colitis, mucosal disease, ileocolic intussusception.

Precautions: Barium should not be used if gastrointestinal perforation is suspected. Barium enemas are not recommended for patients that have had proctoscopy within 12 hours or cleansing enemas within 4 hours before the study.

Contrast Agents	**Dosage**
Barium sulfate 20%	5-7 ml/lb
Air	Volume equal to amount of contrast material removed

Equipment: Enema catheter/Foley catheter, syringe, enema can and adapter with 3-way valve.

Survey: VD and lateral views of the abdomen before enemas.

Patient Preparation: The colon should be free of fecal material. Fast the animal for 24 hours. Give enemas the previous night. General anesthesia is required.

Illustrations for Chapter 10 begin on page 178.

Procedure: Make lateral and ventrodorsal views of the abdomen before administration of the contrast medium. Place the catheter in the rectum and inflate the cuff to prevent leakage. Administer three-fourths of the calculated dose. Radiograph the animal in ventrodorsal position to check the amount of bowel distention. If the colon is not fully distended, add 5 ml of contrast medium and repeat the radiograph. Continue until proper distention is achieved. With proper distention, make a lateral view of the abdomen. With the catheter still in place, remove the contrast medium and replace it with negative-contrast medium. Make lateral and ventrodorsal views of the abdomen. Remove as much of the contrast medium as possible before removing the catheter.

Comments: Air may be used as the medium for a negative-contrast study. Avoid overdistention of the colon. Use higher kVp values for positive-contrast studies. Saline should be used to dilute the contrast medium to a 20% solution.

Urinary Tract Studies

Cystography

Cystography involves use of positive- and/or negative-contrast agents to evaluate the bladder.

Indications: Hematuria, polyuria, dysuria, trauma to caudal abdomen, calculus, neoplasia, mural lesions, determine location of urinary bladder, congenital anomalies, diverticulum, functional abnormalities.

Contrast Agents	Dosage
Water-soluble organic iodides	3-5 ml/lb
Air	3-5 ml/lb

Equipment: Urethral catheter, lubricating jelly, syringe and catheter adapter, 3-way stopcock.

Survey: VD and lateral views of the abdomen, including the entire urinary tract, made after the colon is free of fecal material.

Patient Preparation: Give 1-2 enemas to eliminate fecal material from the colon. Tranquilization or general anesthesia may be necessary to fully inflate the bladder.

Illustrations for Chapter 10 begin on page 178.

Pneumocystogram (Fig 5): Before the contrast study, make lateral and ventrodorsal views centered over the bladder. Place a urinary catheter securely in the bladder. Withdraw all the urine. Inject the negative-contrast medium slowly while palpating the bladder. Terminate the injection if much resistance is met. Make lateral and ventrodorsal views centered over the bladder after the contrast medium has been administered.

Double-Contrast Cystogram (Fig 6): Make lateral and ventrodorsal views centered over the bladder before the contrast study. Place a urinary catheter securely in the bladder. Withdraw all the urine. Inject the negative-contrast medium slowly while palpating the bladder. Terminate the injection if much resistance is met. Make lateral and ventrodorsal views centered over the bladder after the contrast medium has been administered. After the radiographs for the pneumocystogram have been made, slowly inject 3-10 ml of the positive-contrast medium into the bladder. Roll the animal from side to side to coat the bladder wall. Make lateral and ventrodorsal views centered over the bladder. Sometimes it is necessary to make the opposite lateral and a dorsoventral projection to pool the contrast medium in all parts of the bladder.

Positive-Contrast Cystogram (Fig 7): Make lateral and ventrodorsal views centered over the bladder before the contrast study. Place a urinary catheter securely in the bladder. Withdraw all the urine. Inject the positive-contrast medium, which should be diluted 50% with saline, slowly while palpating the bladder. Terminate the injection if much resistance is met. Make lateral and ventrodorsal views centered over the bladder after the contrast medium has been administered.

Comments: If you suspect rupture/perforation, inject only a small quantity of contrast medium and then observe radiographically. A severely diseased urinary bladder could rupture with excessive intralumenal pressure. The dose of contrast varies according to patient size and the ability of the urinary bladder to distend, so always palpate the bladder when distending it with contrast medium. However, it is important to properly distend the bladder. Positive-contrast studies may be performed using contrast medium diluted 50% with

Illustrations for Chapter 10 begin on page 178.

saline. Obtain all urine samples for bacteriologic studies before injection of the contrast medium.

Urethrography

This study is to evaluate the urethra. It can be made using retrograde or voiding methods (Fig 8).

Indications: Dysuria, pelvic fractures, urinary incontinence, hematuria, mucosal defects, displacement/deviation of urethra, calculus, obstruction, evaluation of the prostate gland.

Contrast Agent	**Dosage**
Water-soluble organic iodide	3-5 ml/lb

Equipment: Urinary catheter, lubricating jelly, syringe, stopcock.

Survey: Lateral and ventrodorsal views of the caudal abdomen after enemas.

Patient Preparation: The colon should be free of fecal material. Tranquilization/anesthesia is required.

Voiding Urethrography: Make lateral and ventrodorsal views of the caudal abdomen before the contrast study. Place a urinary catheter securely in the bladder. Inflate the bladder with diluted positive-contrast medium. With the animal in lateral recumbency, a cassette in place and the machine ready, apply external pressure to the bladder. Make an exposure when urine is seen flowing from the urethra.

Retrograde Urethrography: Make lateral and ventrodorsal views of the caudal abdomen before the contrast study. Place a urinary catheter securely in the bladder. Inflate the bladder with diluted positive-contrast medium. With the animal in lateral recumbency, a cassette in place and the machine ready, attach a syringe with an adequate amount of positive-contrast medium to the urinary catheter. Slowly begin to inject the contrast medium. As the contrast medium is injected, slowly withdraw the catheter. When the catheter tip reaches the distal urethra, inject a bolus of contrast medium while the exposure is being made.

Comments: Lateral views are usually adequate.

Illustrations for Chapter 10 begin on page 178.

Excretory Urogram
(formerly Intravenous Pyelogram or IVP)

An excretory urogram gives information relative to renal function and the structure of the kidneys and ureters. The basis for the study is the kidneys' capacity to concentrate and excrete circulating organic iodinated contrast medium. This study contrasts the kidneys, ureters and urinary bladder (Fig 9).

Indications: To identify size, shape, location and margination of the kidneys and ureters. Suspected hydronephrosis, obstruction, renal calculus, congenital anomalies and ureteral rupture can be detected. The excretory urogram also provides a crude estimate of the renal function.

Contrast Agent	**Dosage**
Water-soluble organic iodide	1 ml/lb or 200-400 mg iodide/lb

Equipment: IV catheter, extension set, syringe with heparinized saline, syringe with contrast medium.

Survey: Lateral and ventrodorsal views of abdomen after enemas.

Patient Preparation: The gastrointestinal tract should be free of ingesta. Fast the animal 24 hours before the study. Give enemas the previous night, and 3 hours and 1 hour before the study. A patent cephalic catheter should be securely in place. Tranquilization/anesthesia as needed.

Procedure: Flush cephalic catheter with heparinized saline. With the animal in ventrodorsal position and the machine ready, start injection of the contrast medium. Inject the contrast medium as rapidly as possible. Make an exposure 10-20 seconds from the start of the injection, even if the entire dose has not been given. Flush the catheter with heparinized saline after the contrast injection has been completed. Immediately make ventrodorsal and lateral views of the abdomen. Repeat the radiographs (lateral and ventrodorsal) 5, 15 and 30 minutes postinjection.

Illustrations for Chapter 10 begin on page 178.

Comments: If ectopic ureters are suspected, make oblique views at 30 minutes postinjection. Inject the contrast medium as quickly as possible. Place time markers to label every view. The urinary bladder cannot be completely evaluated from an excretory urogram alone because proper distention cannot be achieved.

Vaginography

This procedure involves administration of contrast medium into the vagina to evaluate vaginal masses and strictures, and urethral problems. If it is impossible to catheterize the bladder, sometimes the vaginogram can be used to introduce contrast medium into the bladder (Fig 10).

Indications: Ectopic ureter, vaginal masses, urethral tumor, obstruction.

Contrast Agent	**Dosage**
Water-soluble organic iodide	1 ml/kg

Equipment: Foley Catheter, syringes, stopcock, tongue forceps.

Survey: Lateral view of the caudal abdomen centered over the bladder, including the pelvis.

Patient Preparation: Anesthesia may be required, depending on temperament of the animal.

Procedure: Place a Foley catheter in the vulva. Inflate the bulb with water or air so the catheter is taught when pulled back. Clamp tongue forceps onto the labia to help prevent the catheter from slipping. Inject the contrast medium slowly. With the animal in lateral recumbency, make an exposure centered over the bladder at the end of the injection.

Comments: Vaginal rupture can occur if excessive pressure is used.

Miscellaneous Studies

Celiography

This study is useful for evaluating the abdominal cavity and the integrity of the diaphragm (Fig 11).

Illustrations for Chapter 10 begin on page 178.

Indications: Diaphragmatic hernia.

Contrast Agent	Dosage
Water-soluble organic iodide	1 ml/lb

Equipment: 20- to 22-gauge, 1-inch needle, syringe.

Survey: Lateral and ventrodorsal views of the abdomen.

Patient Preparation: 8 x 8-cm area clipped and surgically prepped on the ventral midline, caudal to the umbilicus. Tranquilization/anesthesia as needed.

Procedure: With the animal in ventrodorsal recumbency and the site prepped, elevate the abdominal wall and advance the needle cranially into the abdomen, keeping the needle parallel to the abdominal wall. Aspirate to make sure the needle is not in a venous structure. Inject the contrast medium while the needle is being removed. Roll the animal to disperse the contrast medium throughout the abdomen. Make lateral and ventrodorsal views of the abdomen.

Pneumoperitoneography

This study is used to evaluate the abdominal organs in animals with reduced abdominal contrast, either from accumulation of abdominal fluid or lack of abdominal fat (Fig 12).

Indications: To evaluate the size, shape and position of abdominal organs/masses.

Precautions: Do not perform if diaphragmatic hernia is suspected.

Contrast Agents	Dosage
Nitrous oxide	250-2500 ml*
Carbon dioxide	250-2500 ml*
Air	250-2500 ml*

*Give until the abdomen is moderately distended.

Illustrations for Chapter 10 begin on page 178.

Equipment: 20- to 22-gauge needle or plastic catheter with adapter syringe, carbon dioxide or nitrous oxide source with reducing valve, X-ray machine capable of producing a horizontal beam.

Survey: Lateral and ventrodorsal views of the abdomen.

Patient Preparation: 8 x 8-cm area clipped and surgically prepped on the ventral midline, caudal to the umbilicus. Tranquilization/anesthesia as needed.

Procedure: With the animal in ventrodorsal recumbency and the site prepped, elevate the abdominal wall and advance the needle or catheter cranially into the abdomen, keeping the needle parallel to the abdominal wall. Aspirate to make sure the needle is not in a venous structure. Attach the needle or catheter to the gas supply or syringe of air. Slowly infuse the abdomen with the negative-contrast medium until the abdomen is moderately distended. Remove the needle/catheter. Make lateral and ventrodorsal views of the abdomen. Sometimes other views are necessary to demonstrate certain abdominal areas. Remove as much air as possible.

Comments: Remove excessive amounts of fluid in the abdomen before injecting the air. Carbon dioxide and nitrous oxide are more rapidly absorbed than room air. Injecting air puts pressure on the diaphragm, which can cause respiratory distress. This also increases the respiratory rate. Pneumothorax can be created if a diaphragmatic hernia is present and room air is used as the contrast medium. Carbon dioxide is safest to use. Reposition the catheter if subcutaneous emphysema is noted.

Fistulography

The extent and origin of fistulous tracts can be determined by injecting positive-contrast medium into the draining wounds and radiographically documenting the path of the tract (Fig 13).

Indications: Evaluate fistulous tracts of unknown origin or extent, detect radiolucent foreign bodies.

Contraindications: Possible dissemination of infection.

Illustrations for Chapter 10 begin on page 178.

Contrast Agent	**Dosage**
Water-soluble organic iodide	Enough to fill the tract

Equipment: Appropriately sized catheter, syringe, 4 x 4-inch gauze sponges.

Survey: Make 2 views of the area at right angles to each other before injecting the contrast medium.

Patient Preparation: The area of interest should be clean and dry.

Procedure: Insert a catheter filled with contrast medium into the tract as far as possible. Pack the skin around the wound with 4 x 4-inch gauze sponges. Inject part of the contrast medium, then slowly withdraw the catheter while injecting the rest of the medium. Inject enough so that contrast medium fills the entire tract. Massage the area to work the contrast medium into deeper tracts. Wipe any contrast medium from the skin. Make at least 2 radiographic views of the area at right angles to each other.

Myelography

This procedure is done to evaluate the location and nature of lesions of the spinal cord. The myelogram is performed by injection of contrast medium into the subarachnoid space.

Indications: Suspected intervertebral disk disease, neoplasms, vertebral instability/malformations, fractures.

Contraindications: Evidence of infection in the cerebrospinal fluid or unless the neurologic deficit appears reversible.

Contrast Agents	**Dosage**
Same dosage for all 3 contrast agents.	
Metrizamide (analytic grade)	0.3 ml/kg for cervical or lumbar areas only
Iohexol	
Iopamidol	0.45 ml/kg for whole spine dose

Illustrations for Chapter 10 begin on page 178.

Equipment: Drape, sterile gloves, 0.22-μ Millipore Filter (Millex-GS: Millipore Products Division), 1.5- to 3.5-inch spinal needle (depends on size of animal), 18-gauge, 1-inch needle, syringe for contrast medium, extension set, 3-ml syringe to collect cerebrospinal fluid, tubes for cerebrospinal fluid analysis.

Survey: Lateral and ventrodorsal views centered and collimated over the area of interest, *eg,* cervical, thoracic, thoracolumbar (T-L) or lumbar vertebrae.

Patient Preparation: General anesthesia is required. Clip the hair over the cervical or the lumbar area, followed by 3 surgical scrubs. For cervical injection, insert the needle in the atlantooccipital joint. For lumbar injection, insert the needle between the 5th and 6th lumbar vertebrae.

Cervical Myelography (Fig 14): Depending on the preference of the myelographer, the patient is placed in sternal recumbency with neck flexed or in lateral recumbency also with the neck in a flexed position. The area is clipped and surgically prepped. A drape is placed over the clipped site. The needle is then inserted into the atlantooccipital joint and cerebrospinal fluid is withdrawn. The contrast medium is injected into the cisterna magna and then the needle is removed. The head should remain elevated for a few minutes to allow the contrast medium to flow caudally. The neck may also need to be massaged to aid flow of contrast medium. Lateral and ventrodorsal views of the cervical spine are made.

Lumbar Myelography (Fig 15): The patient is placed in lateral recumbency. The spine may also be flexed, with the rear limbs placed between the front limbs to help open the vertebral spaces. The area is clipped and surgically prepped. A drape is placed over the clip site. Once the needle is in the subarachnoid space, cerebrospinal fluid is collected and the contrast medium is slowly injected. With the needle in place, a lateral view is made. Then the needle is withdrawn and a ventrodorsal view is made.

Comments: Deliver the contrast medium slowly. Oblique, flexed or extended views may be necessary. After cervical myelography, keep the head elevated to decrease the chance of seizures.

Illustrations for Chapter 10 begin on page 178.

Sialography

Sialography is performed to visualize the salivary ducts and glands (Fig 16).

Indications: Suspected salivary mucocele.

Contrast Agents	Dosage
Water-soluble organic iodide	0.5-1 ml
Propyliodone in peanut oil	0.1-0.3 ml

(Dionosil oily: Glaes)

Equipment: Blunt cannula (lacrimal), blunted 22-, 25- and 26-gauge needles, tissue forceps, syringe, mouth gag.

Survey: Lateral and ventrodorsal views of the skull.

Patient Preparation: General anesthesia is required.

Procedure: Four ducts can be canulated and injected with contrast medium. These are the parotid, zygomatic, mandibular and sublingual ducts. After the duct of interest has been identified, the cannula is then inserted into the duct up to the hub. The contrast medium is then injected. Lateral and ventrodorsal views of the skull are then made.

Comments: A lot of time, patience and experience are required to perform sialograms.

Arthrography

Arthrography involves introduction of contrast medium, either positive or negative, into the synovial fluid to contrast the articular surfaces and joint capsule (Fig 17).

Indications: Outlines articular cartilage defects and joint capsule abnormalities.

Contrast Agent	Dosage
Water-soluble organic iodide	4-5 ml

Illustrations for Chapter 10 begin on page 178.

Equipment: 20-gauge, 1-inch needle, 2 6-ml syringes.

Survey: Two views, mediolateral and craniocaudal or caudocranial, are necessary before administration of the contrast medium.

Patient Preparation: General anesthesia is required. An 8 x 8-cm area is clipped, surgically scrubbed and draped.

Procedure: A 20-gauge needle with the syringe attached is inserted into the joint. Aspiration of synovial fluid confirms correct placement of the needle. The syringe is then removed and replaced with the second syringe filled with 4-5 ml of contrast medium. The contrast medium is injected with a slight amount of pressure and then the needle is withdrawn. The joint should then be flexed and extended to allow the contrast medium to mix with the synovial fluid. Two views, mediolateral and craniocaudal or caudocranial, of the joint are then made.

Comments: Radiographic views should be made within one minute after injection, as some of the contrast medium may be absorbed if an extended period has elapsed after injection. This procedure may also be performed on horses or cattle, using a larger needle and more contrast medium.

Nonselective Angiocardiography

This procedure requires injection of contrast medium into a cephalic or jugular catheter to obtain information about cardiac abnormalities (Fig 18).

Indications: May be useful in detecting some congenital diseases, such as right-to-left shunts and pulmonic stenosis. Cardiomyopathy in cats, right atrial or ventricular masses and pericardial diseases may also be seen.

Precautions: Problems could arise if the patient is allergic to the contrast medium.

Contrast Agent	**Dosage**
Water-soluble organic iodide	1 ml/kg

Equipment: Cephalic or jugular catheter, syringe.

Illustrations for Chapter 10 begin on page 178.

Patient Preparation: Sedation or anesthesia is usually necessary to obtain adequate images. A cephalic or jugular catheter should be securely placed.

Procedure: Place the animal in lateral recumbency and set the technique on the machine. Have as many cassettes as possible for ready use. Administer a bolus injection of contrast medium. Make the first radiograph while the injection is being made. Make radiographs 1 second apart for 9 seconds.

Comments: Selective angiocardiography is rarely performed by veterinarians in practice because of the specialized equipment required.

Recommended Reading

Bettmann MA: Angiographic contrast agents: Conventional and new media compared. *Am J Radiol* 139:787-794, 1982.

Douglas SW *et al: Principles of Veterinary Radiography.* 4th ed. Bailliere Tindall, London, 1987. pp 241-286.

Fischer HW: Catalog of intravascular contrast media. *Radiol* 159:561-563, 1986.

Morgan JP and Silverman S: *Techniques of Veterinary Radiography.* 3rd ed. Veterinary Radiology Associates, Davis, CA, 1982. pp 255-291.

Ticer JW: *Radiographic Technique in Veterinary Practice.* 2nd ed. Saunders, Philadelphia, 1984.

Widmer WR *et al:* Iohexol and iopamicol myelography in the dog: A clinical trial comparing adverse effects and myelographic quality. *Vet Radiol Ultrasound* 33:327-333, 1992.

Notes

Illustrations for Chapter 10 begin on page 178.

Figure 1. Lateral projection of a normal canine esophagagogram.

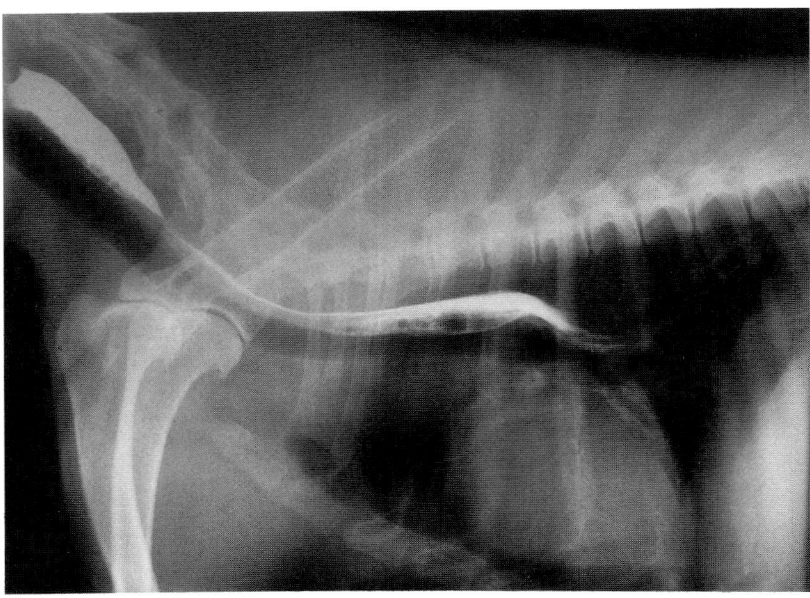

Figure 2. Normal feline upper gastrointestinal series. Image A is a lateral view made 15 minutes after barium administration.

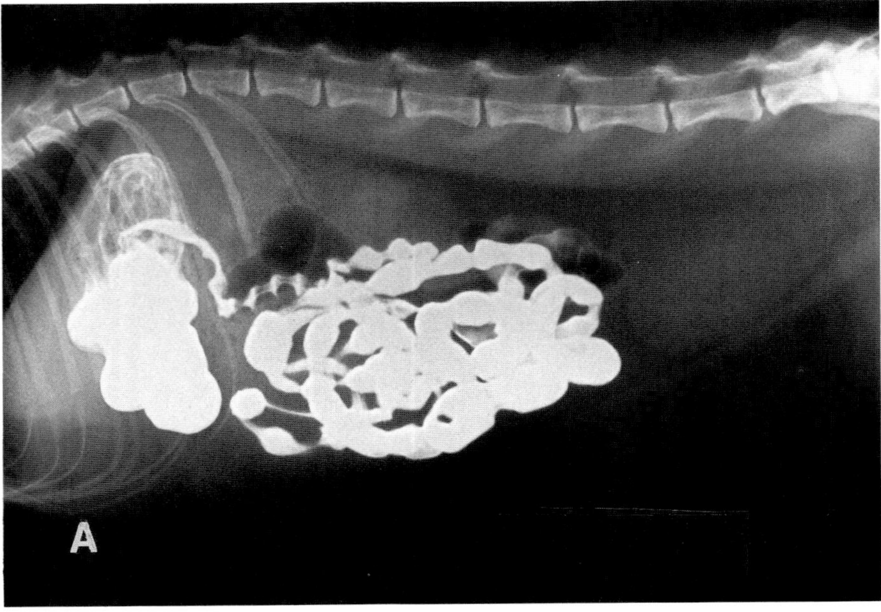

Figure 2, continued. Image B is a ventrodorsal view made 15 minutes after barium administration. Images C and D are lateral and ventrodorsal views made 3 hours after barium administration. The study is complete at this point because the barium has reached the colon.

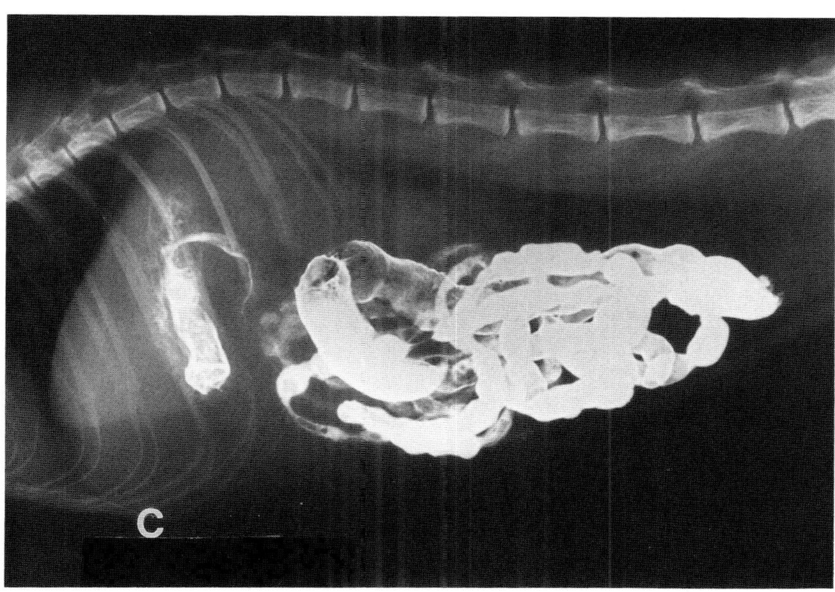

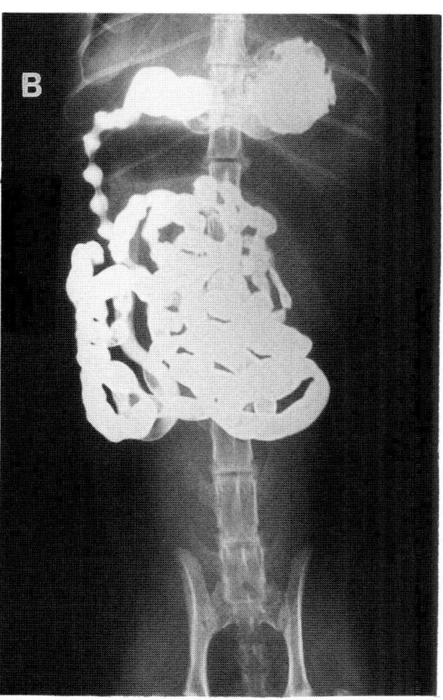

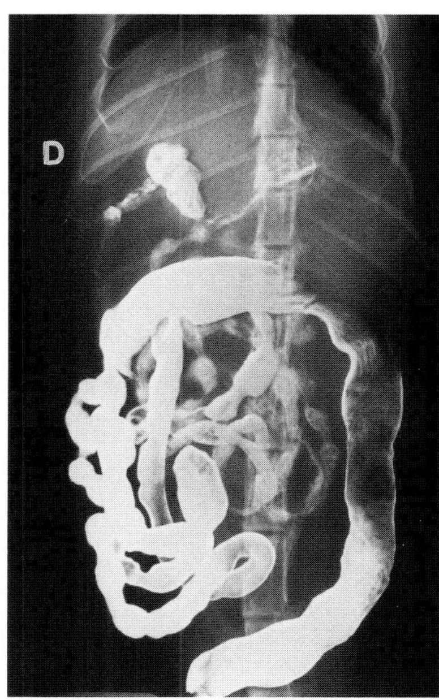

Figure 3. Lateral (A) and ventrodorsal (B) projections of a normal canine double-contrast gastrogram.

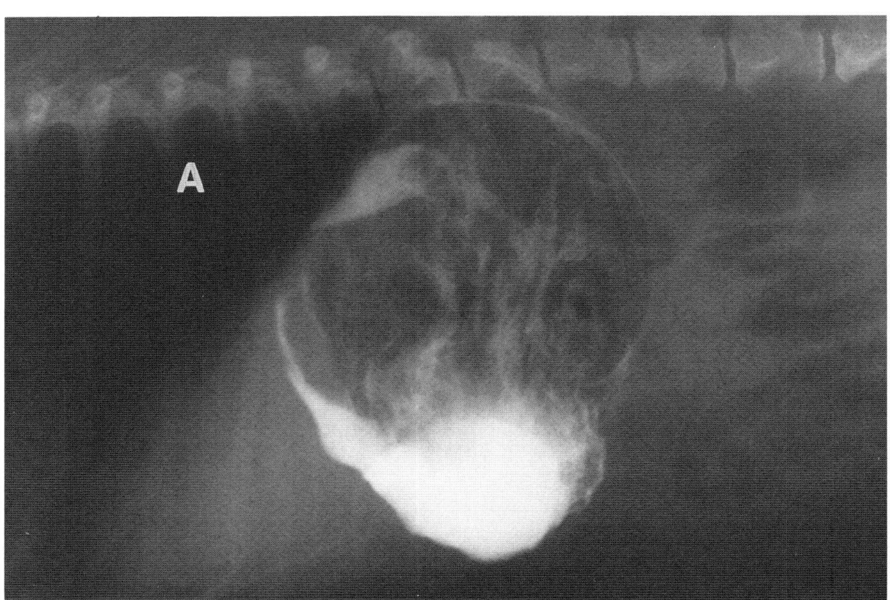

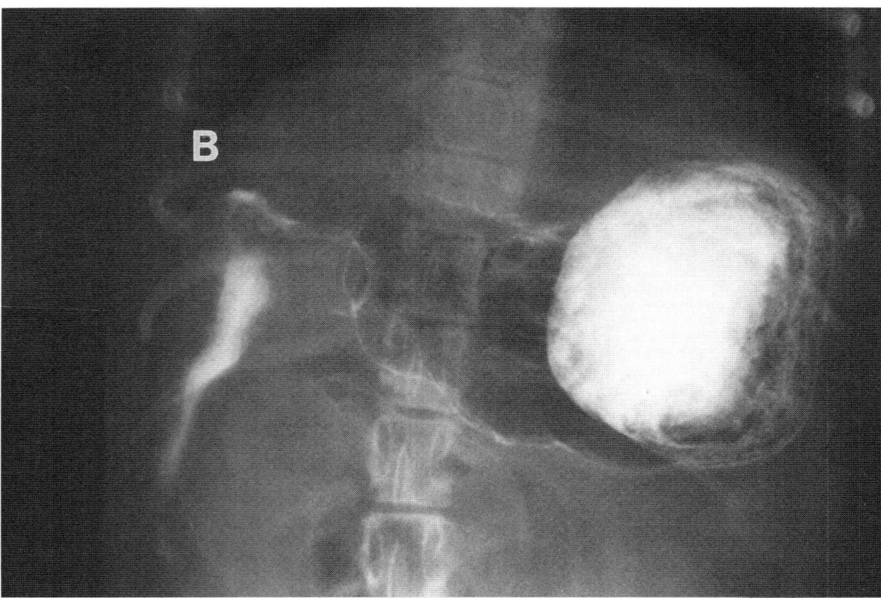

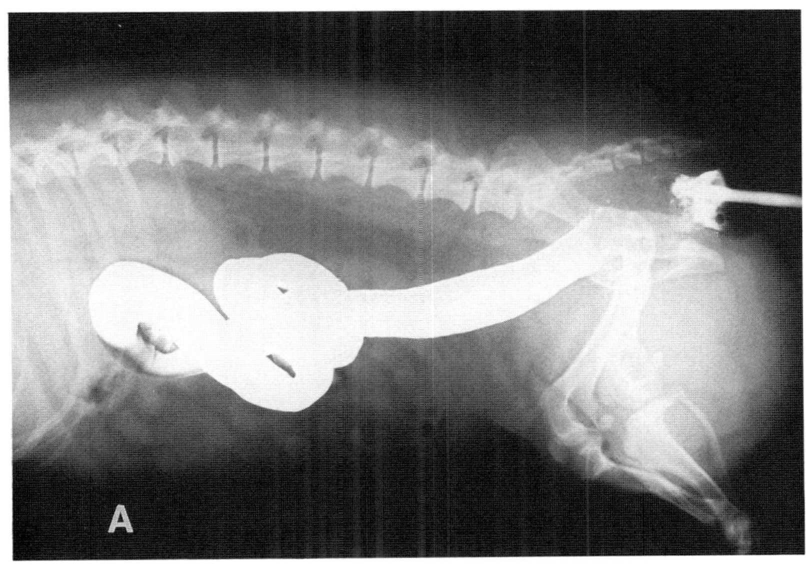

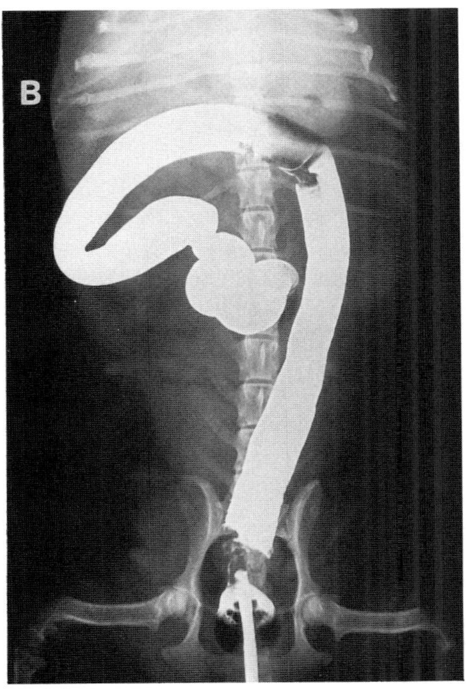

Figure 4. Normal canine barium enema. Lateral (A) and ventrodorsal (B) views. After imaging with the positive-contrast medium in the colon, remove as much of the contrast medium as possible. Replace the removed positive-contrast medium with an equal amount of air and make lateral and ventrodorsal projections.

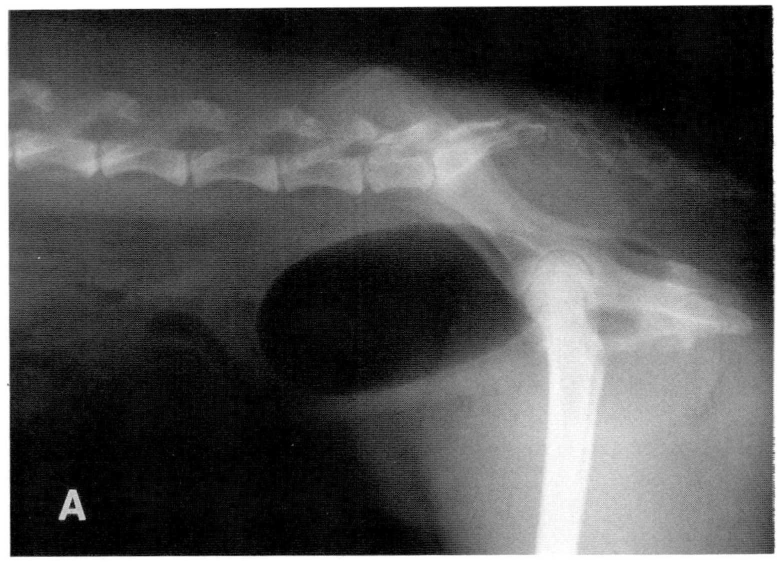

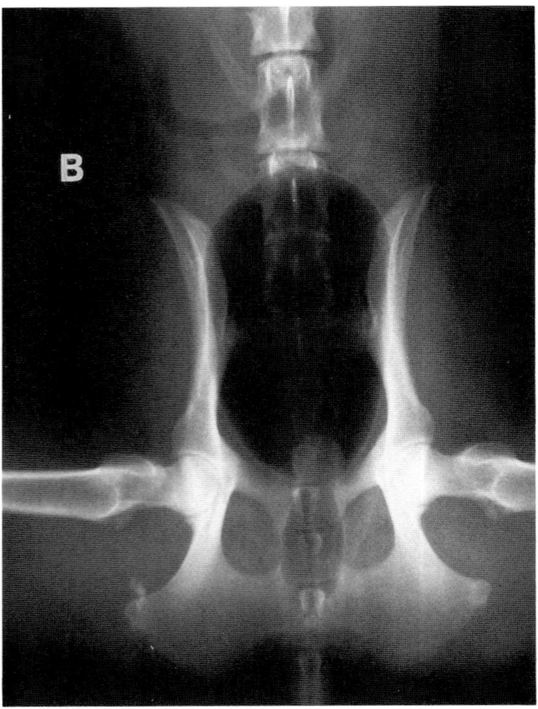

Figure 5. Lateral (A) and ventrodorsal (B) projections of a normal canine pneumo-cystogram. Notice the complete distention of the urinary bladder.

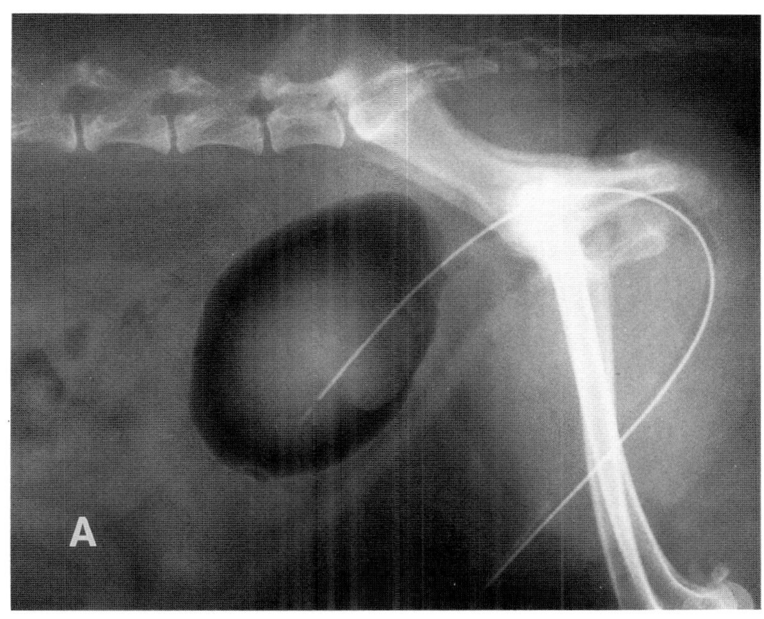

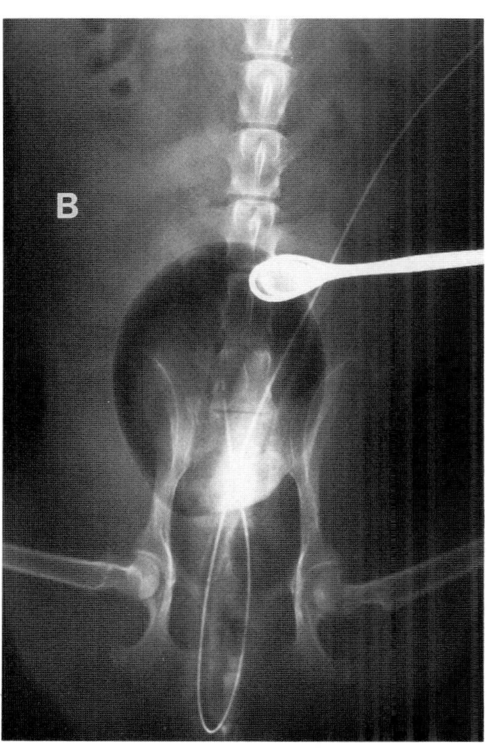

Figure 6. Canine double-contrast cystogram with transitional-cell carcinoma of the bladder wall. On the lateral projection (A), a lesion is outlined in the vertex and trigone of the bladder. In the ventrodorsal view (B), a tongue forceps is placed on the prepuce to prevent expulsion of air from the bladder.

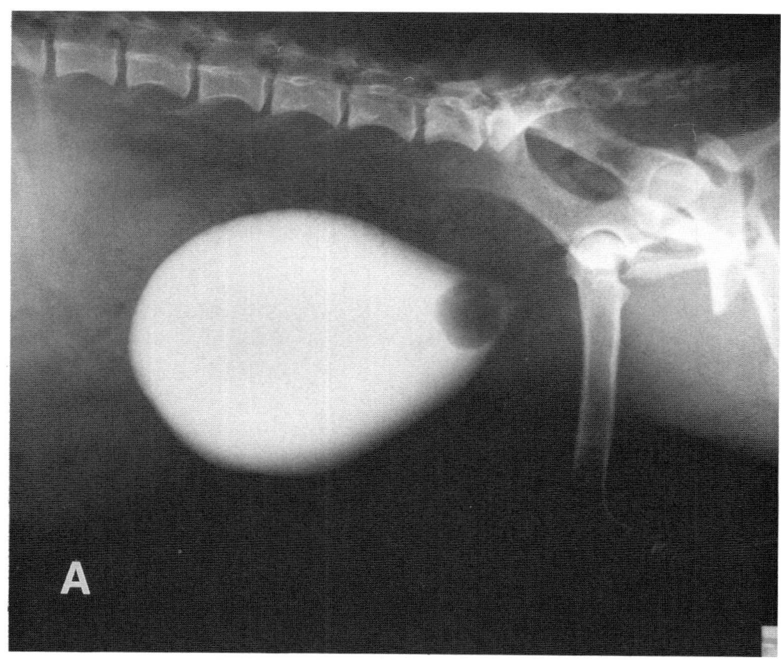

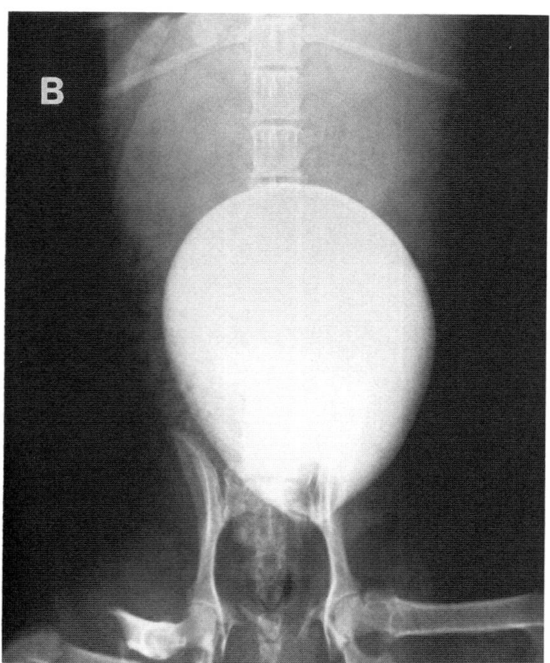

Figure 7. Canine positive-contrast cystogram. Lateral (A) and ventrodorsal (B) projections. This animal had been hit by a car, sustaining pelvic and femoral fractures. It was feared the urinary bladder had ruptured, so this was an emergency procedure forgoing the normal patient preparation.

Figure 8. Lateral projection of a normal canine retrograde urethrogram.

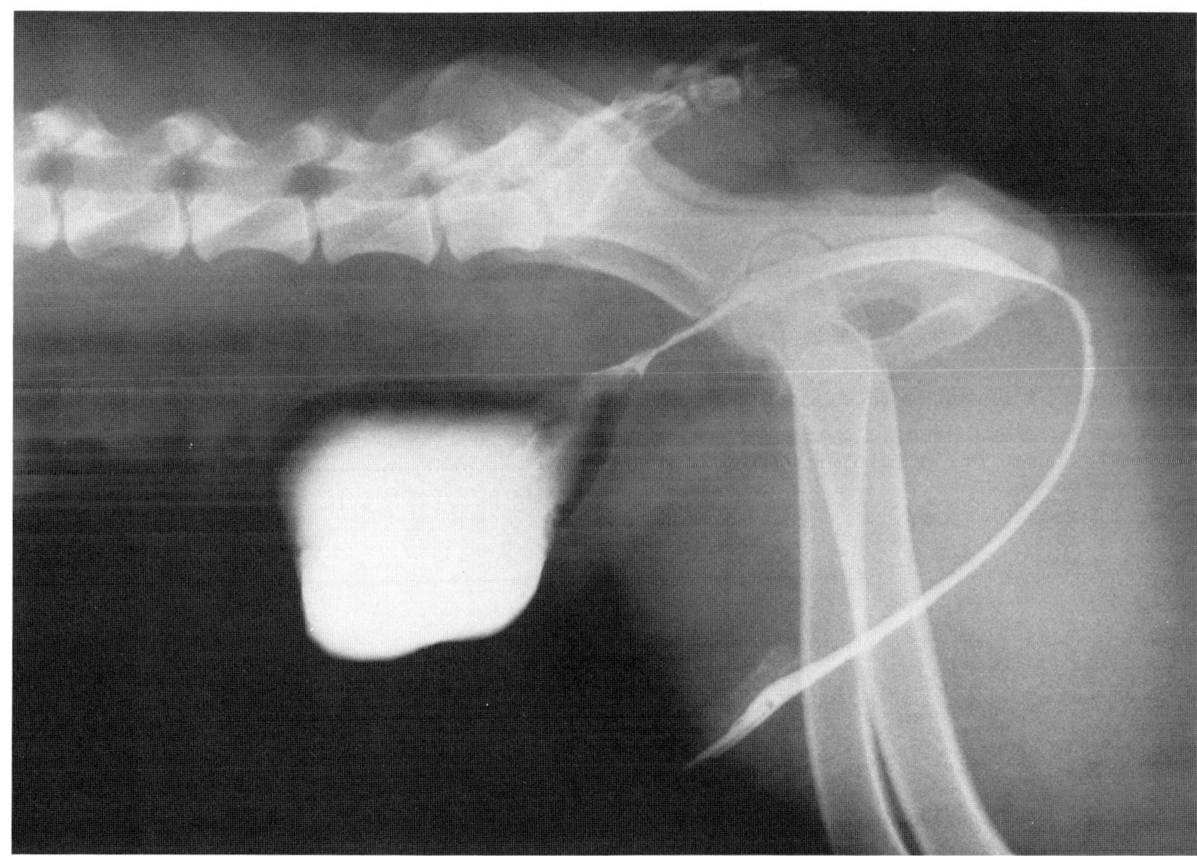

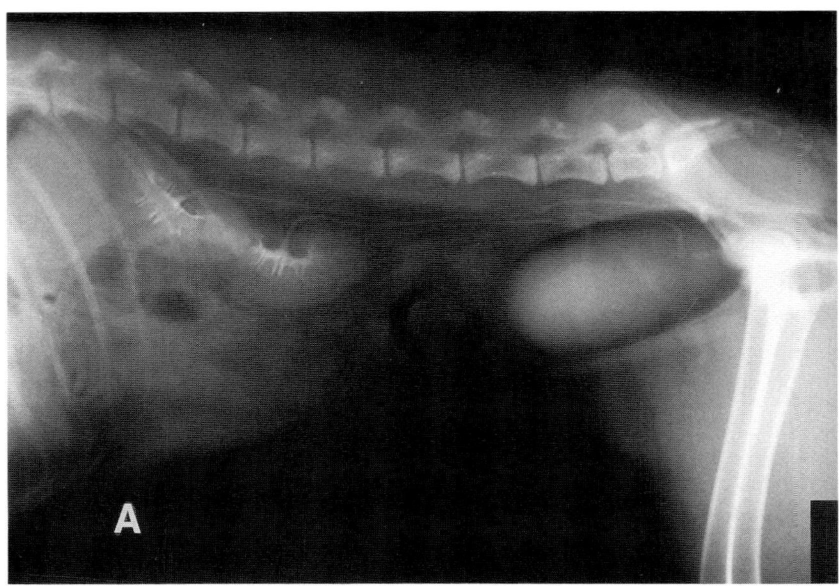

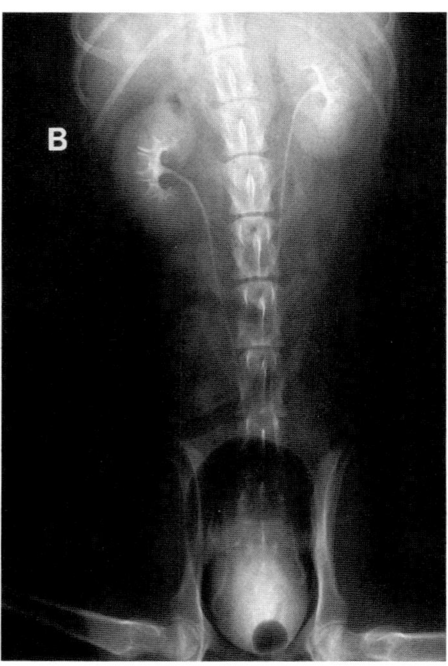

Figure 9. Canine
excretory urogram.
Lateral (A) and ventro-
dorsal (B) projections at
15 minutes after
injection of positive-
contrast medium.

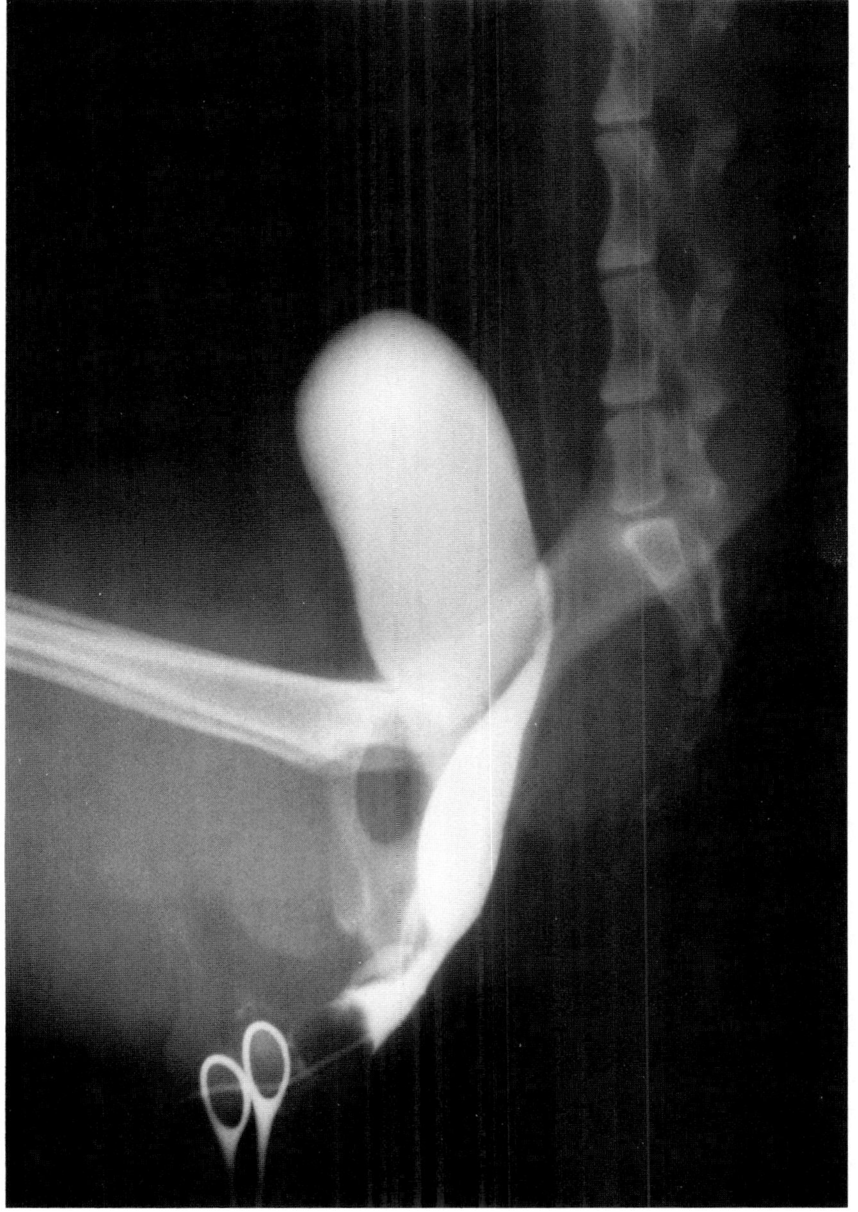

Figure 10. Lateral projection of a canine vaginogram.

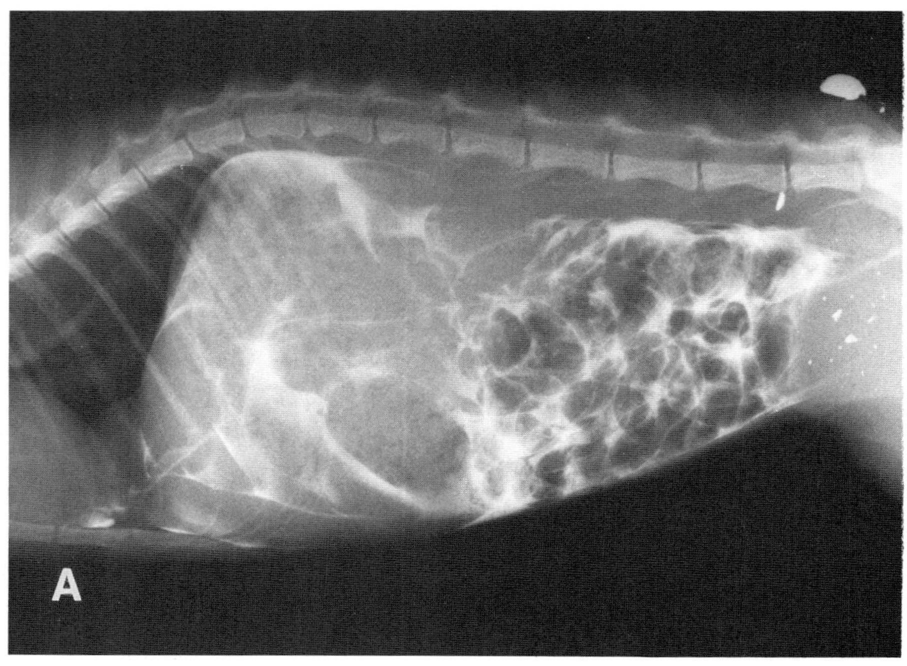

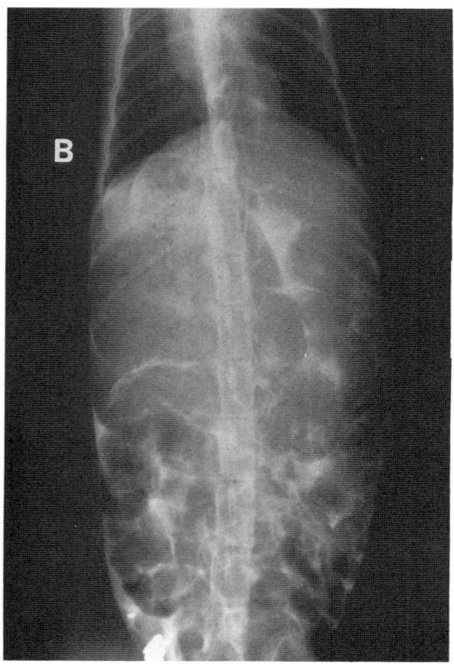

Figure 11. Lateral (A) and ventrodorsal (B) projections of a celiogram for a cat with a traumatic diaphragmatic hernia. Notice the contrast medium in the thoracic cavity on both projections.

Figure 12. Lateral projection of a canine pneumoperitoneogram.

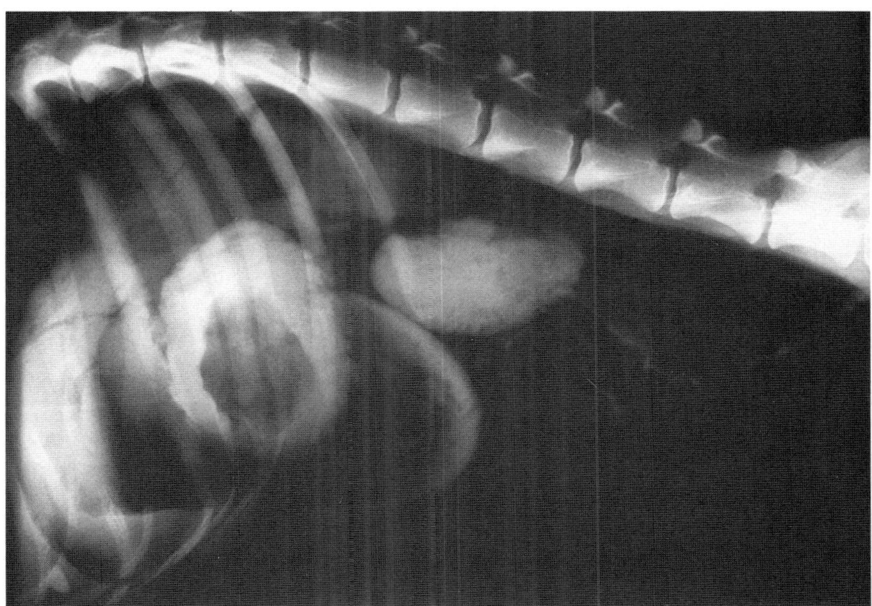

Figure 13. Lateral (A) and craniocaudal (B) projections of a fistulogram performed on the canine elbow area.

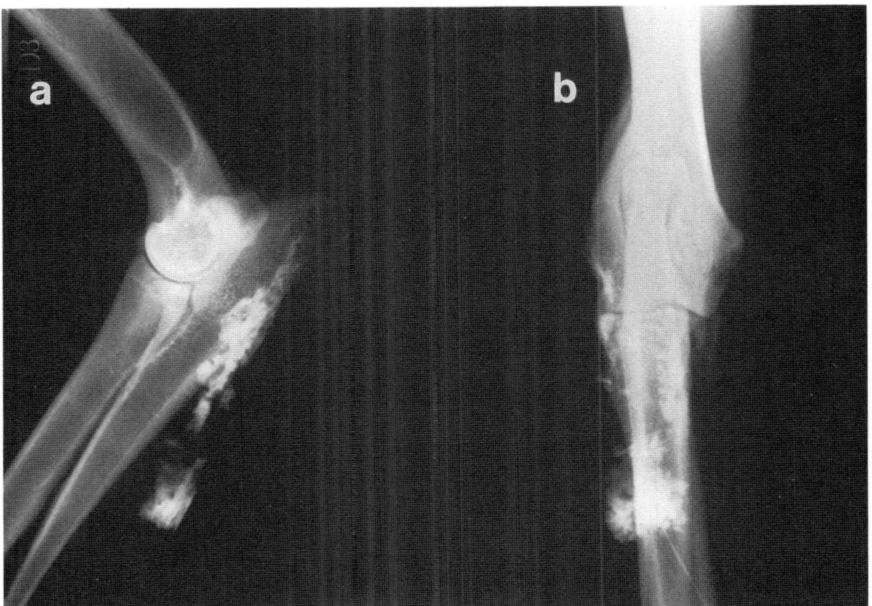

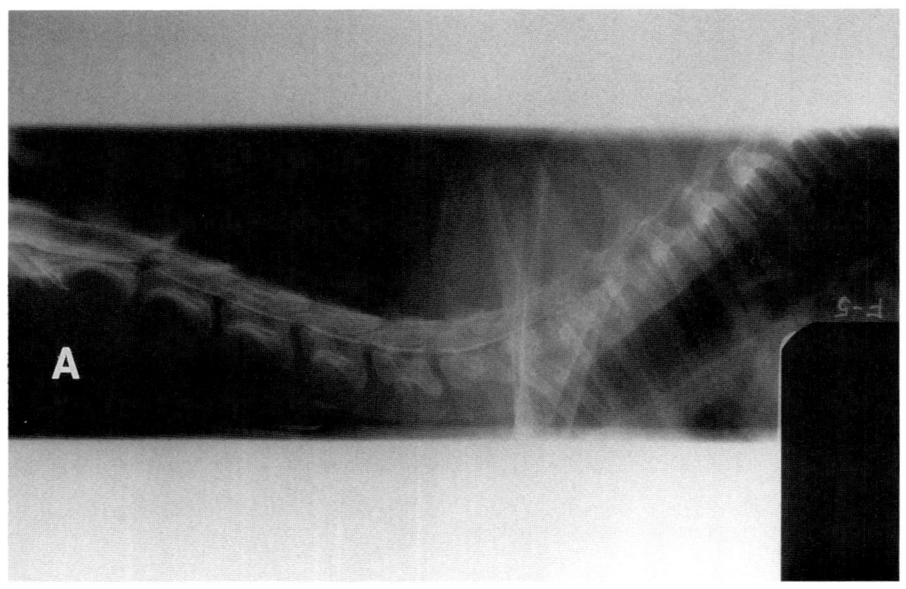

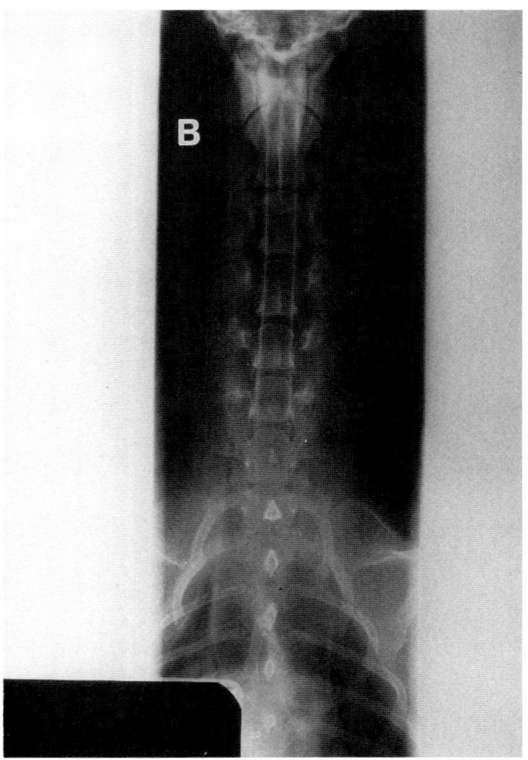

Figure 14. Lateral (A) and ventrodorsal (B) projections of a canine cervical myelogram.

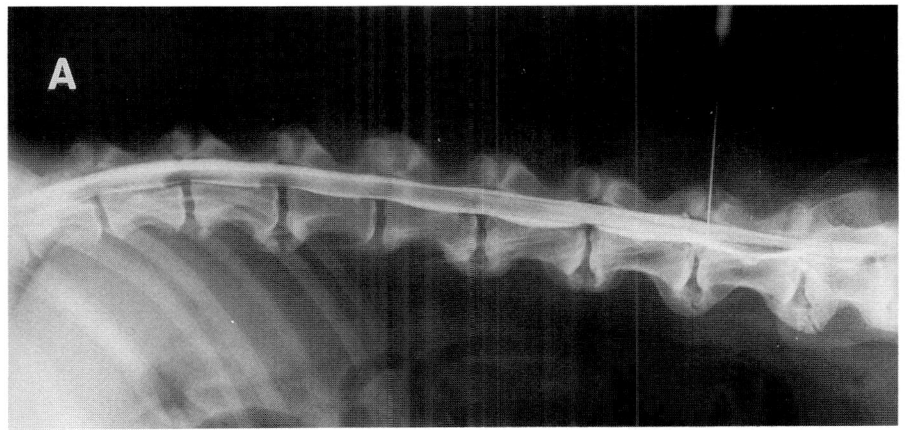

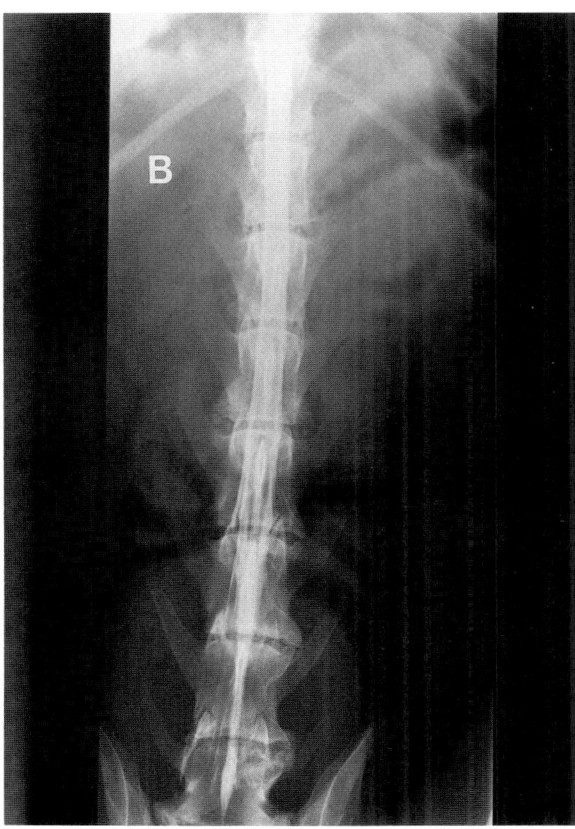

Figure 15. Lateral (A) and ventrodorsal (B) projections of a canine lumbar myelogram. Notice that the needle remains in place for the lateral projection but is removed for the ventrodorsal projection.

Figure 16. Lateral projection of a canine sialogram.

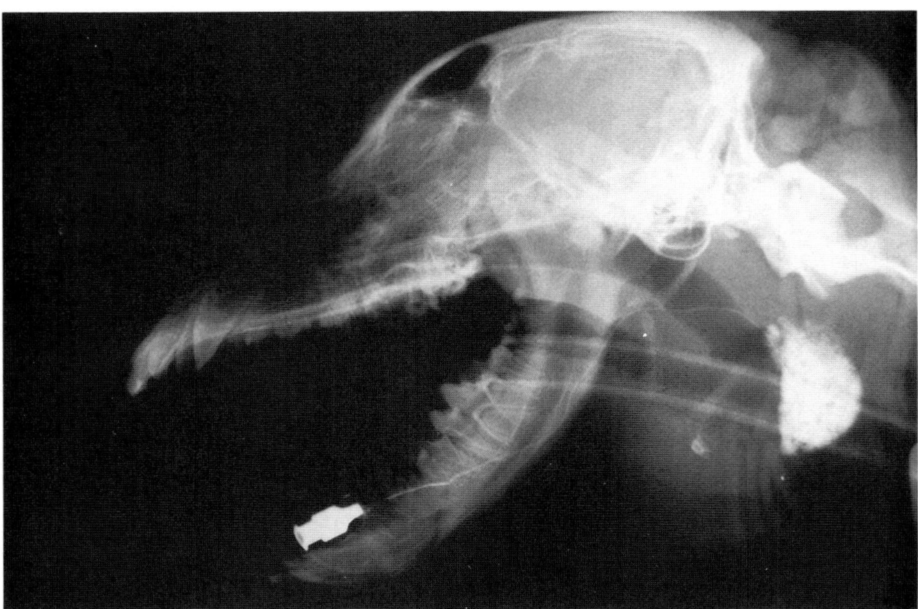

Figure 17. Lateral projection of an arthrogram of a canine shoulder joint.

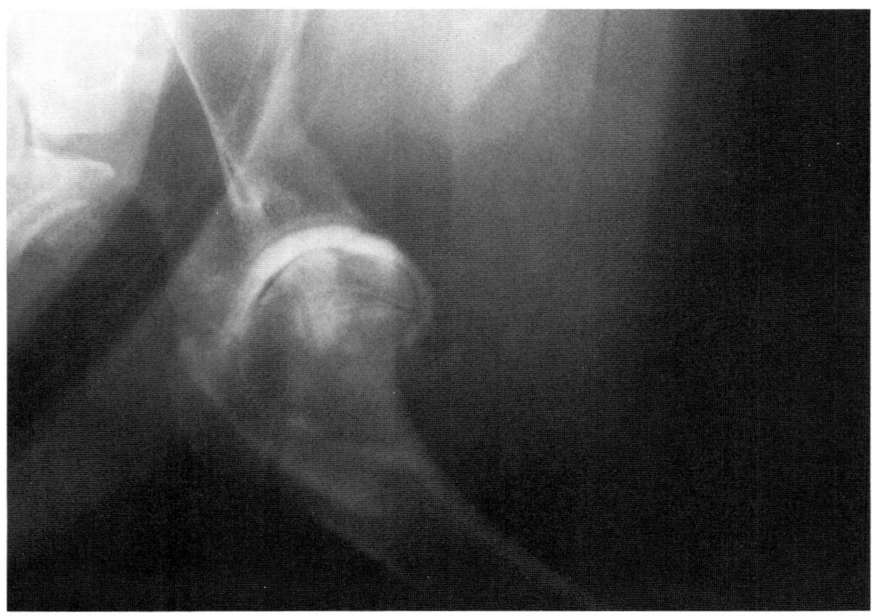

Figure 18. Lateral projection of a nonselective angiocardiogram.

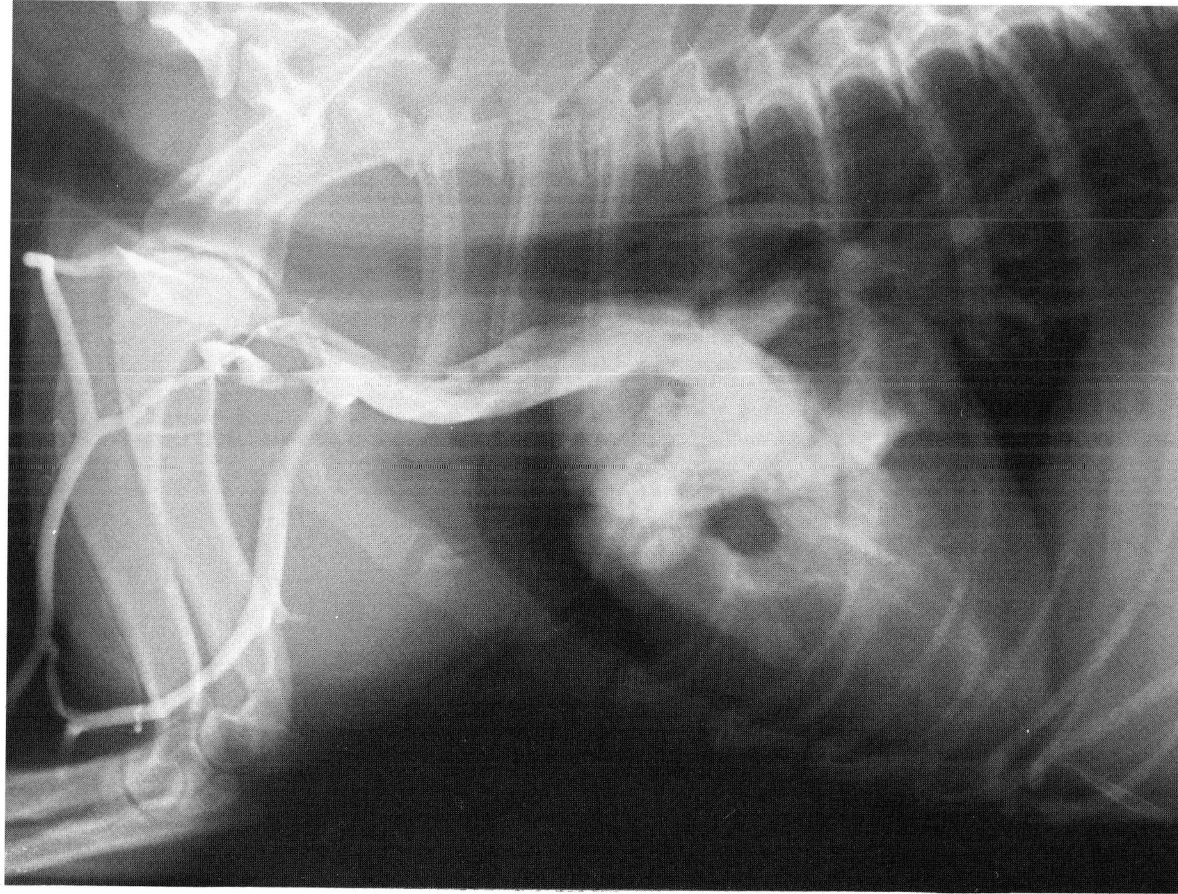

Notes

11

Large Animal Radiographic Positioning

The techniques described in this chapter are focused on positioning of horses. However, they are easily adapted to cattle, sheep, goats and pigs. The descriptions are limited to the extremities because of the limited capability of portable or mobile x-ray machines. Views involving the skull, pelvis and thorax require a machine with high mA capabilities and are beyond the scope of this text.

As with small animals, patient positioning is very important for accomplishing diagnostic radiographs in large animals. The horse should be positioned squarely so that weight is evenly distributed on each limb. If the weight is not evenly distributed, the joint spaces may be inaccurately interpreted.

Radiographic Aids

Radiographic aids used for large animal radiography can be custom made or items found around the farm.

Wooden Blocks

Wooden blocks are necessary to obtain certain positioning. They should be constructed so that they are solid and large enough for the entire hoof to fit on it comfortably. Also, you must elevate the foot high enough so when imaging the distal phalanx, the cassette can be placed distal to the palmar/plantar surface of the hoof. When using blocks to elevate a foot, the contralateral limb should also be elevated to the same height to ensure proper weight distribution.

Cassette Tunnel

The cassette tunnel is another aid that can be made (Fig 1). It is a protective sleeve made of a radiolucent material, such as Plexiglas, that can withstand a horse's weight. Carbon sandpaper can be glued to the surface of the tunnel to prevent the hoof from slipping.

Navicular Box

A navicular box is useful when imaging the distal sesamoid bone (Figs 2, 39). It is a box constructed to support the hoof in a position so the dorsal aspect of the hoof is perpendicular to the floor and the

Figure 1. Cassette tunnel.

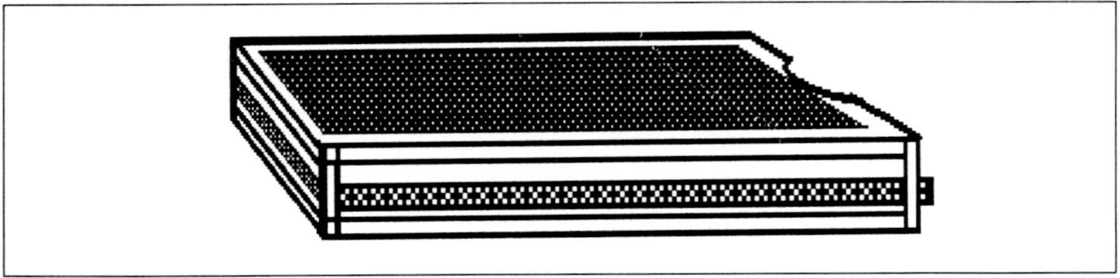

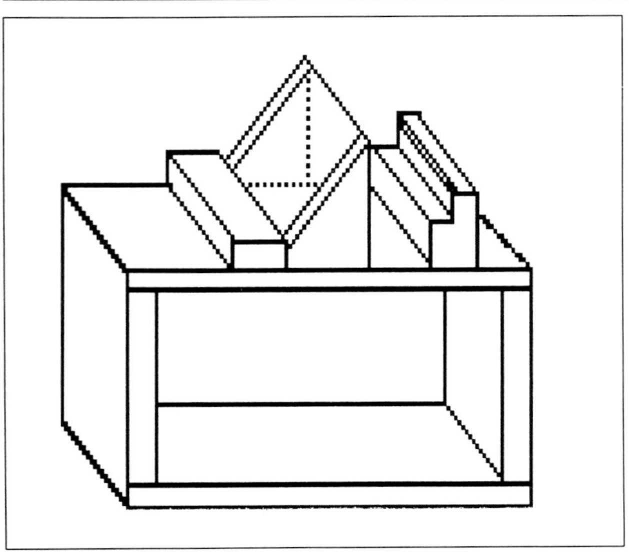

Figure 2. Navicular box (see also Figure 39, page 223).

palmar/plantar surface is parallel to the cassette. The part of the box supporting the hoof is made of Plexiglas, and the image is made through this surface.

Carpal Views

Position the horse squarely so that both feet are together and the leg being imaged is perpendicular to the ground.

Dorsopalmar

Hold the cassette against the palmar aspect of the carpus. Position the primary beam parallel to the floor and center on the middle of the carpal joint. The image should include the area from the distal radius to the proximal metacarpus. A true dorsopalmar view is achieved when the intercarpal space between the radial and intermediate carpal bones has no other bones superimposed (Figs 3, 4).

Lateromedial

Hold the cassette against the medial aspect of the leg. Position the primary beam parallel to the floor and center on the middle of the carpal joint. The image should include the area from the distal radius to the proximal metacarpus. A true lateromedial view is achieved when all the carpal bones are completely superimposed over one another. This allows the dorsal surface of the carpus to be viewed (Figs 3, 5).

Dorsolateral-Palmaromedial Oblique

Hold the cassette against the palmaromedial aspect of the leg. Position the primary beam parallel to the floor and center on the middle of the carpal joint, 30 degrees off of true lateromedial. The image should include the area from the distal radius to the proximal metacarpus. This oblique allows for a clear view of the dorsomedial and palmarolateral surfaces of the carpal bones (Figs 3, 6).

Dorsomedial-Palmarolateral Oblique

Hold the cassette against the palmarolateral aspect of the leg. Position the primary beam parallel to the floor and center on the middle of the carpal joint, 30 degrees off of true mediolateral. The image should include the area from the distal radius to the proximal metacarpus. This oblique allows for a clear view of the dorsolateral and palmaromedial surfaces of the carpal bones (Figs 3, 7).

Flexed Lateromedial

Flex the limb approximately 60 degrees, keeping the metacarpus parallel and the radius perpendicular to the ground. Hold the cassette against the medial surface of the carpal joint. It is important that the horse stands squarely on the remaining 3 limbs, allowing the flexed limb to be positioned perpendicular to the ground. Position the primary beam parallel to the floor and center on the space between the proximal and distal rows of carpal bones so that the interarticular spaces can be visualized (Figs 8, 9).

Figure 3. Positioning for standard projections of the carpus.

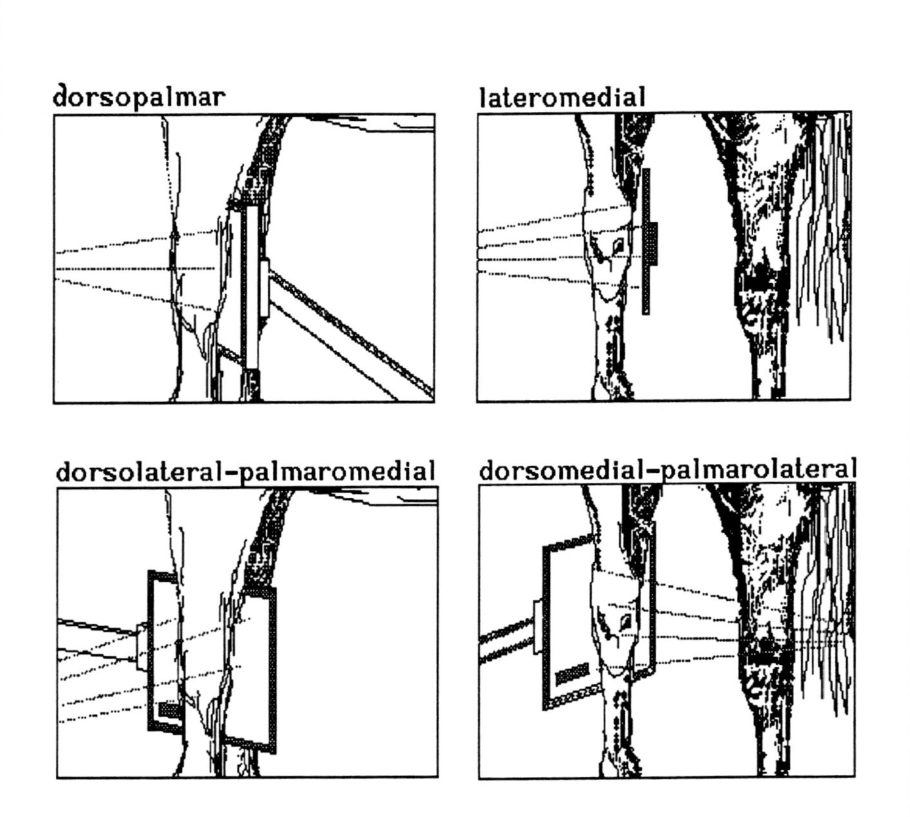

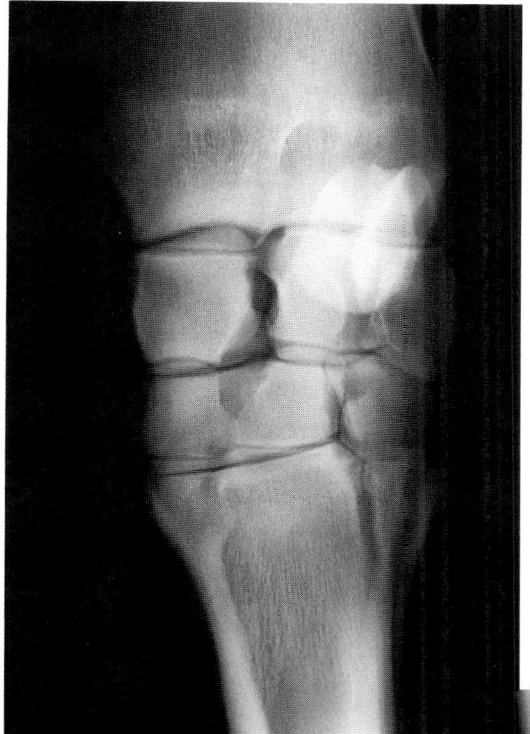

Figure 4. Dorsopalmar projection of the carpus (left).

Figure 5. Lateromedial projection of the carpus (right).

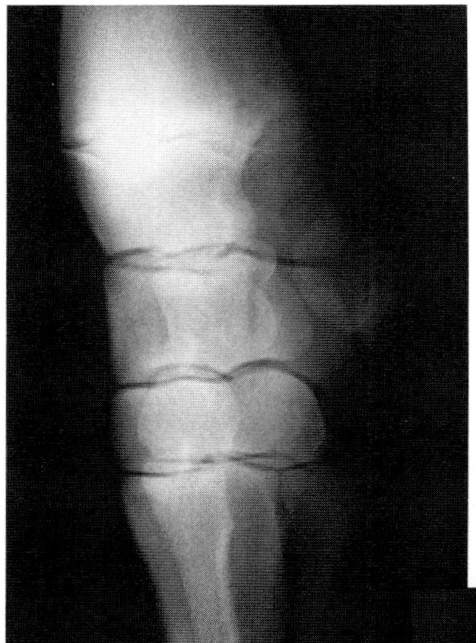

Figure 6. Dorsolateral-palmaromedial projection of the carpus (left).

Figure 7. Dorsomedial-palmarolateral projection of the carpus (right).

Dorsoproximal 60 Degrees – Dorsodistal Oblique

Flex the limb pushing the carpal joint cranially. Place the cassette on the dorsodistal aspect of the limb and parallel to the floor. Angle the primary beam 60 degrees in a proximal to distal direction, centering on the carpal joint. Because the cassette is not truly perpendicular to the primary beam, there will be some elongation of the carpal joint. This view is used to visualize the proximal row of carpal bones (Figs 8, 10).

Dorsoproximal 20 Degrees – Dorsodistal Oblique

Flex the limb, pushing slightly cranially and keeping the metacarpus parallel to the ground. Place the cassette on the dorsodistal aspect of the limb and parallel to the floor. Angle the primary beam 20 degrees in a proximal to distal direction, centering on the carpal joint. Because the cassette is not truly perpendicular to the primary beam,

Figure 8. Positioning for additional projections of the carpus.

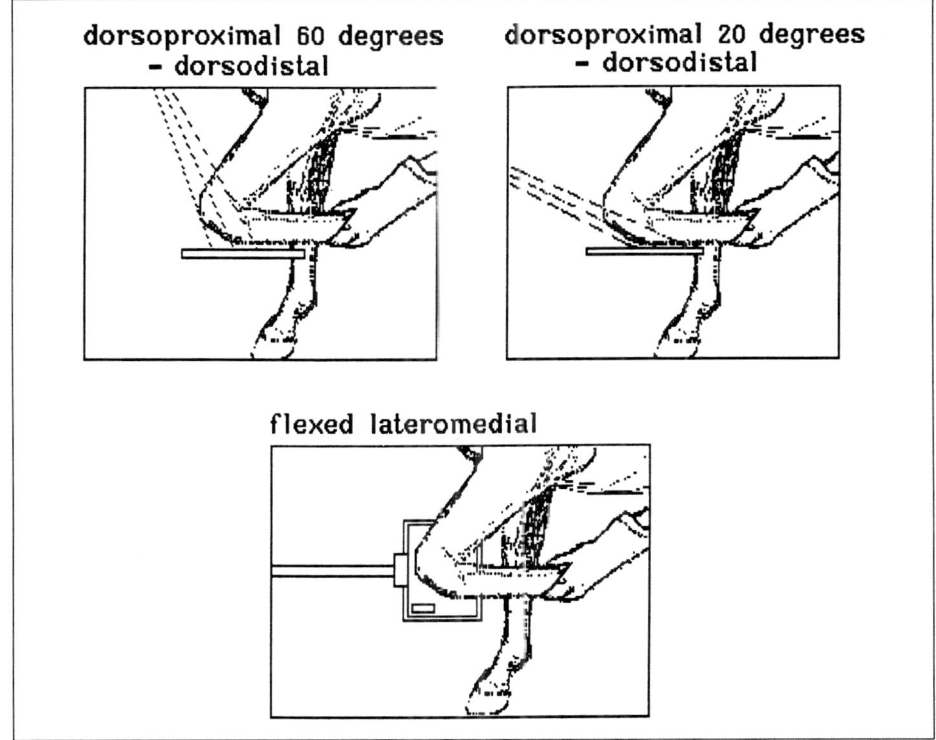

there will be some elongation of the carpal joint. This view is used to visualize the distal row of carpal bones (Figs 8, 11).

Tarsal Views

Position the horse with its weight evenly distributed on all 4 legs. Position the limb so the metatarsus is perpendicular to the ground.

Dorsoplantar

Position the horse so the limb of interest has a slight lateral rotation, making it possible for the primary beam to travel in a true dorsoplantar direction. If the horse is standing squarely, its body will obstruct the positioning of the x-ray tube. Hold the cassette on the plantar surface of the tarsal joint. Position the primary beam parallel to the floor and center on the proximal intertarsal space. The image should include the area from the distal tibia to the proximal metatarsus (Figs 12, 13).

Lateromedial

Place the cassette on the medial surface of the tarsal joint. Position the primary beam parallel to the floor and center on the proximal intertarsal joint. The image should include the area from the distal

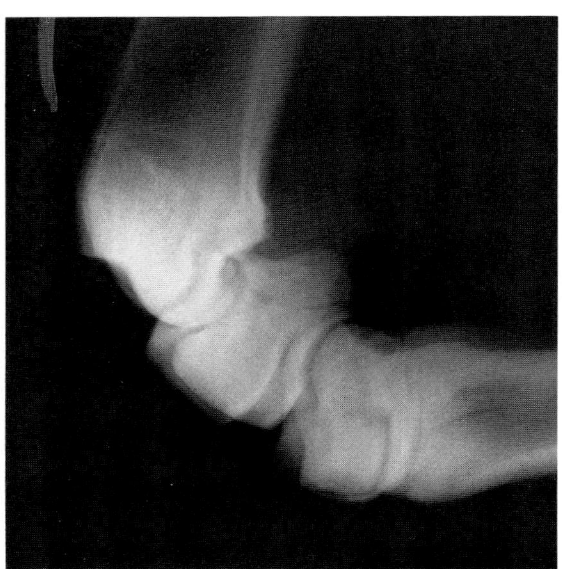

Figure 9. Flexed lateromedial projection of the carpus.

tibia to the proximal metatarsus. A true lateromedial view shows the trochlea of the talus superimposed so that only one trochlear ridge is visible (Figs 12, 14).

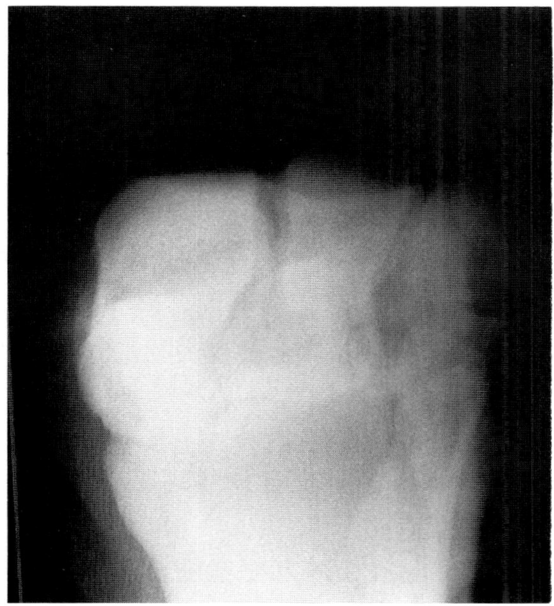

Figure 10. Dorso-proximal 60-degree dorsodistal projection of the proximal row of carpal bones.

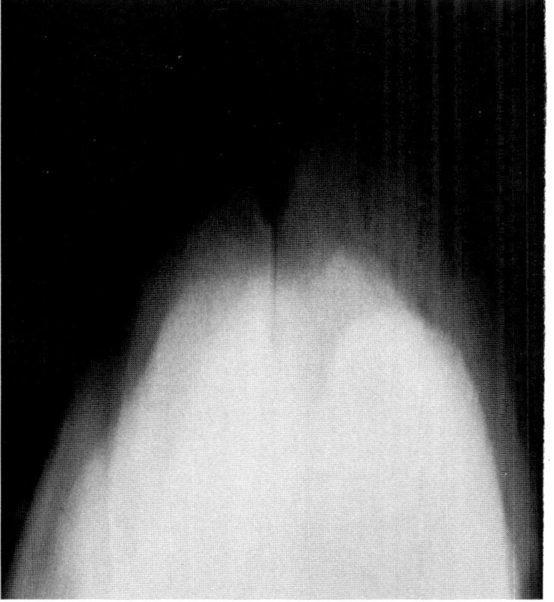

Figure 11. Dorso-proximal 20-degree dorsodistal projection of the distal row of carpal bones.

Dorsolateral-Plantaromedial Oblique

Place the cassette on the plantaromedial aspect of the tarsus. Position the primary beam parallel to the floor and center on the proximal intertarsal joint, 45 degrees off of true lateromedial. The image should include the area from the distal tibia to the proximal metatarsus. It is used to visualize the dorsomedial and plantarolateral surfaces of the tarsal bones (Figs 12, 15).

Dorsomedial-Plantarolateral Oblique

Place the cassette on the plantarolateral aspect of the tarsus. Position the primary beam parallel to the floor and center on the proximal intertarsal joint, 45 degrees off of true mediolateral. The image should include that area from the distal tibia to the proximal metatarsus. It is used to visualize the dorsolateral and plantaromedial surfaces of the tarsal bones (Figs 12, 16).

Figure 12. Positioning for standard projections of the tarsus.

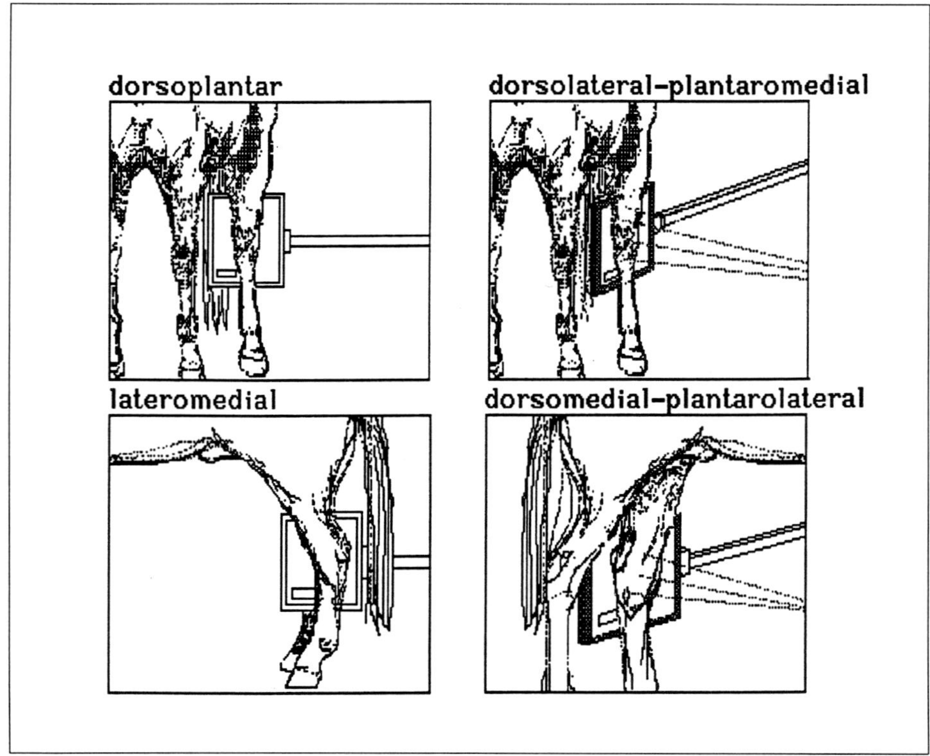

Dorsoplantar (Flexed)

Flex the limb so that the metatarsus is parallel to the ground, pushing the whole limb caudally. Place the cassette on the distoplantar surface of the tarsus. Project the primary beam in a plantarodorsal direction at a 60-degree angle. This image isolates the calcaneus without superimposition of the tarsal bones (Figs 17, 18).

Metacarpal Views

Position the horse squarely, with its weight evenly distributed on all 4 limbs. The limb of interest should be perpendicular to the ground.

Dorsopalmar

Place the cassette on the palmar surface of the metacarpus, keeping it parallel to the limb. Position the primary beam parallel to the floor and center midway between the carpal and metacarpo-

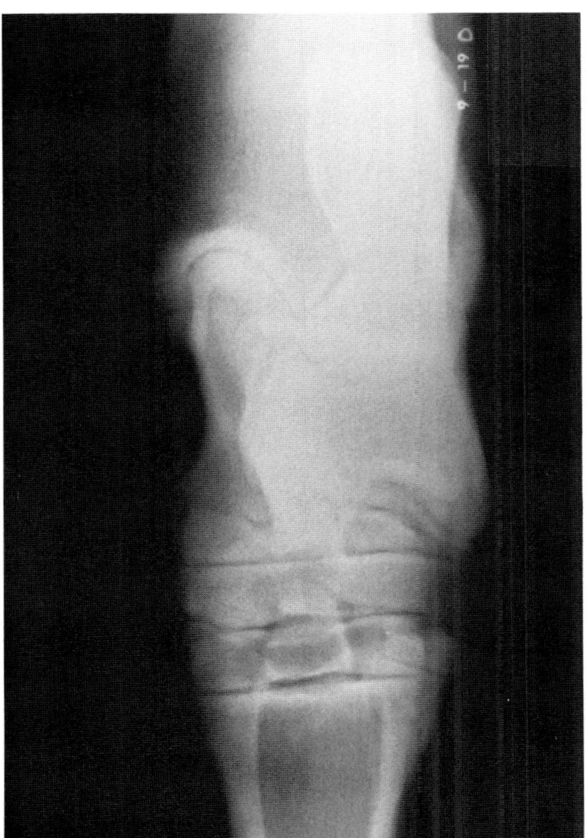

Figure 13. Dorsoplantar projection of the tarsal joint.

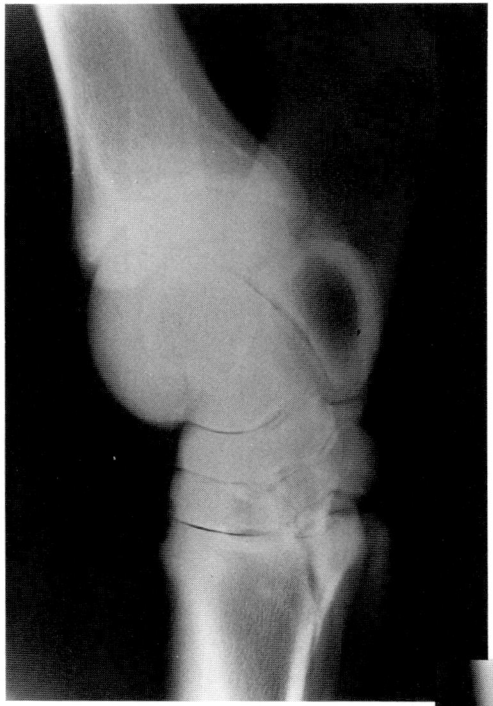

Figure 14. Lateromedial projection of the tarsal joint (left).

Figure 15. Dorsolateral-plantaromedial projection of the tarsal joint (right).

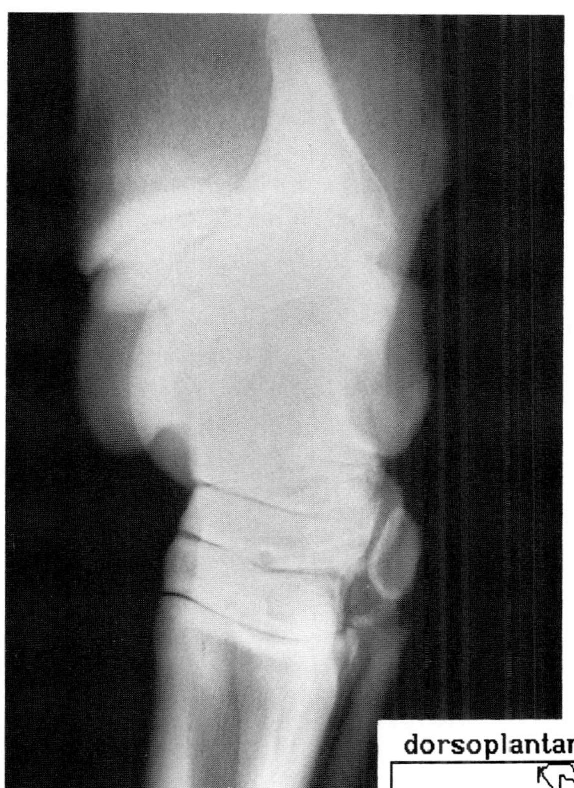

Figure 16. Dorsomedial-plantarolateral projection of the tarsal joint (left).

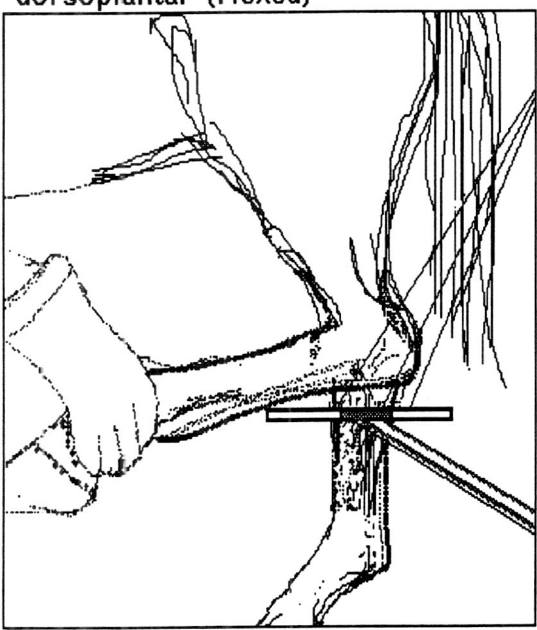

Figure 17. Positioning for an additional projection of the tarsus (right).

phalangeal joints. The image should include the carpal and meta-carpophalangeal joints. A 7 x 17-inch cassette is necessary to image the entire metacarpal region (Figs 19, 20).

Lateromedial

Place the cassette on the medial aspect of the metacarpus, keeping it parallel to the limb. Position the primary beam parallel to the floor and center midway between the carpal and metacarpophalangeal joints. The image should include the carpal and metacarpophalangeal joints. A 7 x 17-inch cassette is necessary to image the entire meta-carpal region. The true lateromedial image shows the second and fourth metacarpal bones superimposed over one another (Figs 19, 21).

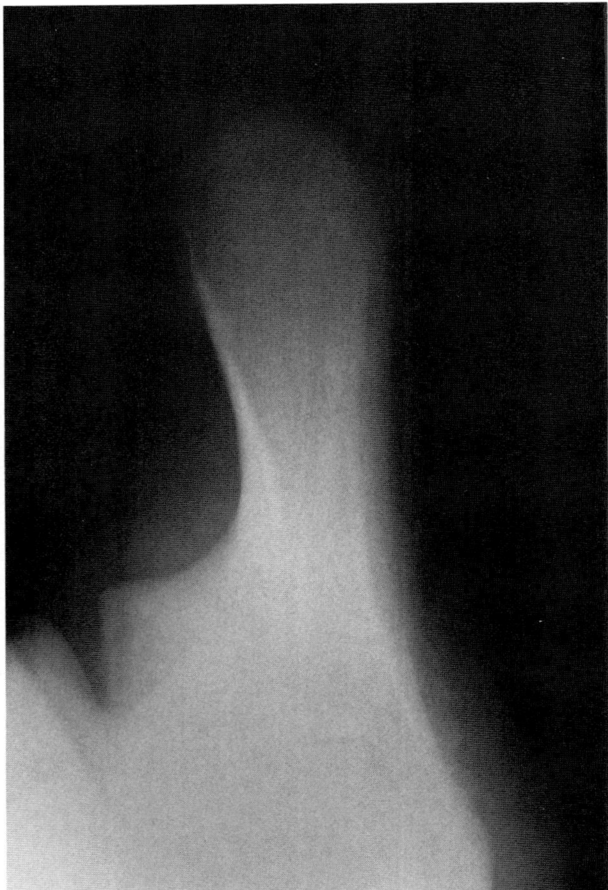

Figure 18. Dorsoplantar (flexed) projection of the tarsus.

Dorsolateral-Palmaromedial Oblique

Place the cassette on the palmaromedial aspect of the metacarpus, keeping it parallel to the limb. Position the primary beam parallel to the floor and center midway between the carpal and metacarpophalangeal joints. Direct the primary beam dorsolaterally, 35-45 degrees off of a true dorsopalmar projection. The image should include the carpal and metacarpophalangeal joints. This image shows the fourth metacarpal bone without superimposition (Figs 19, 22).

Dorsolateral-Palmarolateral Oblique

Place the cassette on the palmarolateral aspect of the metacarpus, keeping it parallel to the limb. Position the primary beam parallel to the floor and center midway between the carpal and metacarpophalangeal joints. Direct the primary beam dorsomedially, 35-45 degrees off of a true dorsopalmar projection. The image should include

Figure 19. Positioning for standard projections of the metacarpus.

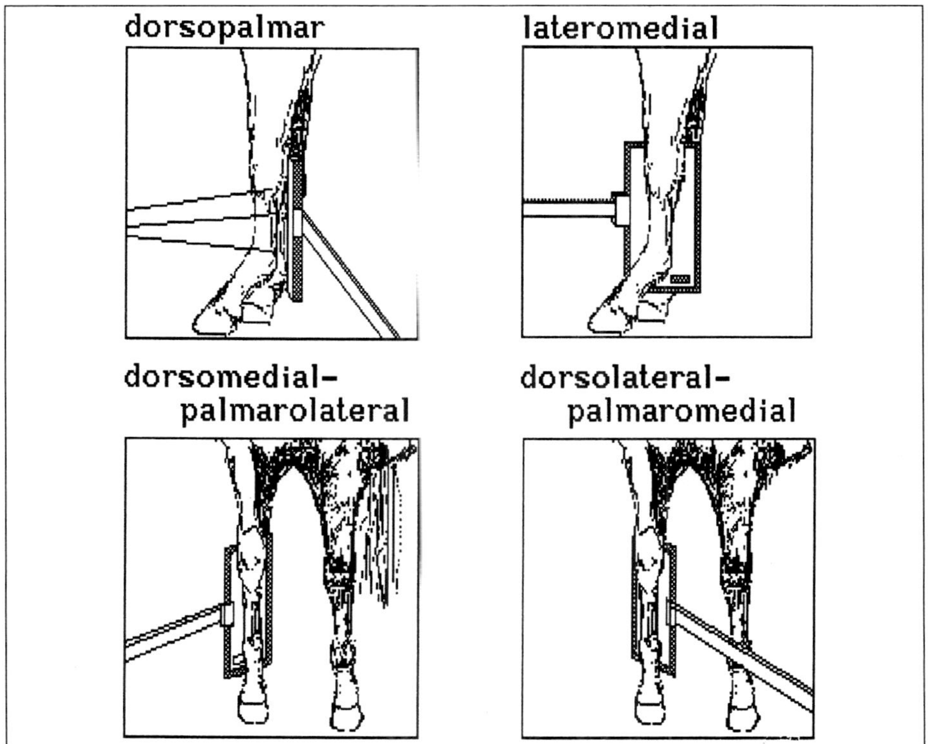

the carpal and metacarpophalangeal joints. This image shows the second metacarpal bone without superimposition (Figs 19, 23).

Metatarsal Views

Positioning for this area is identical to that for the metacarpus, with the exception that the term *palmar* is replaced with *plantar* when referring to the rear limb. It is also important that the radiographs be labeled correctly as those of a rear limb, using LR (left rear) and RR (right rear).

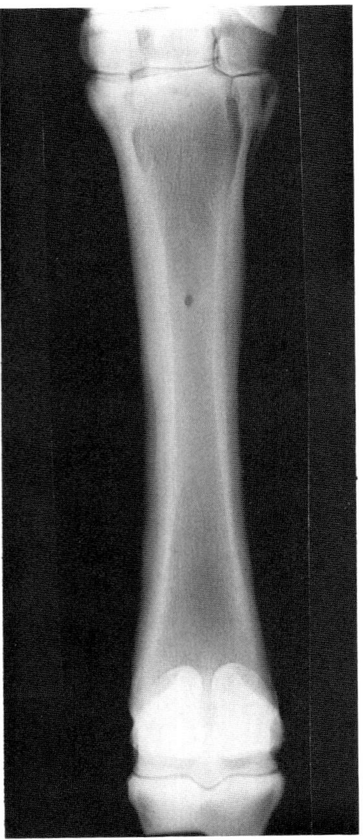

Figure 20. Dorsopalmar projection of the metacarpus.

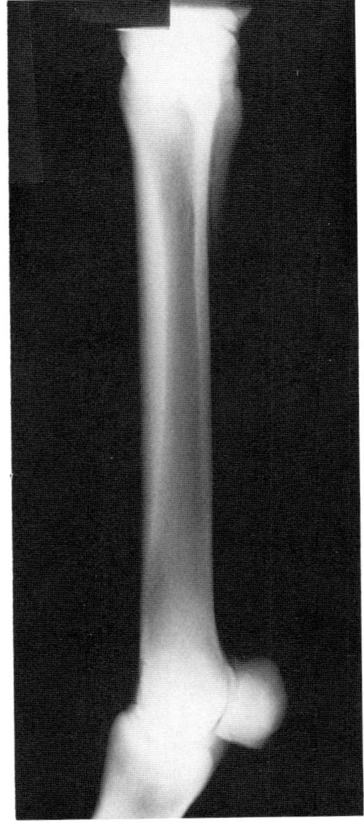

Figure 21. Lateromedial projection of the metacarpus.

Views of the
Metacarpophalangeal Joint
(Fetlock Joint)

Position the horse squarely, with its weight distributed evenly on both front legs. It is important that the leg be perpendicular to the ground in a normal weight-bearing position. It may be necessary to place the horse on blocks of wood if the x-ray machine cannot be moved close to the ground. When this is the case, both feet should be placed on blocks to ensure that they are evenly bearing weight.

Figure 22. Dorsolateral-palmaromedial projection of the metacarpus.

Figure 23. Dorsomedial-palmarolateral projection of the metacarpus.

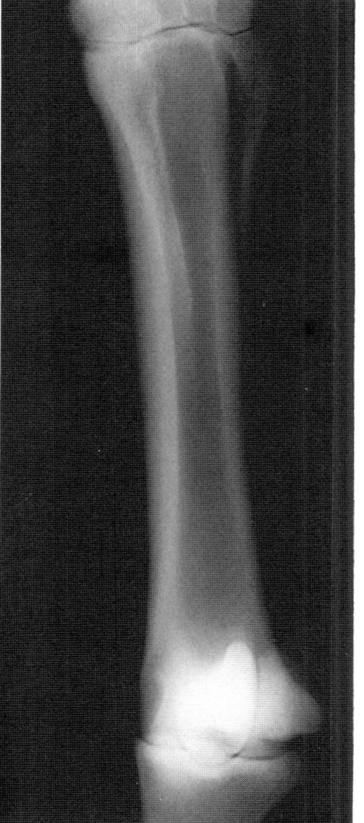

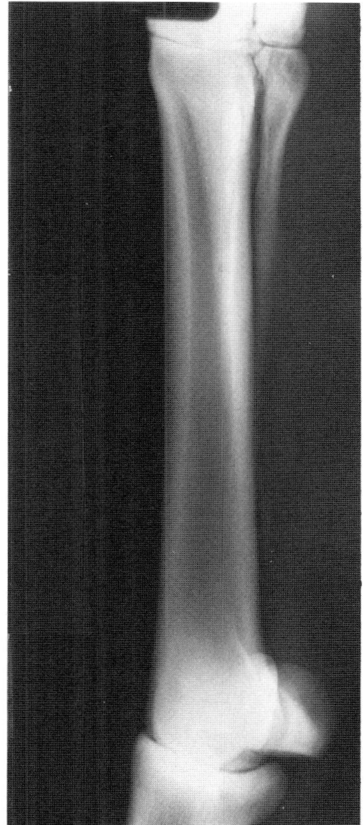

Dorsopalmar

Angle the primary beam 20 degrees proximal to distal and center on the midsagittal plane of the metacarpophalangeal joint. Place the cassette against the palmar surface of the limb and position it so that it is perpendicular to the primary beam. This view projects the sesamoids dorsal to the metacarpophalangeal joint space (Figs 24, 25).

Lateromedial

Place the cassette on the medial aspect of the joint. Direct the primary beam parallel to the floor and center on the metacarpophalangeal joint. A true lateromedial view displays the metacarpal condyles and the sesamoids superimposed, and a visible joint space (Figs 24, 26).

Figure 24. Positioning for standard projections of the metacarpophalangeal joint (fetlock).

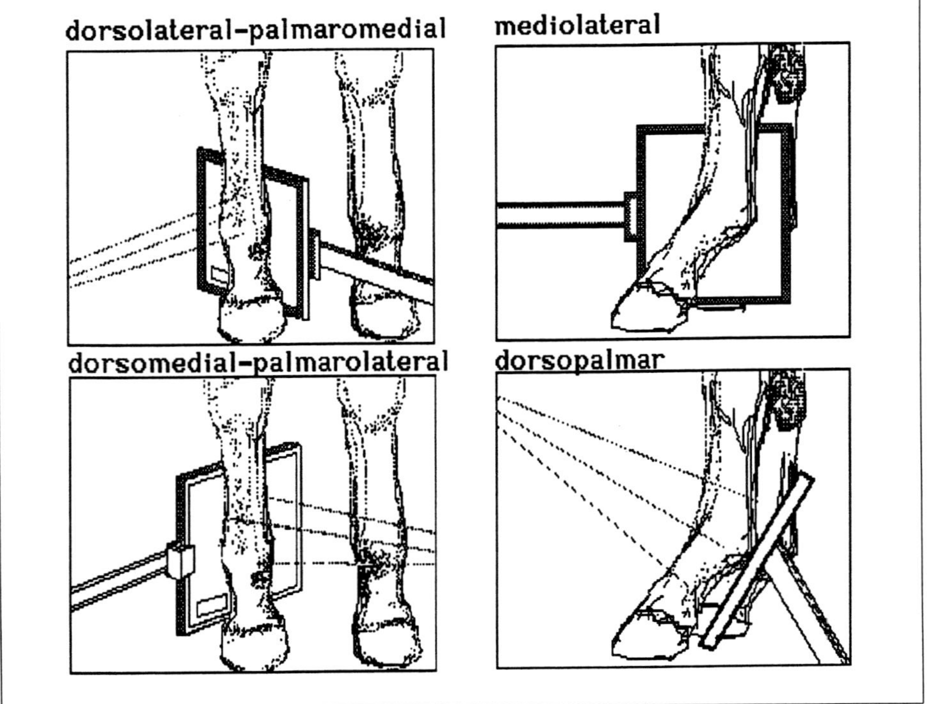

Dorsolateral-Palmaromedial Oblique

Place the cassette on the palmaromedial aspect of the joint. Position the primary beam parallel to the floor and center on the metacarpophalangeal joint. Direct the primary beam dorsolaterally, 45 degrees off of a true dorsopalmar projection. This allows the lateral sesamoid to be visualized without the medial sesamoid bone superimposed (Figs 24, 27).

Dorsomedial-Palmarolateral Oblique

Place the cassette on the palmarolateral aspect of the joint. Position the primary beam parallel to the floor and center on the metacarpophalangeal joint. Direct the primary beam dorsomedially, 45 degrees off of a true dorsopalmar projection. This allows the medial sesamoid bone to be visualized without the lateral sesamoid bone superimposed (Figs 24, 28).

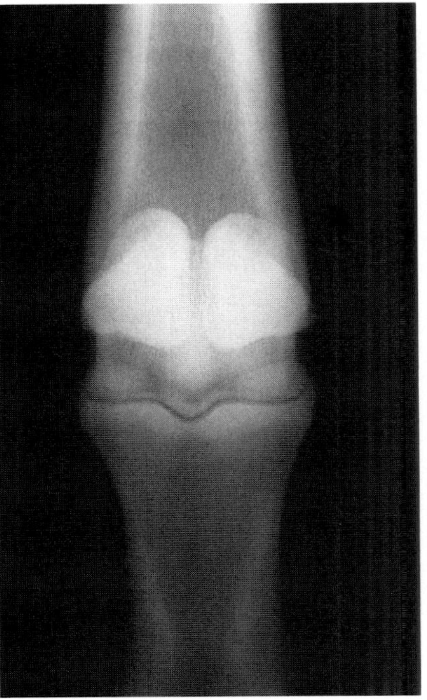

Figure 25. Dorsopalmar projection of the metacarpophalangeal joint (fetlock).

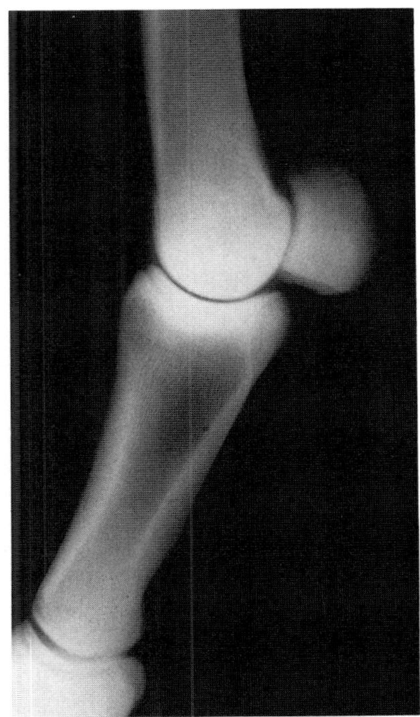

Figure 26. Lateromedial projection of the metacarpophalangeal joint (fetlock).

Views of the
Metatarsophalangeal Joint
(Fetlock Joint)

Positioning for this joint is identical to that for the metacarpophalangeal joint, with the exception that the term *palmar* is replaced with *plantar* when referring to the rear limb. Because the anatomy is the same, it is important that the radiographs be labeled correctly as those of a rear limb, using LR (left rear) and RR (right rear).

Proximal Interphalangeal Joint
(Pastern Joint)

Position the horse squarely, with its weight distributed evenly on both legs. It is important that the leg be perpendicular to the ground in a normal weight-bearing position. It may be necessary to place the horse on blocks of wood if the x-ray machine cannot be moved close to the ground. When this is the case, both feet should be placed on blocks to ensure that they are evenly bearing weight.

Figure 27. Dorsolateral-palmaromedial projection of the metacarpophalangeal joint (fetlock).

Figure 28. Dorsolateral-palmarolateral projection of the metacarpophalangeal joint (fetlock).

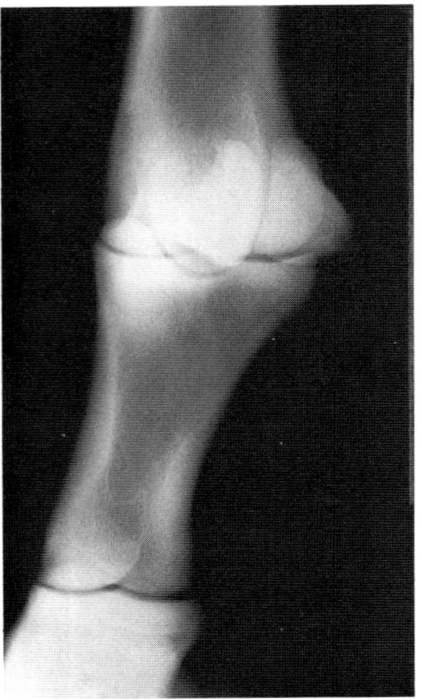

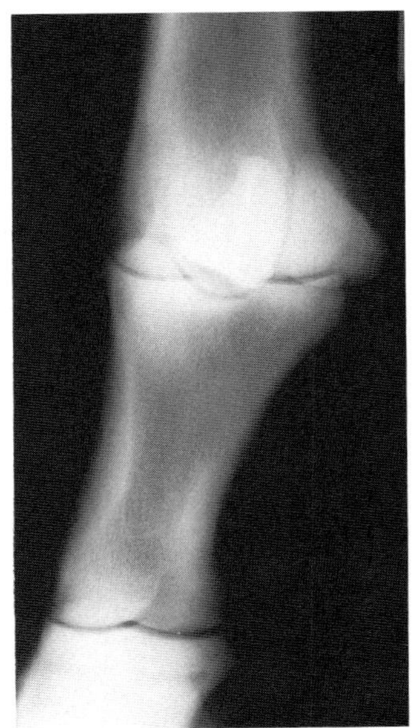

Dorsopalmar

Angle the primary beam 15-20 degrees proximal to distal and center on the proximal interphalangeal joint. When positioning the horse, place the foot being imaged on the caudal aspect of the wooden block. This allows the cassette to be rested on the ground, perpendicular to the primary beam. Place the cassette on the palmar surface of the limb. This image shows the proximal and middle phalanges (Figs 29, 30).

Lateromedial

Place the cassette on the medial aspect of the joint. Position the primary beam parallel to the floor and center on the proximal interphalangeal joint. This image shows the proximal and middle phalanges (Figs 29, 31).

Views of the Distal Phalanx
(Coffin Bone)

Lateromedial

Position the horse with the foot of interest and the contralateral limb on blocks of wood. This raises the distal limb off the floor so that

Figure 29. Positioning for standard projections of the proximal interphalangeal joint (pastern).

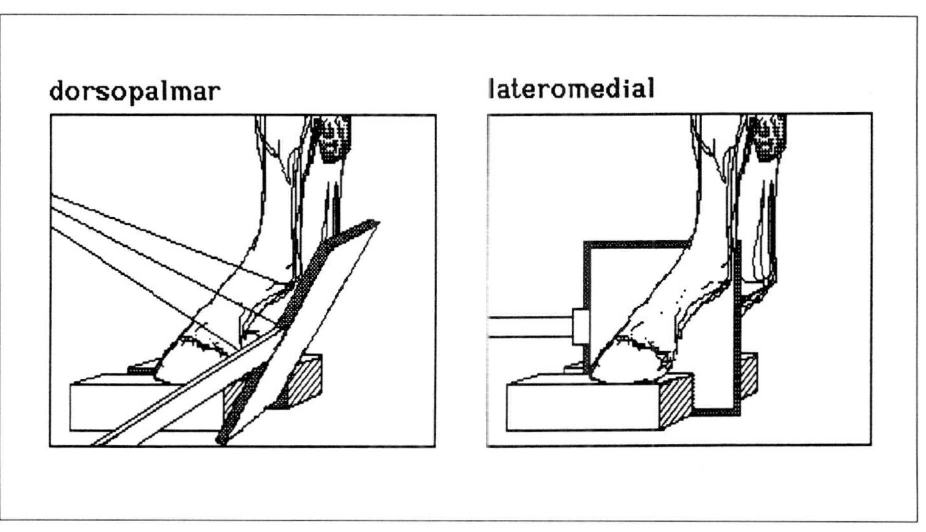

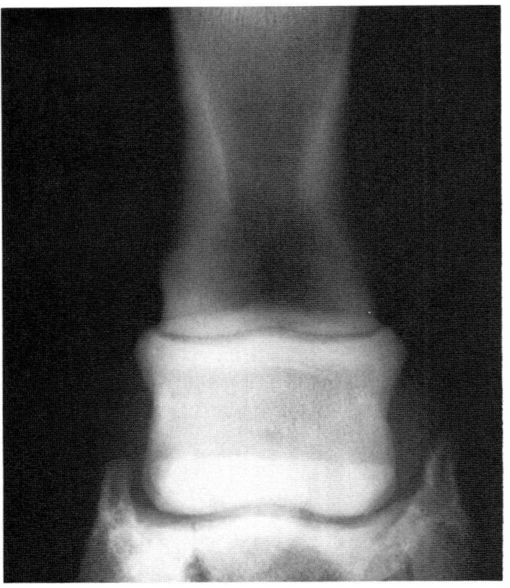

Figure 30. Dorsopalmar projection of the proximal interphalangeal joint (pastern).

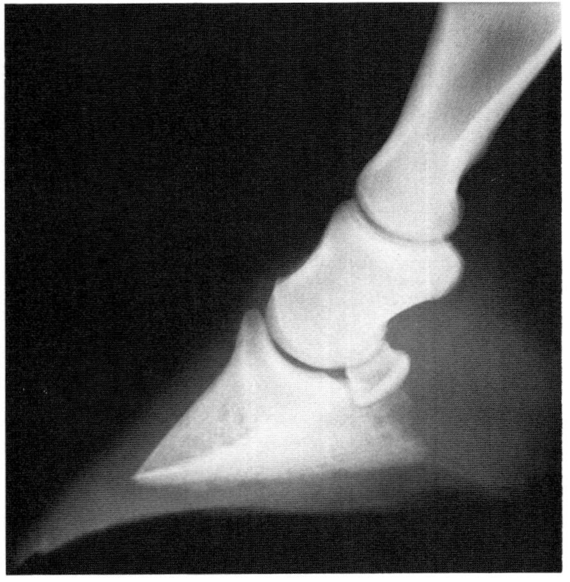

Figure 31. Lateromedial projection of the proximal interphalangeal joint (pastern).

the entire phalanx may be radiographed. Place the cassette on the medial aspect of the hoof, making sure to include the bulbs of the heel and the entire toe to evaluate rotation of the distal phalanx. Position the primary beam parallel to the floor and center on the coronary band. This view includes the proximal, middle and distal phalanx. The wings of the coffin bone and the navicular bone should be superimposed over one another (Figs 32, 33).

Preparation

If horseshoes are present, they should be pulled. The hoof should then be cleaned and trimmed to new sole. This prevents ingrained debris from causing artifacts on the finished radiograph. Air trapped in the sulcus of the hoof may also cause an artifact. To prevent this, the sulcus should be packed with a radiolucent material, such as soft soap, petroleum jelly or modeling clay. Place a paper towel or dry

Figure 32. Positioning for standard projections of the distal phalanx (coffin bone).

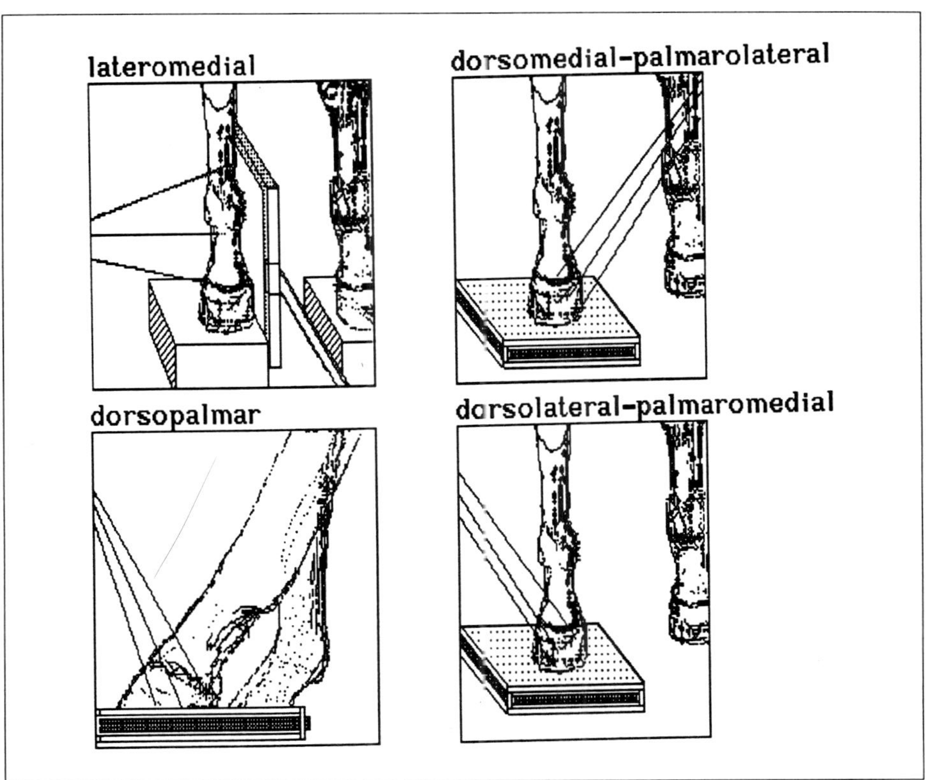

gauze over the bottom of the hoof to protect the packing (Figs 34, 35, 36).

Dorsopalmar

Extend the limb cranially and place it on the cassette tunnel. Angle the primary beam proximodistally 60 degrees and center just distal to the coronary band. Because it is impossible to have the cassette perfectly perpendicular to the beam, there will be some distortion of the coffin bone on the radiograph. The resulting view should show equal proportions of each wing of the coffin base (Figs 32, 37).

Dorsolateral-Palmaromedial Oblique

Place the cassette in the cassette tunnel. Extend the limb cranially and place it on the cassette tunnel. Angle the primary beam 60 degrees proximodistally so that it is perpendicular to the hoof wall. Then direct the primary beam dorsolaterally, 45 degrees off of a true dorsopalmar projection and center just distal to the coronary band. This view is used to visualize the lateral wing of the coffin bone (Figs 32, 38).

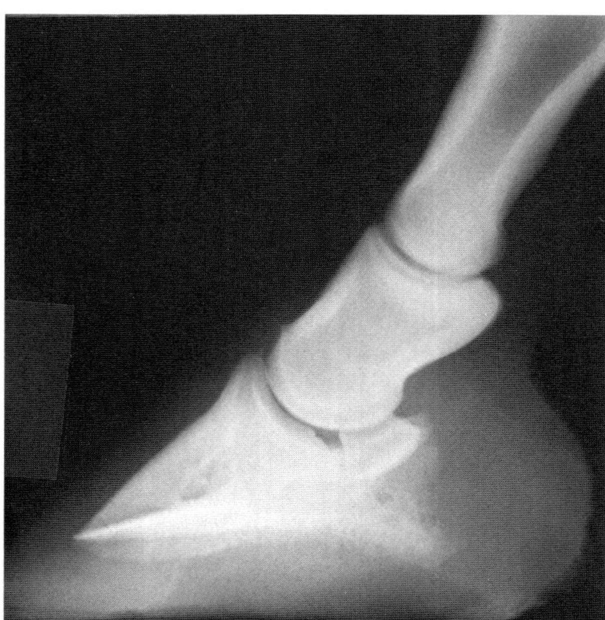

Figure 33. Lateromedial projection of the distal phalanx (coffin bone).

Dorsomedial-Palmarolateral Oblique

Place the cassette in the cassette tunnel. Extend the limb cranially and place it on the cassette tunnel. Angle the primary beam 60 degrees proximodistally so that it is perpendicular to the hoof wall. Then direct the primary beam dorsomedially, 45 degrees off of a true dorsopalmar projection and center just distal to the coronary band. This view is used to visualize the medial wing of the coffin bone (Fig 32).

Views of the
Distal Sesamoid
(Navicular Bone)

Preparation

If horseshoes are present, they should be pulled. The hoof should then be cleaned and trimmed to new sole. This prevents ingrained debris from causing artifacts on the finished radiograph. Air trapped in the sulcus of the hoof may also cause an artifact. To prevent this,

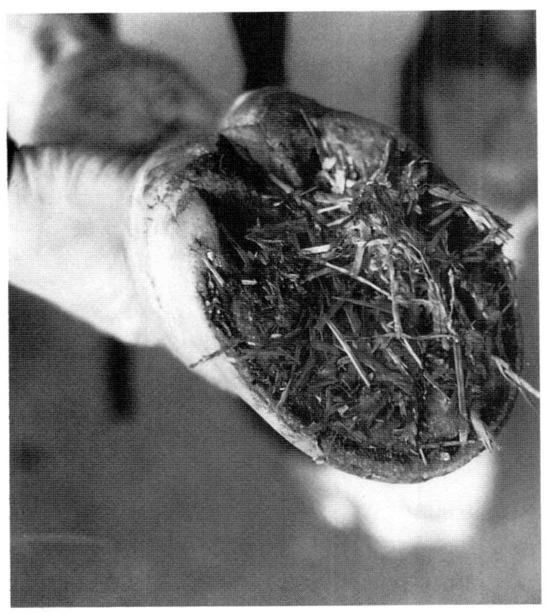

Figure 34. The hoof must be prepared before imaging the distal phalanx and distal sesamoid. Pull the shoe, then clean and trim the foot to a new sole.

the sulcus should be packed with a radiolucent material, such as soft soap, petroleum jelly or modeling clay. Place a paper towel or dry gauze over the bottom of the hoof to protect the packing (Figs 34, 35, 36).

Dorsoproximal-Palmarodistal Oblique (Upright Pedal)

Have the horse bear weight on the opposite limb, while the limb that is being radiographed is placed in a navicular box. This box has a groove to hold the hoof in an upright position, so that the dorsal hoof wall is perpendicular to the floor. Position the primary beam parallel to the floor and center on the coronary band. Place the cassette in the box behind the hoof so that it lies parallel to the dorsal hoof wall. This position projects the navicular bone dorsal to the coffin joint for better evaluation (Figs 39, 40).

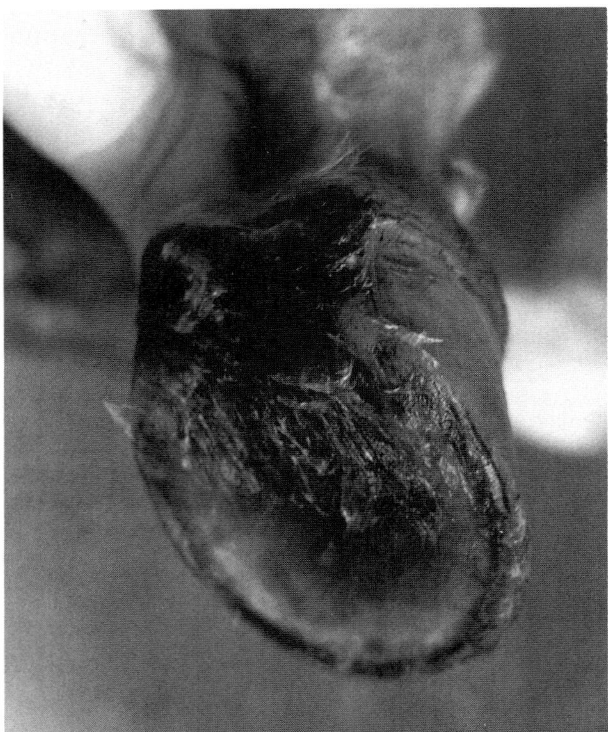

Figure 35. Pack the hoof with a radiolucent material to remove air in the sulcus.

Palmaroproximal-Dorsodistal Oblique (Caudal Tangential)

Place the cassette in the cassette tunnel. Have the horse stand on the cassette tunnel with the limb of interest positioned caudally, while the horse is still bearing weight equally on all 4 limbs. Angle the x-ray machine 45 degrees proximodistally and position it underneath the horse's abdomen so that the beam may be directed in a palmar to dorsal direction. Center the primary beam between the bulbs of the heel. This image allows the palmar surface of the navicular bone to be visualized (Figs 39, 41).

Views of the Rear Feet

The views and positioning for the rear feet are identical to those for the front feet, except that the term *palmar* is replaced with *plantar* in all view descriptions. It is also important that the radiographs be labeled correctly as those of a rear limb, using LR (left rear) and RR (right rear).

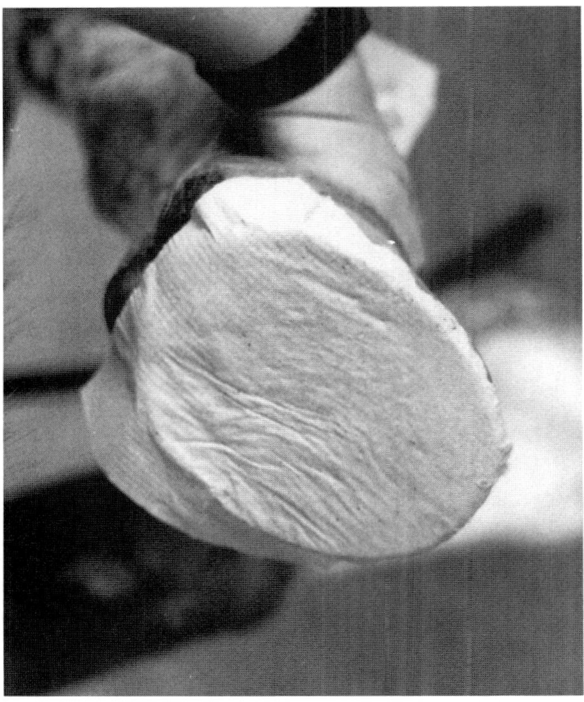

Figure 36. Place a paper towel or dry gauze over the packing for protection.

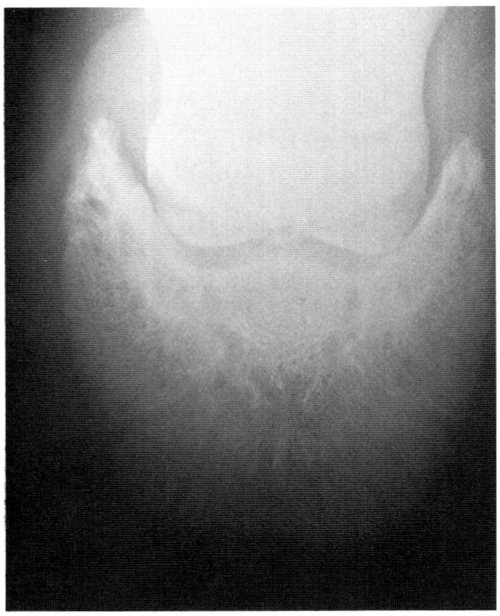

Figure 37. Dorsopalmar projection of the distal phalanx (coffin bone).

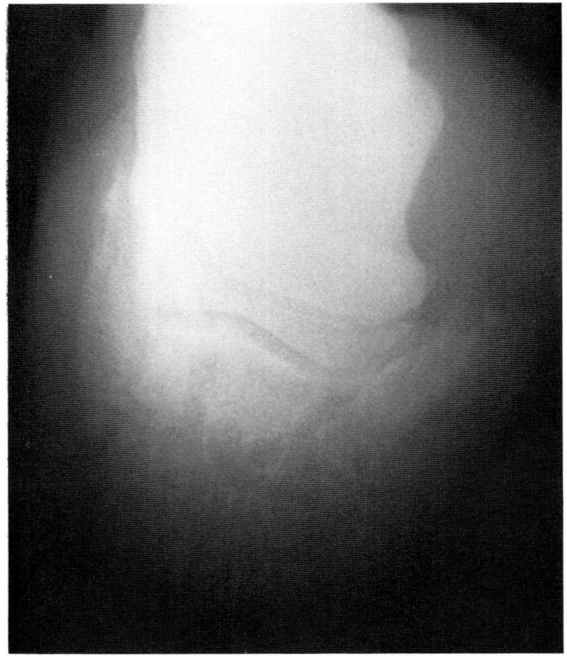

Figure 38. Dorsolateral-palmaromedial projection of the distal phalanx (coffin bone).

Views of the Femorotibial Joint
(Stifle Joint)

Have the horse stand squarely, with its weight evenly distributed on all 4 legs. Caution should be used when radiographing this area, as it is a very sensitive area for a horse. The cassettes should be held in place with a cassette holder. Place the cassette firmly against the horse. A light touch is more irritating than a firm one.

Caudocranial

Place the cassette against the cranial aspect of the joint. Because of the position of the joint, angle the primary beam slightly proximodistally. It is important to note that the femorotibial joint deviates laterally. This should be kept in mind when positioning the x-ray tube. Direct the primary beam toward the midsagittal plane of the limb and center on the joint. The resulting view visualizes the femoral condyles, proximal tibia and patella (Figs 42, 43).

Figure 39. Positioning for standard projections of the distal sesamoid (navicular bone).

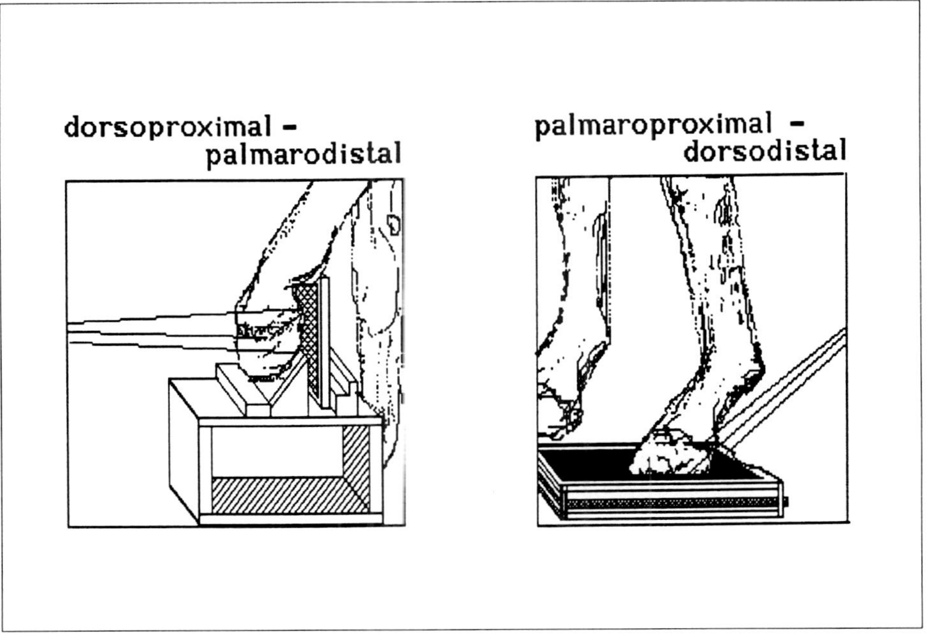

Lateromedial

Place the cassette against the medial aspect of the joint as high (dorsal) in the flank as possible. Position the primary beam parallel

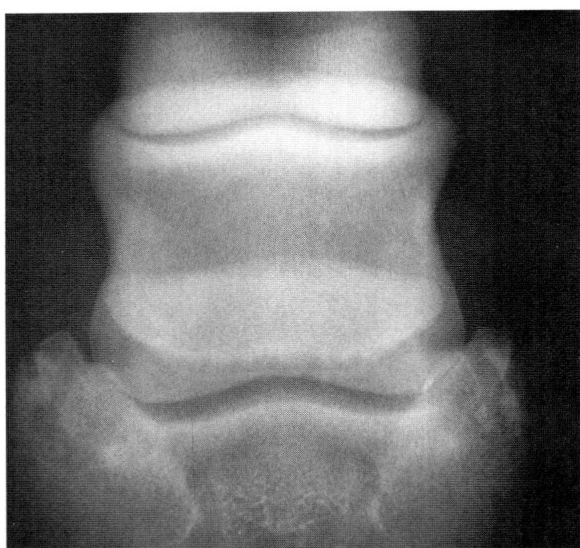

Figure 40. Dorso-proximal-palmarodistal projection of the distal sesamoid (navicular bone).

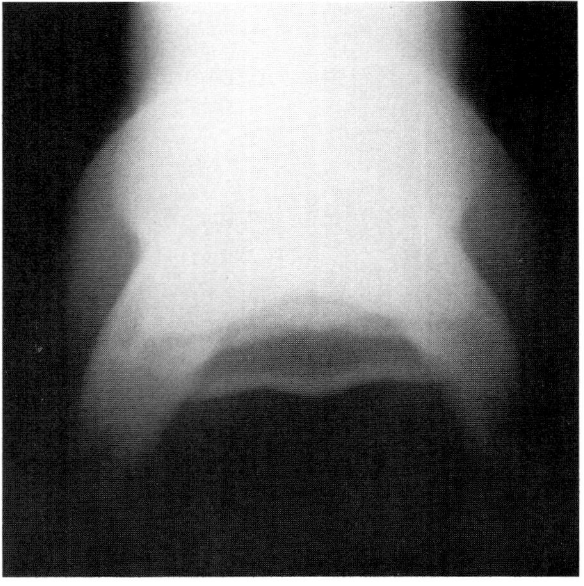

Figure 41. Palmaro-proximal-dorsodistal projection of the distal sesamoid (navicular bone).

to the floor and center on the joint. This image includes the femorotibial joint, proximal tibia and patella. The femoral condyles should be superimposed so that only 1 condyle is visualized (Figs 42, 44).

Views of the
Brachioantebrachial Joint
(Elbow Joint)

Craniocaudal

Position the horse with the front limbs slightly abducted to separate the elbow from the thoracic musculature. Place the cassette diagonally on the caudal surface of the joint. Angling the cassette allows a larger portion of the medial surface to be captured on the radiograph. Position the primary beam parallel to the floor and center

Figure 42. Positioning for standard projections of the femorotibial joint (stifle).

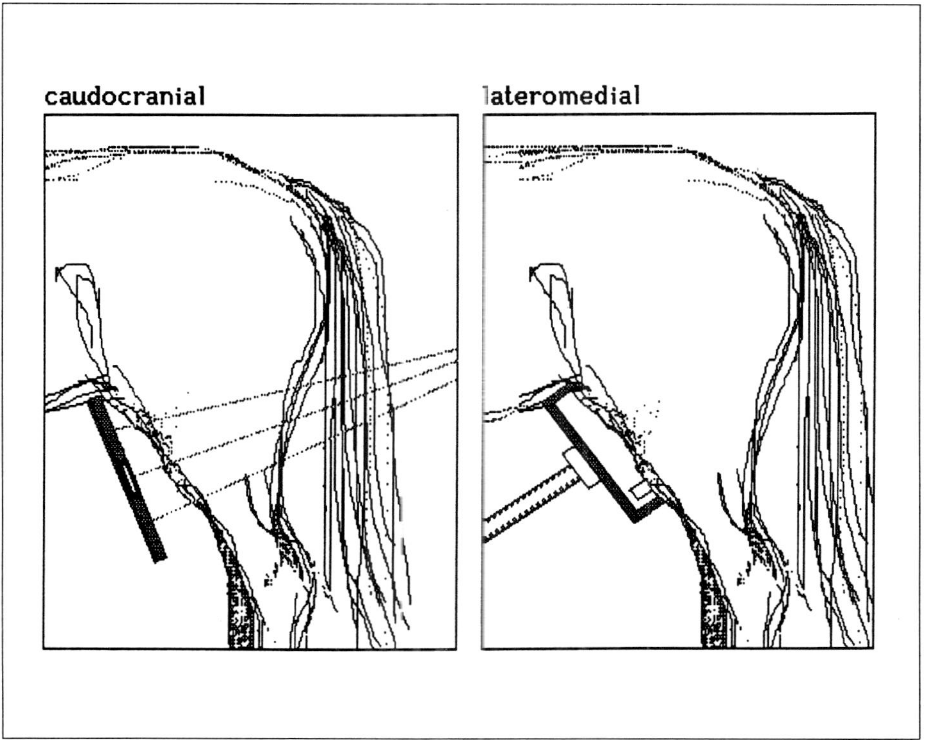

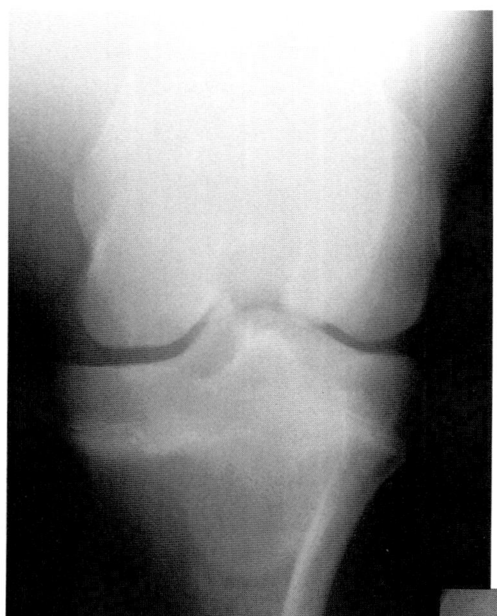

Figure 43. Caudocranial projection of the femoro-tibial joint (stifle).

Figure 44. Lateromedial projection of the femorotibial joint (stifle).

Figure 45. Positioning for standard projections of the brachioantebrachial joint (elbow).

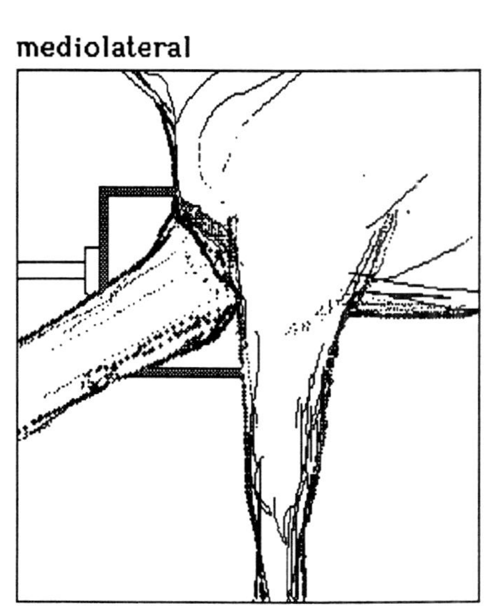

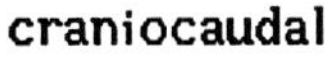

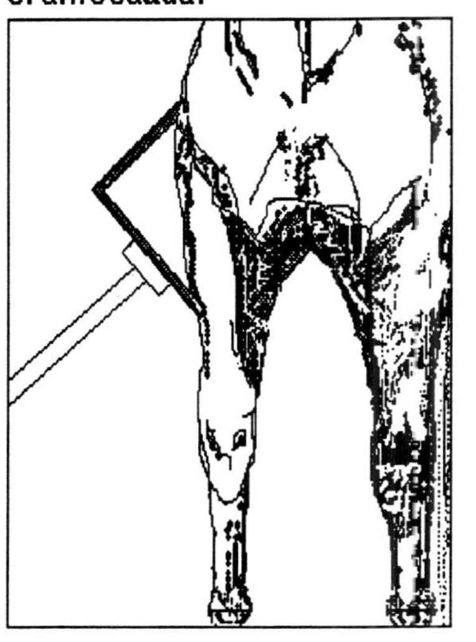

on the joint. The resulting view should contain distal humerus, brachioantebrachial joint and proximal radius (Figs 45, 46).

Mediolateral

Extend the limb of interest cranially and have it held by an assistant. This minimizes the overlap of the pectoral muscles, improving the image. Place the cassette on the lateral aspect of the joint, parallel to the limb. Position the primary beam parallel to the floor and center on the joint. This image visualizes from the distal humerus to the proximal radius (Figs 45, 47).

Recommended Reading

Douglas SW *et al: Principles of Veterinary Radiography.* 4th ed. Bailliere Tindall, London, 1987. pp 287-339.

Feeney DA *et al:* A 200 centimeter focal spot – film distance (FFD) technique for equine radiography. *Vet Radiol* 23:13-19, 1982.

Mendenhall A and Cantwell HD: *Equine Radiographic Procedures.* Lea & Febiger, Philadelphia, 1988.

Morgan JP and Silverman S: *Techniques of Veterinary Radiography.* 3rd ed. Veterinary Radiology Associates, Davis, CA, 1982. pp 194-238.

Ticer JW: *Radiographic Technique in Veterinary Practice.* 2nd ed. Saunders, Philadelphia, 1984. pp 404-498.

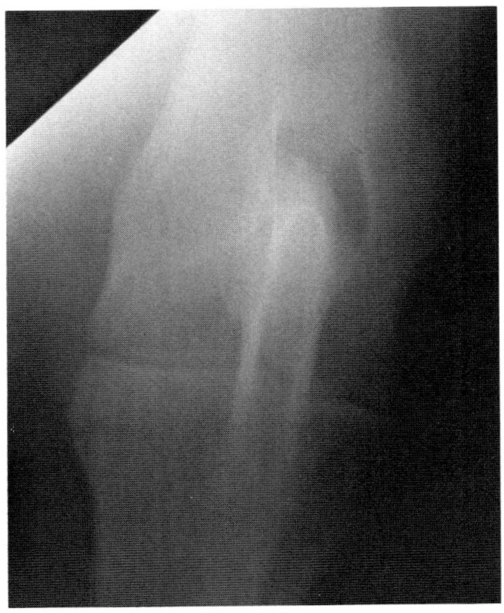

Figure 46. Cranio-caudal projection of the brachioantebrachial joint (elbow).

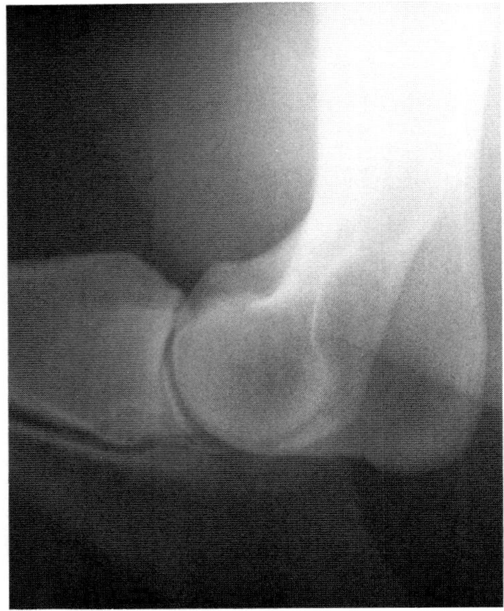

Figure 47. Medio-lateral projection of the brachioantebrachial joint (elbow).

Notes

Notes

12

Diagnostic Ultrasonography

Diagnostic ultrasonography is used in veterinary medicine for noninvasive imaging of soft tissue. A transducer sends low-intensity, high-frequency sound waves into soft tissues, where they interact with the tissue interfaces. Some of the sound waves are reflected back to the transducer and some are transmitted into deeper tissues. Sound waves that are reflected back to the transducer (*echoes*) are then analyzed by computer to produce a gray-scale image.

Use of ultrasonography in conjunction with radiography gives the veterinarian an excellent diagnostic tool. Radiographs demonstrate the size, shape and position of the organs. Sonograms display the findings found on the radiographs, as well as the soft tissue textures and the dynamics of some of the organs (*eg*, motility of the bowel).

Basic Physics

Sound waves are classified by wavelength, frequency and velocity.

Wavelength

Ultrasound wave forms are similar to audible sound, but ultrasound has a shorter wavelength. As ultrasound travels through tissues, it forms longitudinal waves consisting of compressions and rarefactions. The areas of compression force the molecules closer together and the areas of rarefaction place them farther apart (Fig 1).

Sound waves can be compared with a transverse wave form (sine wave). With the pressure starting at zero, compression causes the pressure to rise to a peak, then fall back to zero. During rarefaction, the pressure falls to a negative value before returning to zero. A *wavelength* is the distance from one band of compression or rarefaction to the next.

Frequency

The *frequency* of a sound wave is the number of complete wave forms (*cycles*) per unit of time (Fig 2). Frequency and wavelength are inversely related. As the frequency increases, the wavelength decreases. Ultrasound uses high-frequency sound waves. The upper range of sound audible to people has a frequency of approximately

Figure 1. Ultrasound waves traveling through the tissues form waves of compression and rarefaction of the tissue molecules. The areas of compression can be compared with the positive half of a sine wave. Rarefaction can be compared with the negative half of a sine wave.

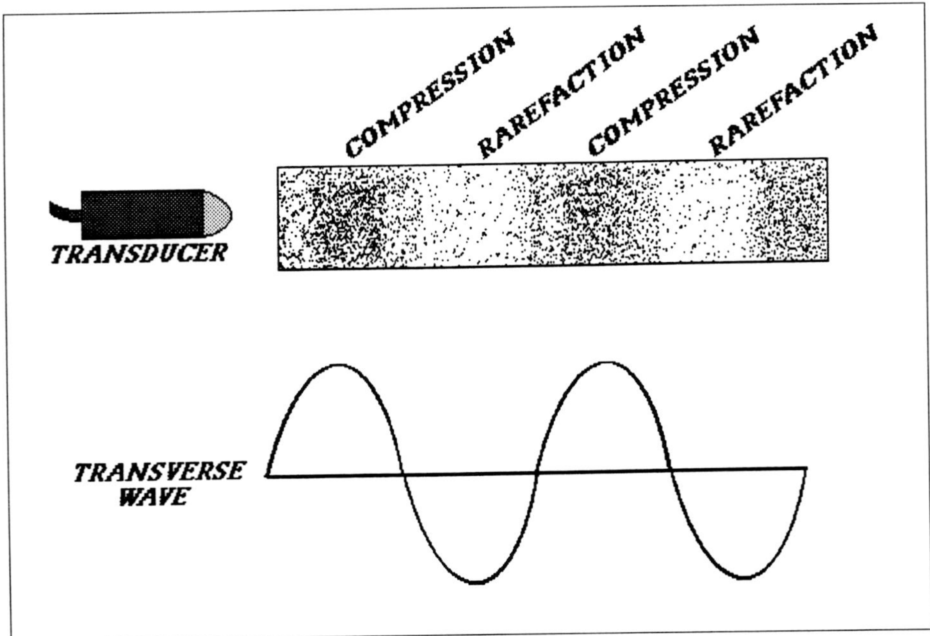

20,000 Hertz (cycles/second, Hz). The frequency of ultrasound waves varies from 2 to 10 million Hz, or 2-10 megaHertz (mHz).

Velocity

Velocity is the speed at which sound travels through a medium. The velocity of ultrasound is similar for all types of soft tissues. A velocity of 1,540 m/sec (average speed in living tissue) is used by the computer software. The computer measures the time each sound wave takes to return to the transducer. It calculates the depth to where the sound was reflected and displays it accordingly on the monitor.

Acoustic Impedance

Acoustic impedance is the ability of living tissue being imaged to resist or impede the transmission of sound. The interface between tissues with different acoustic impedance becomes a reflective surface for the sound waves.

Acoustic impedance varies slightly among most tissues, depending upon the density and elasticity of the tissue (Fig 3). Even though the

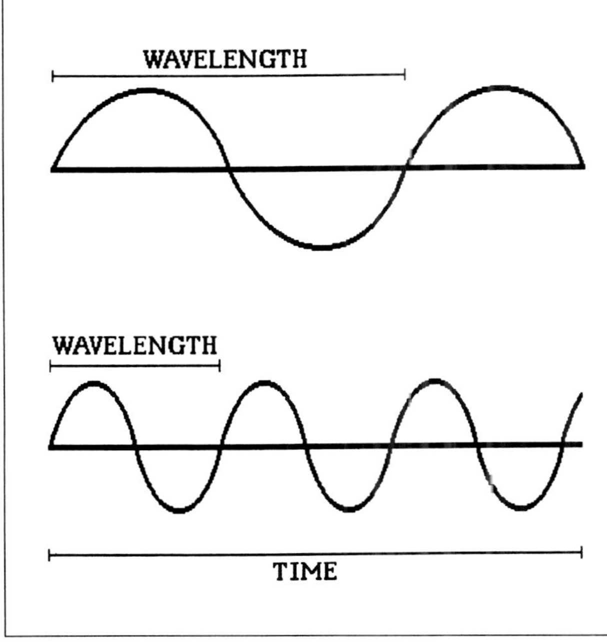

Figure 2. Frequency and wavelength are inversely related. As the wavelength increases, the frequency decreases.

impedance of most tissues varies only slightly, the difference allows one tissue type to be distinguished from another while transmitting some sound through to reflect off of deeper tissues. It is when the acoustic impedance varies greatly that the reflector becomes nearly perfect. For example, interfaces between soft tissue and air, or soft tissue and bone vary greatly in acoustic impedance, thus reflecting nearly all sound. This means that air-filled structures and bony structures are barriers to ultrasound waves.

Attenuation

As ultrasound travels through tissues, it loses intensity or *attenuates*. The attenuation occurs through scatter and absorption. *Scattering* occurs when the sound reflects in many directions off the different tissue interfaces. Some of the sound is reflected in directions so that it never reaches the transducer. *Absorption* occurs from molecular friction created when the sound passes through the tissues, producing heat. The molecular friction is caused by the compressions and rarefactions of the sound waves. The progressive loss of energy in the form of heat can eventually result in total absorption of the sound wave.

Sound that travels into and out of the tissues is subject to attenuation. This limits the depth of tissues that can be imaged. The amount

Figure 3. Acoustic impedance of different tissue types.

Tissue Type	Acoustic Impedance (Rayls)
Fat	1.38×10^5
Water	1.48×10^5
Blood	1.61×10^5
Kidney	1.62×10^5
Soft tissue (average)	1.63×10^5
Liver	1.65×10^5
Muscle	1.70×10^5
Bone	7.80×10^5
Air	0.0004×10^5

of attenuation depends upon the frequency of the transducer. Sound emitted from a high-frequency transducer attenuates faster than sound emitted from a lower-frequency transducer. Thus, a lower-frequency transducer can image tissues deeper than a higher-frequency transducer can.

Transducers

Ultrasound transducers emit a series of sound pulses and receive the returning echoes. A weak electrical current applied to the piezoelectric crystals incorporated in the transducer causes the crystals to vibrate and produce sound waves. After sending a series of pulses, the crystals are dampened to stop further vibrations. When struck by the returning echoes, the crystals vibrate again. This time the crystals convert these echoes into electrical energy.

Scan Plane

Transducers are available in different configurations, which are mechanical or electronic. The scan plane can either be a *sector scan* (wedge-shaped image) or a *linear-array scan* (rectangular image). A mechanically driven sector scan can be produced by a belt and pulley used to wobble a single crystal or rotate multiple crystals across a scan plane. Another method of producing a sector scan is with the use of *phased-array* or *annular-array* configurations. With phased array, the crystals are pulsed sequentially with a built-in delay to create a "pseudo-sector" scan plane. Annular array arranges the crystals in concentric rings. By using electronic phasing of the many crystals, annular-array transducers produce a 2-dimensional image by steering the entire array through a sector arc.

Sector scanners are useful when imaging areas that are limited by ribs, gas-filled bowels or lungs. The narrow near field and wide far field enable the transducer scan plane to be positioned in between or around these structures. The linear-array scanner produces a scan plane by alternately firing groups of crystals in sequence. The pulsing of each group of crystals occurs so rapidly that individual pulses cannot be observed by the human eye. Linear-array scanners are useful in areas with unrestricted window size. The rectangular scan plane is ideal for equine tendons or large or small animal transrectal imaging.

Frequency and Resolution

The frequency of the transducer determines the amount of detail or resolution of the image. The higher the frequency, the shorter the wavelength. The shorter the wavelength, the better the resolution of the image.

There are 2 types of resolution: *axial* and *lateral*. *Axial resolution* refers to the ability to differentiate between 2 reflecting interfaces that lie along the axis of the transmitted sound beam. If the wavelength of the sound is longer than the distance between the 2 interfaces, these are displayed as a single object. If the wavelength of the sound is shorter than the distance between the 2 interfaces, these are displayed as 2 separate objects.

Lateral resolution refers to the ability to differentiate between 2 reflecting interfaces that lie in a plane perpendicular to the transmitted sound beam. Lateral resolution depends on the width of the sound beam. With a wide sound beam, 2 separate reflective interfaces that lie within the width of that beam are displayed as only 1 reflection.

A sound beam naturally diverges, with a loss of lateral resolution in the far field. A method to compensate for this is to focus the sound beam in one area, known as the *focal zone*. The sound beam can be focused by using an acoustic lens or by electronically transmitted means. Either way, the resolution is improved in the focal zone.

Transducer Care

Transducers are expensive and the most fragile part of the ultrasound equipment. Care must be taken when handling them. Avoid hard impacts that can severely damage the sensitive crystals. It is also advisable to prevent exposure to extreme temperature changes. Some transducers are sensitive to certain types of cleaning agents. Always refer to the manufacturer's instructions for appropriate cleaning products.

Display Modes

There are 3 different display modes: *A-mode* (amplitude mode), *B-mode* (brightness mode) and *M-mode* (motion mode).

A-Mode

A-mode was the first form of ultrasound used and is the simplest as far as computer software. With A-mode, the returning echoes are displayed as a series of peaks on a graph. The higher the intensity of the returning sound, the higher the peak at that tissue depth. A-mode is not used in showing tissue motion or anatomy. The main use in veterinary medicine is to measure the amount of subcutaneous fat in pigs.

B-Mode

B-mode uses bright pixels, or dots, on a screen, where A-mode uses peaks on a graph (Fig 4). A dot appears on the screen corresponding to the depth at which the echo was formed. The dot's degree of brightness is proportional to the intensity of the returning echo. The greater the intensity, the brighter the dot. The image that is generated is a 2-dimensional anatomic slice that is continually updated. This mode is currently used for diagnostic applications.

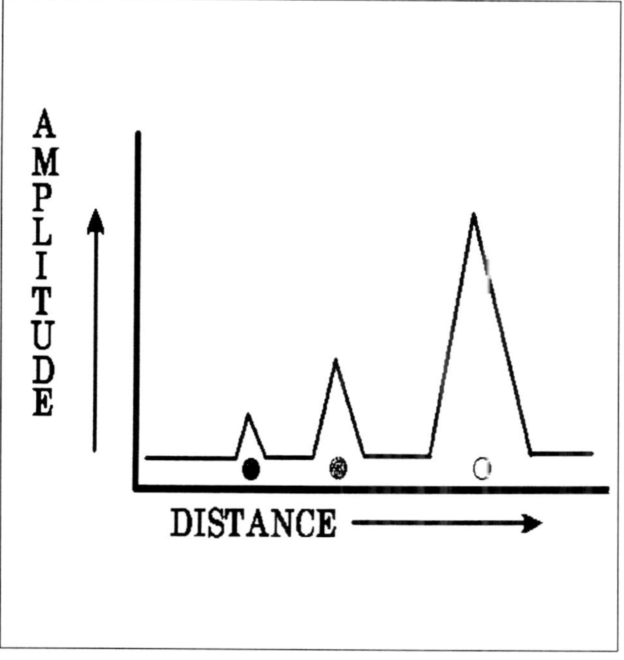

Figure 4. Where A-mode uses peaks on a graph to depict the strength of the returning echoes, B-mode uses bright pixels, or dots, on a monitor. The brighter the pixel, the stronger the returning echo.

M-Mode

M-mode is the continuous display of a thin slice of an organ over time. M-mode projects the echoes from a thin beam of sound over a time-oriented baseline (Fig 5). The main use is with echocardiography to assess the size of the chambers and the motion of the cardiac valves and walls.

Terminology Describing Echotexture

The terminology used to describe tissue texture within an ultrasound image is simple. *Echogenic* or *echoic* means that most of the sound is reflected back to the transducer. Echogenic areas appear white on the screen. *Sonolucent* means that most of the sound is transmitted to the deeper tissues, with only a few echoes reflected back to the transducer. Sonolucent areas appear dark on the screen. *Anechoic* is used to describe the tissue that transmits all the sound through to deeper tissues, reflecting none of the sound back to the transducer. Anechoic areas appear black on the screen and are generally fluid-filled structures (Fig 6).

Figure 5. M-mode displays the motion of a thin slice of an organ over time.

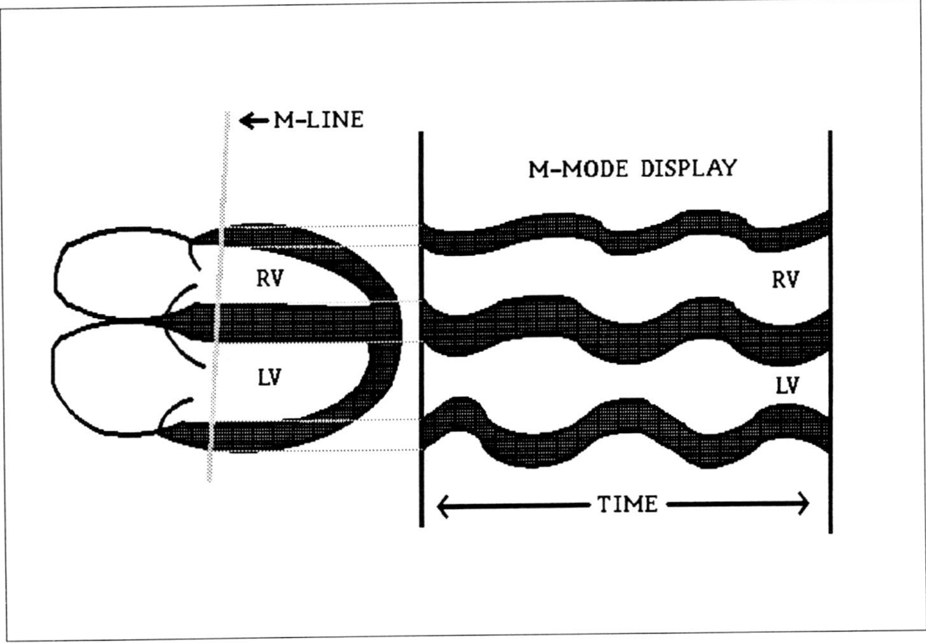

The soft tissues are not only represented as black or white, but also as many shades of gray in between. Additional terminology has been established to describe these areas. *Hyperechoic* is used to describe tissues that reflect more sound back to the transducer than do surrounding tissues. Hyperechoic areas appear brighter than surrounding tissues. *Hypoechoic* is used to describe tissues that reflect less sound back to the transducer than do surrounding tissues. Hypoechoic areas appear darker than surrounding tissues. *Isoechoic* is used to describe tissue that appears to have the same echotexture as surrounding tissues (Fig 7).

So that various findings can be verbally pointed out and discussed during ultrasonography, the ultrasound unit screen has been divided into 9 zones, with each zone having its own label (Fig 8). In this way, the sonographer can verbally point out the area of interest (*eg*, midfield or near field left).

Patient Preparation

To achieve an optimal acoustic window giving the best-quality image, the transducer must closely contact the skin. Hair or fur must be clipped and, in some cases, shaved. Occasionally, thin-coated

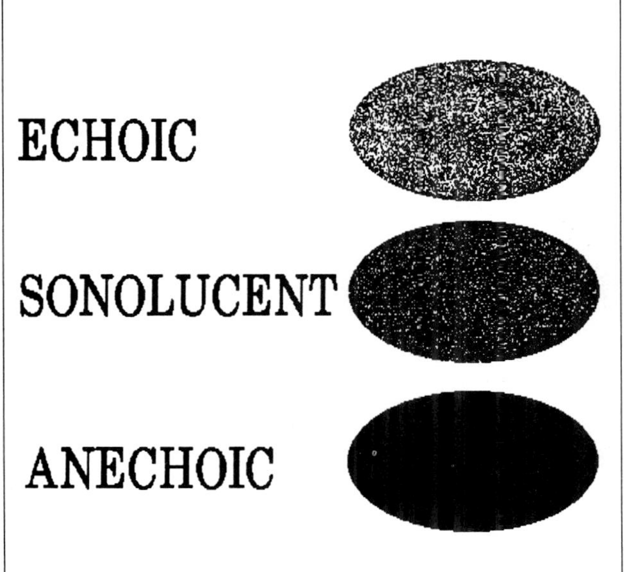

Figure 6. Echoic tissue appears bright or white on the monitor. Sonolucent tissue appears dark on the monitor. Anechoic tissue appears completely black on the monitor.

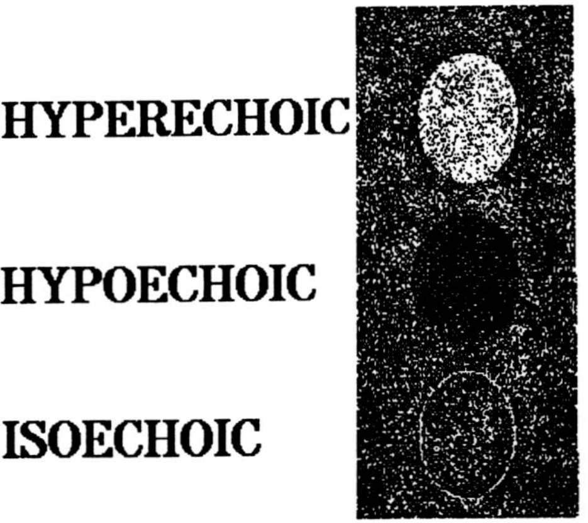

Figure 7. An area within an organ or the whole organ that is brighter or whiter than surrounding tissue is described as hyperechoic. Areas that are darker than surrounding tissue are described as hypoechoic. Areas that are the same as surrounding tissue are described as isoechoic.

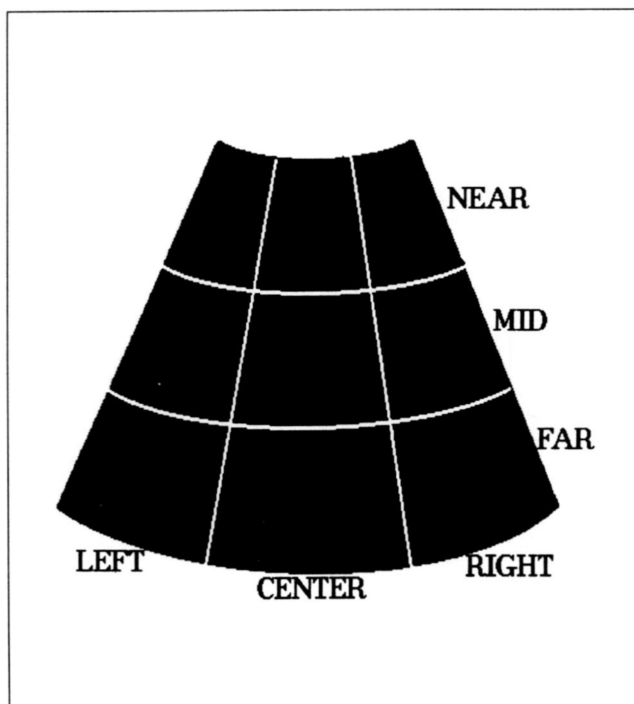

Figure 8. The 9 scan zones used to point out an area on the screen.

animals can be imaged with minimal preparation. An acoustic coupling gel is used in all cases to eliminate the air interface and improve the acoustic window. Before applying the acoustic coupling gel, the area should be wiped with alcohol or generous amounts of soapy water to remove any loose hairs, dirt and skin oils.

Fasting of small animals before abdominal ultrasonography is recommended. The ingesta and gas in the bowel decrease the amount of the abdomen that can be visualized.

Equipment Controls

Ultrasound equipment has many controls for adjusting the image. Improper adjustment of any of these can greatly decrease the quality of the image.

Brightness and Contrast

The television monitor has controls to adjust the brightness and contrast of the image on monitor. If the brightness has been adjusted too high or too low on the monitor, compensating with any other control cannot correct the brightness or darkness. Most machines have a gray bar that displays the gray-scale capability. This capability varies from 1,664 to 128 shades of gray. The brightness and contrast should be adjusted so that black, white and all intermediate shades of gray can be seen.

Depth

The depth allows for adjustment of the amount of tissue being displayed on the monitor. The depth from the surface of the transducer is measured in centimeters. The area of interest (*eg*, kidney, heart) should cover at least two-thirds of the screen. By decreasing the amount of depth being displayed, the area in the near field becomes larger (Fig 9).

Gain and Power

Gain (overall) and *power* (output) can affect the overall brightness of the image (Fig 10). Gain and power are 2 ways to compensate for attenuation of the sound beam as it travels through the tissues.

Figure 9. The depth control affects the amount of tissue that is being displayed. The area of interest should cover at least two-thirds of the screen. Image A displays 8 cm of depth, where Image B displays 6 cm of depth.

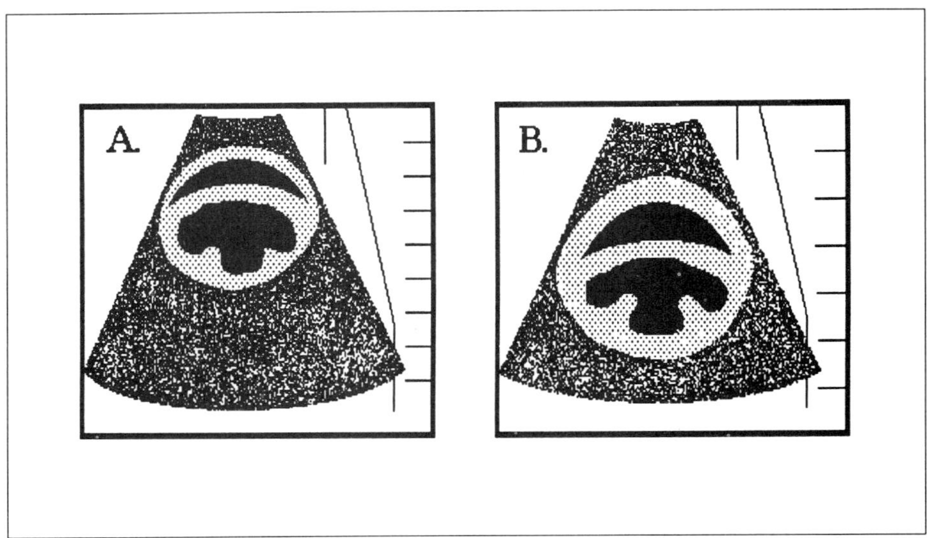

Figure 10. The gain and power controls affect the overall brightness of the screen. The higher the overall gain or the power, the brighter the image on the screen. Images A and C display an adequate overall brightness, while Images B and D (next page) display increased brightness overall.

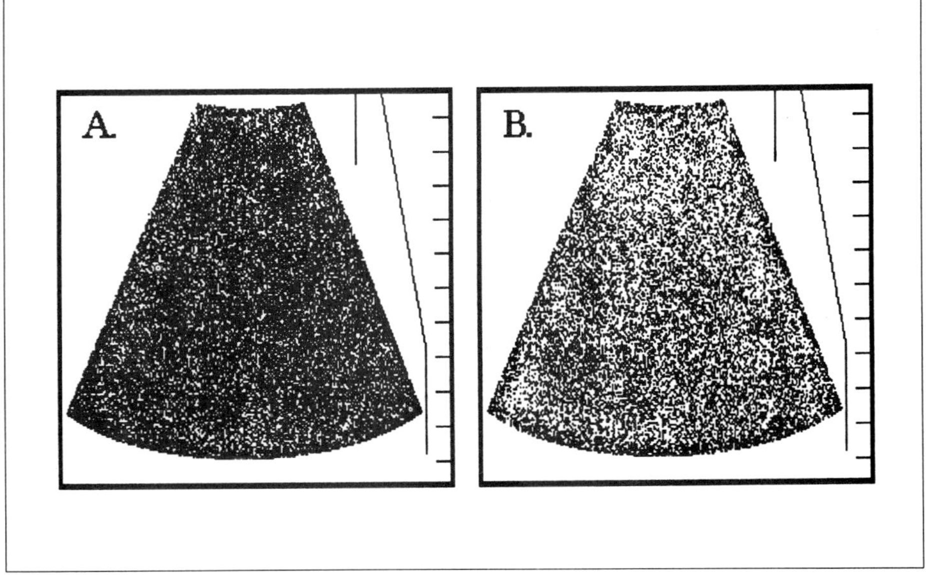

Figure 10, continued. Image C (top) and Image D (bottom).

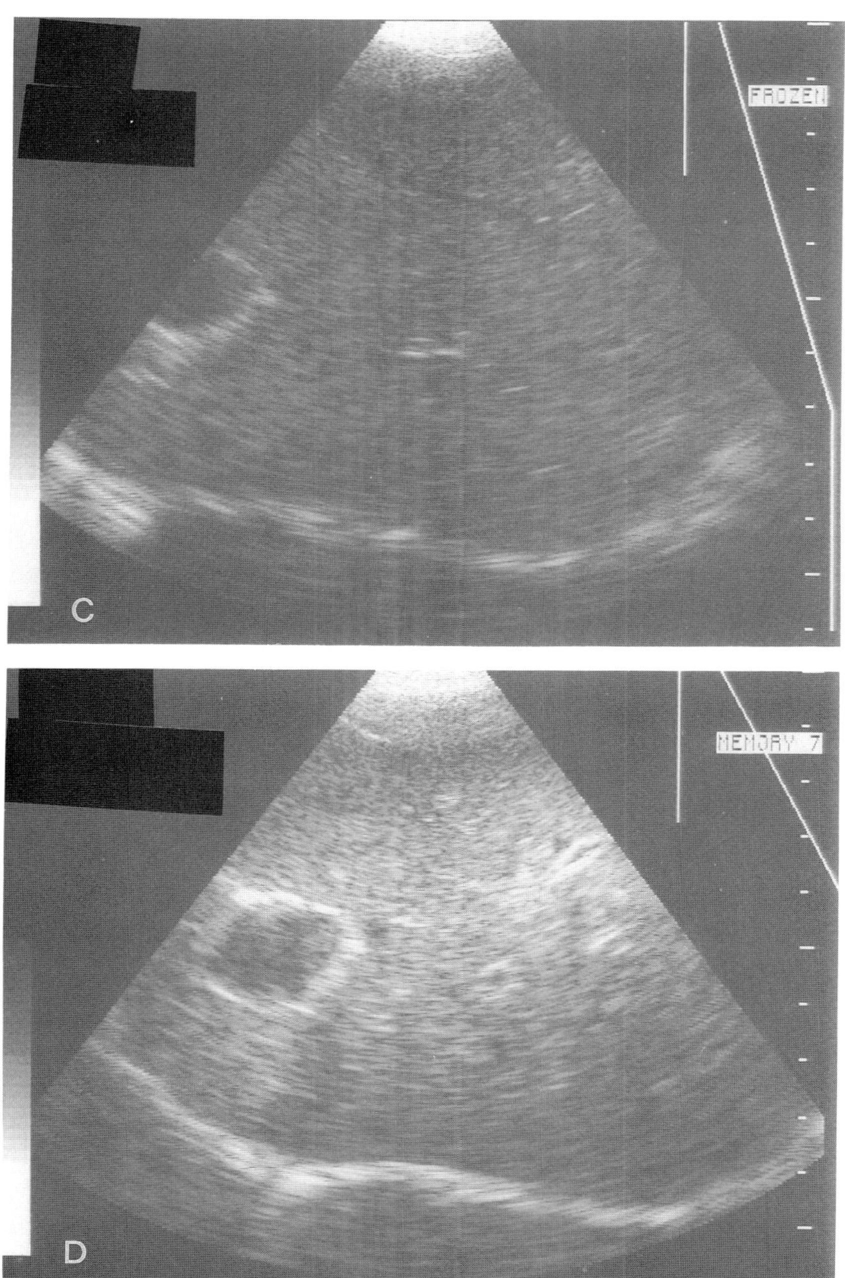

Increasing the gain increases the sensitivity of the transducer to receiving the returning echoes. This can be compared with the volume on a hearing aid. Turning the volume up increases the person's ability to hear incoming sounds.

The power controls the intensity of the sound generated by the transducer. Increasing the power increases the intensity of the sound wave leaving the transducer. The sound is attenuated at the same rate; however, a higher-intensity sound wave transmitted into the tissues results in higher-intensity sound waves returning to the transducer.

Time Gain Compensation

The controls that make up the time gain compensation (TGC) are the most important and most often improperly set. The purpose of the TGC is to make like tissues look alike. The intensity of the sound decreases progressively as it returns from deeper tissues. When imaging the liver, for example, 3 similar reflectors located at 4 cm, 6 cm and 8 cm of depth should have the same brightness on the monitor. However, because of attenuation of the echoes returning from deeper tissues, the brightness gradually decreases (Fig 11A). To compensate for loss of energy, TGC adds increasing amounts of electronic gain to the returning echoes (Fig 11B). This causes the 3 echoes returned from different depths to have the same brightness on the monitor (Fig 11C).

Three typical controls that make up the TGC are *near-field gain, far-field gain* and *delay*. The near-field gain controls the amount of electronic gain added to the sound returning from the near field (Fig 12). This should be set so that the echoes blend uniformly with those displayed in the mid field.

The far-field gain controls the amount of electronic gain added to the echoes returning from the far field (Fig 13).

Delay (also called break point or starting point) controls the depth at which the gain is first applied (Fig 14). This control is only used when imaging areas containing fluid in the near field (*eg*, ascites, pleural fluid). Because sound is not attenuated much when traversing fluid, deeper structures appear too bright. Delaying the point at which the electronic gain is started compensates for the lack of attenuation through the fluid. When scanning normal tissues, there is no need to apply any delay in the TGC.

Adjustments

If proper brightness cannot be achieved, the following things should be verified. First, check the brightness and contrast of the monitor. If the brightness and contrast controls on the monitor are incorrectly set, changing the TGC cannot compensate for this error. Next, check the power setting to make sure it is not too low. If all the controls are set correctly, the next step is to attempt to improve the acoustic contact with the skin. This can be done by applying more coupling gel or shaving the clipped area with a razor. If none of these work, change to a lower-frequency transducer. Some resolution will

Figure 11. Time gain compensation (TGC) makes similar tissues look alike. Chart A shows the decreasing intensity of returning echoes caused by attenuation of the sound beam from the deeper tissues. To compensate for the loss in intensity, electronic gain or intensity is added in increasing amounts to the returning echoes (Chart B). The results are shown in Chart C, where the echoes at all the depths have the same intensity and appear to have equal brightness.

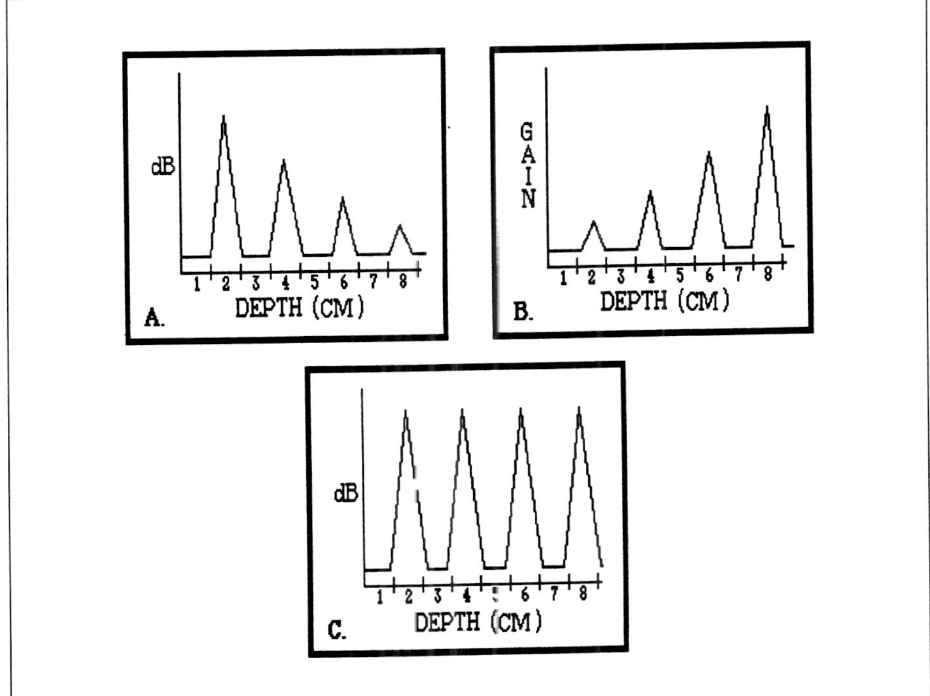

Figure 12. Increasing the near-field gain increases the brightness in the near field. Images A and C (bottom) display adequate brightness in the near field, while Images B and D (next page) display increased brightness in the near field.

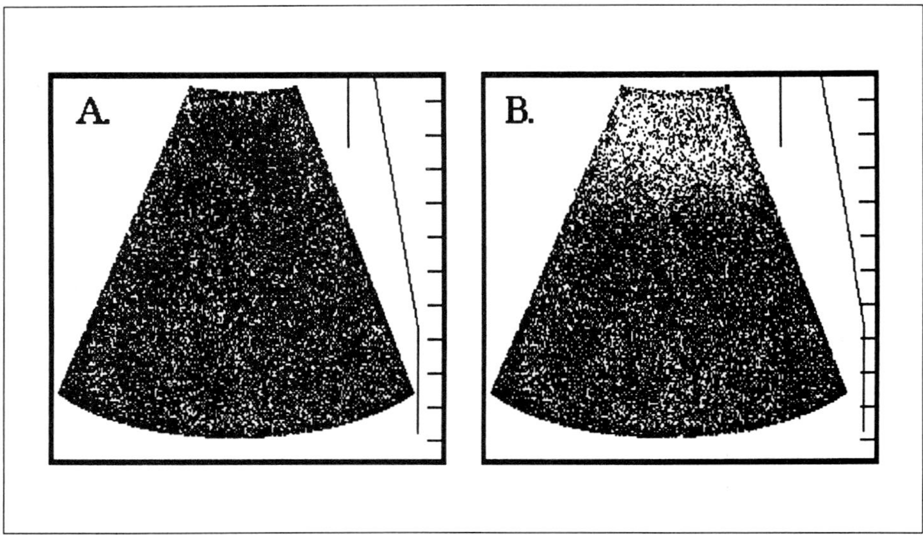

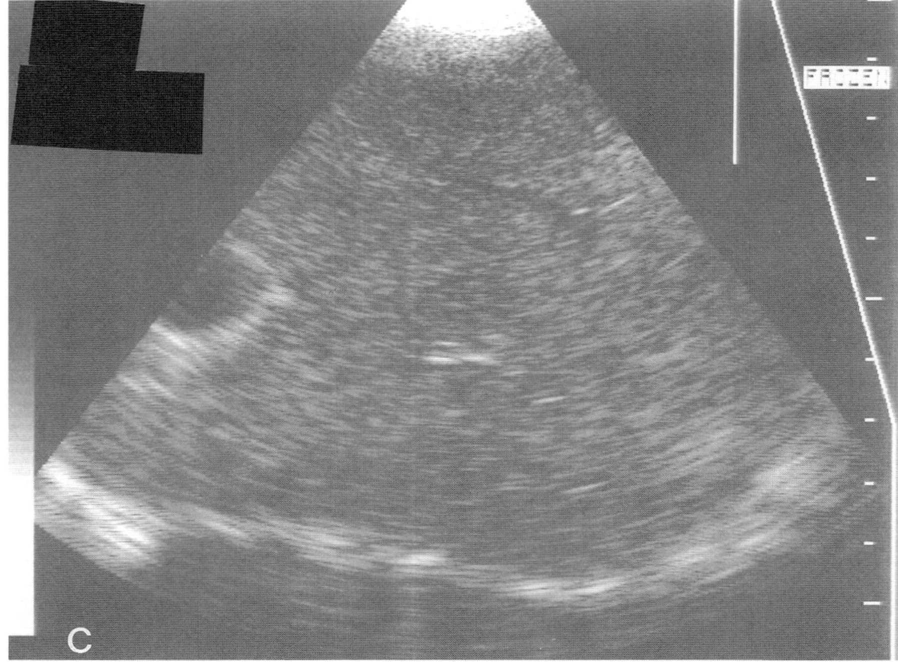

Figure 12, continued. Image D.

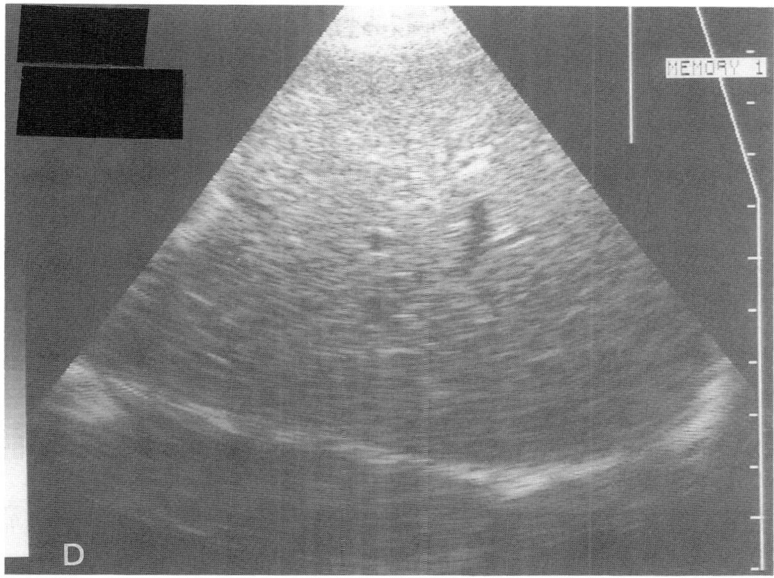

be lost, but it is a necessary tradeoff when brightness cannot be achieved.

Artifacts

Artifacts can occur during any ultrasound study. Proper identification of these artifacts is important to prevent confusion or misinterpretation. Some artifacts can aid in making a diagnosis. Two such artifacts include *acoustic shadowing* and *distant enhancement*. Others, if not readily identified, can be confused as part of the anatomy or a disease process.

Acoustic Shadowing

Acoustic shadowing occurs when the sound is attenuated or reflected at an acoustic interface (Fig 15). This prevents the sound from being transmitted to deeper tissues, resulting in fewer or no returning echoes from those areas.

Structures that can cause acoustic shadowing include bone, calculi, mineralization and occasionally fat. For acoustic shadowing to occur, the interface must be in the focal zone of the transducer. If not, the

Figure 13. Increasing the far-field gain increases the brightness in the far field. Images A and C (bottom) display adequate brightness in the far field, while Images B and D (next page) display decreased brightness in the far field.

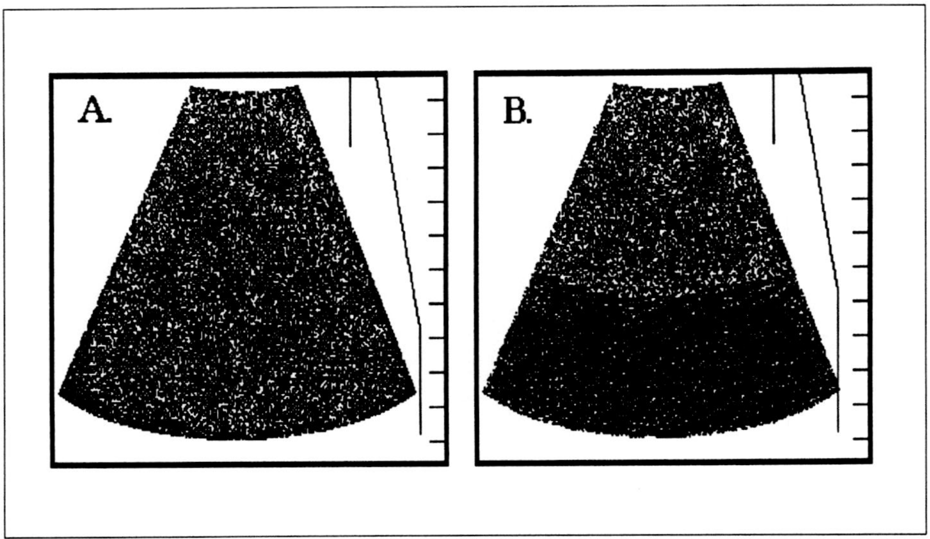

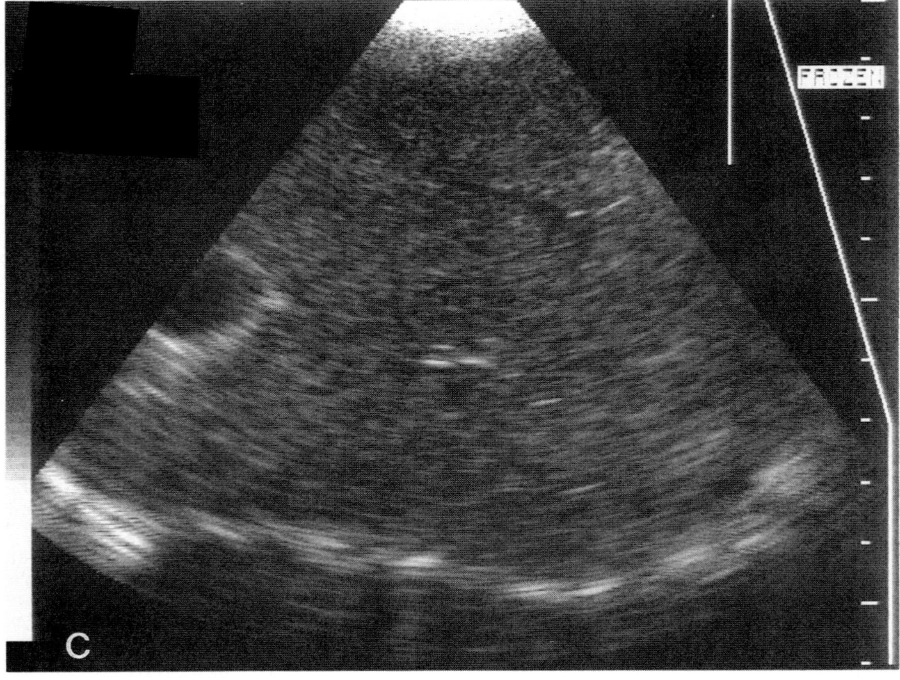

Figure 13, continued. Image D.

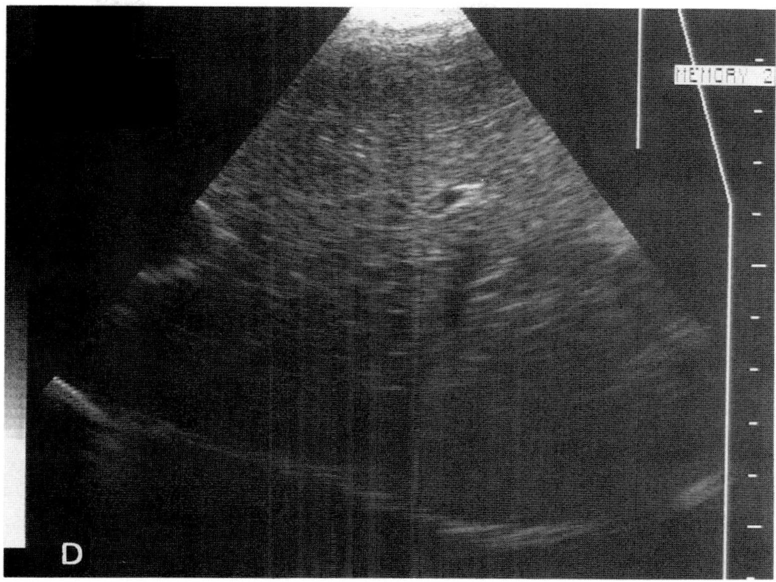

shadowed area may be filled in with echoes from the surrounding tissues as the sound beam diverges. This artifact is more pronounced with higher-frequency transducers.

Distant Enhancement

Distant enhancement occurs when the sound beam traverses a cystic structure (Fig 16). The tissues deep to the cystic structure appear brighter than surrounding tissues. The enhancement occurs because sound traveling through the fluid-filled areas is less attenuated than in surrounding tissues. This artifact is useful in establishing that an anechoic or hypoechoic structure is in fact fluid-filled.

Slice Thickness

Many artifacts have no diagnostic usefulness and, if not identified as artifacts, can lead to confusion. One of these includes the *slice thickness* artifact. This artifact occurs when imaging an anechoic or hypoechoic structure. Echoes are added when the transducer receives echoes with different amplitudes from the same area at the same depth. The computer then averages these amplitudes and incorpo-

Figure 14. The delay control affects the point to which the gain is first applied. This is usually used when imaged areas contain large amounts of fluid. With Images A and C (bottom), no delay has been added. For Images B and D, delay has been added. C and D (next page) are images of small intestines surrounded by abdominal fluid. Notice the increase in echogenicity of the intestines in Image C as compared with Image D, where delay has been applied.

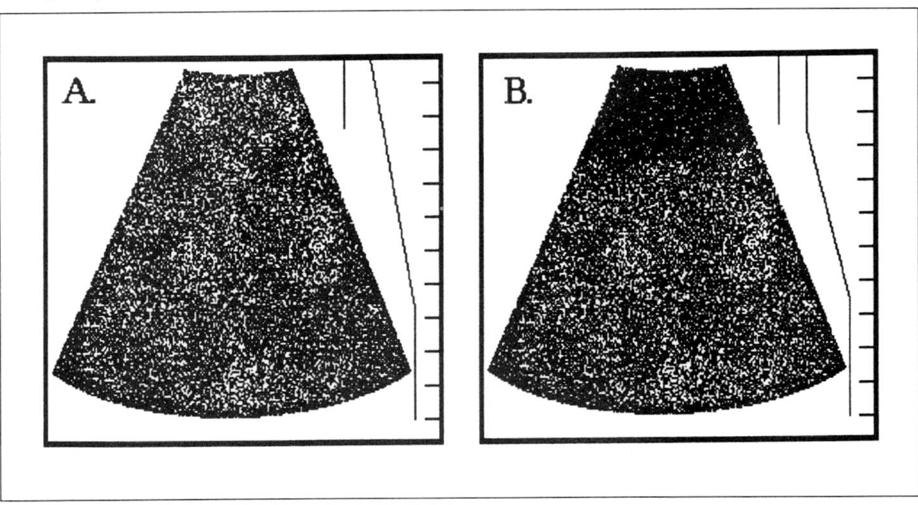

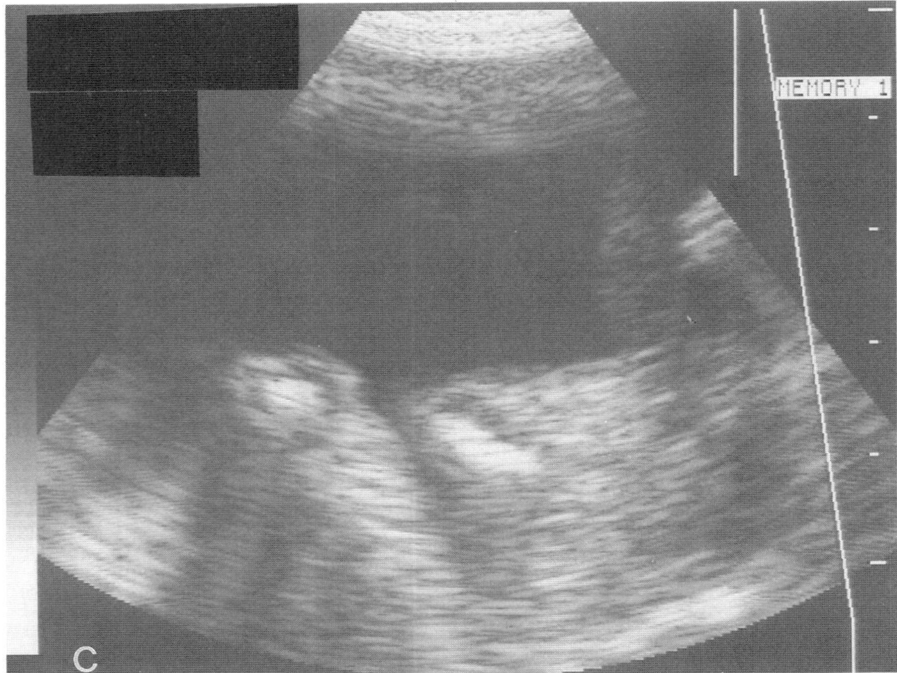

Figure 14, continued. Image D.

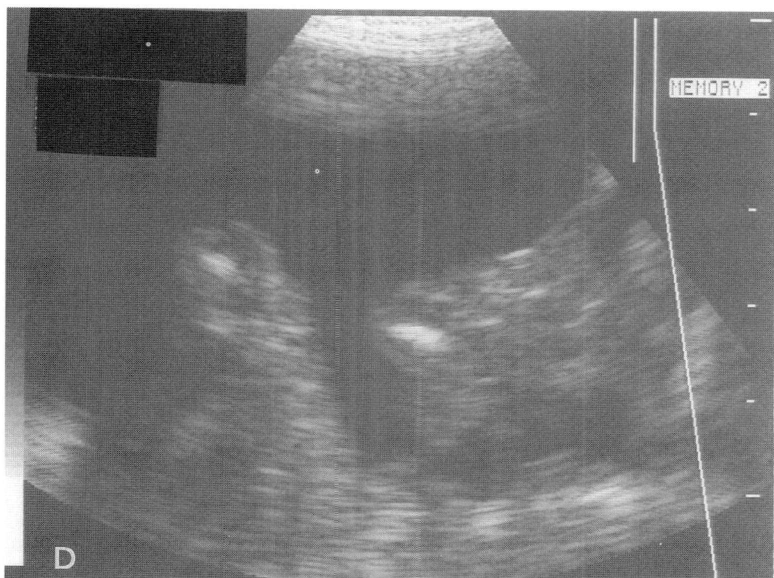

rates them in the 2-dimensional image (Fig 17). This artifact can be minimized by decreasing the overall gain; however, it will not totally eliminate it.

Reverberation

Reverberation occurs when sound is reflected off a highly reflective interface (*eg,* soft tissues to air or soft tissues to bone/metal) and then reflected back into the tissues by the surface of the transducer (Fig 18). This bouncing back and forth can continue until the sound energy has been completely attenuated. Each time the sound returns to the transducer, it produces an image at a location on the screen that is proportional to the time of travel between the transducer and the reflective interface. This creates a series of lines that are equidistant on the screen.

Mirror Image

A *mirror-image* artifact can be produced in areas with strongly reflective interfaces. This artifact creates the illusion of liver on the thoracic side of the diaphragm or the appearance of a second heart

Figure 15. Acoustic shadowing from a calculus in the urinary bladder. The white arrow indicates the highly reflective surface of the calculus. The black arrows indicate shadowing caused by the calculus.

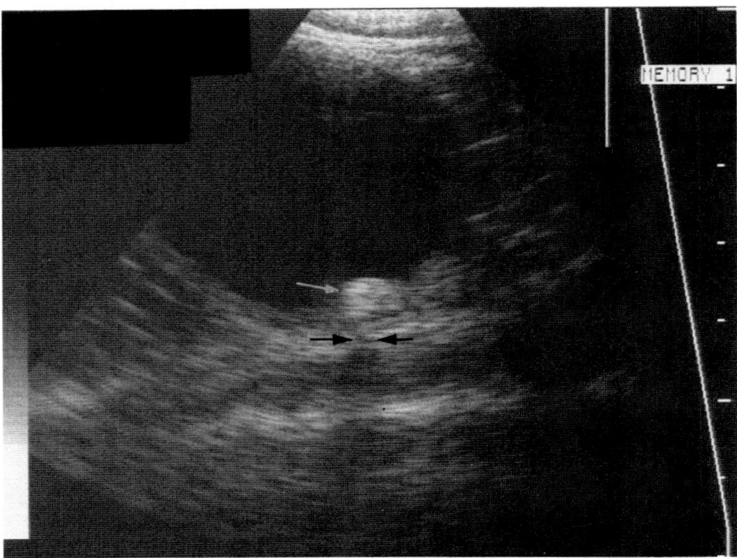

Figure 16. Distance enhancement in the liver is caused by sound waves passing through the fluid-filled gallbladder.

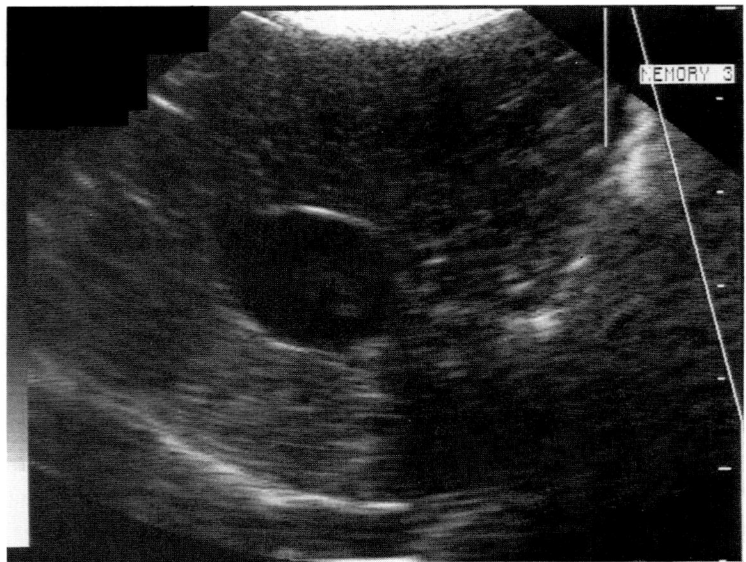

Figure 17. Urinary bladder containing a slice of thickness artifact on the far wall of the bladder (white arrows).

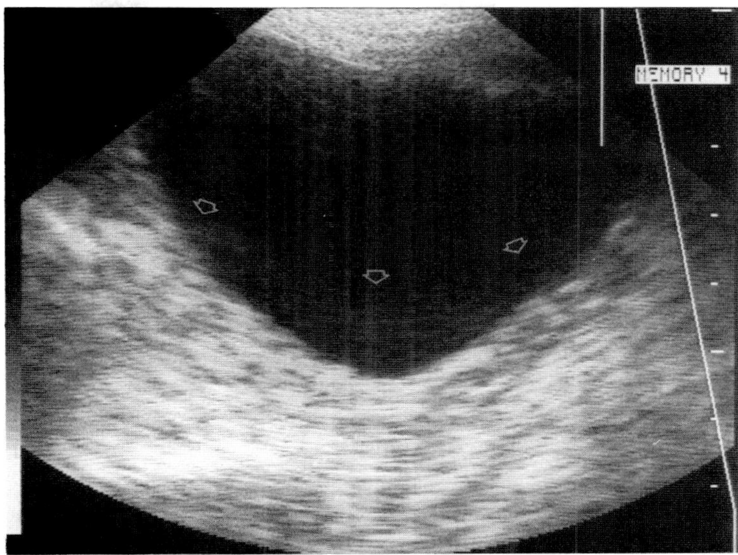

Figure 18. Reverberation artifact caused by a metal hemostatic clip in a dog's abdomen. Notice the equally spaced echoic lines (white arrows) trailing from the white interface created by the metal clip.

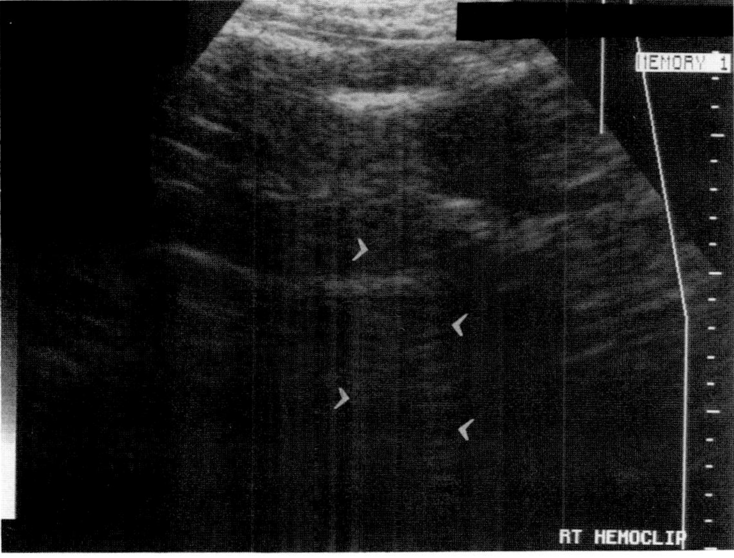

beyond the lung interface (Fig 19). Sound transmitted into the liver is reflected off the diaphragm. Some of those echoes are not reflected directly toward the transducer, but back into the liver. In the liver, some of the misdirected echoes are reflected back to the diaphragm and then to the transducer. The computer sees the misdirected echoes as being reflected from the other side of the diaphragm. One way this artifact can be minimized is by decreasing the depth to include only the area of interest.

Refraction

Refraction artifact is produced when the transmitted sound is refracted at an interface between 2 tissues of different acoustic impedance. When a sound wave strikes an interface that is perpendicular, part is reflected back to the transducer and part is transmitted in a straight path into the deeper tissues. If the sound wave

Figure 19. Mirror-image artifact. The black arrows indicate the liver/diaphragm to lung interface. In the near field to this line is the actual liver. The far field represents the mirror image of the liver.

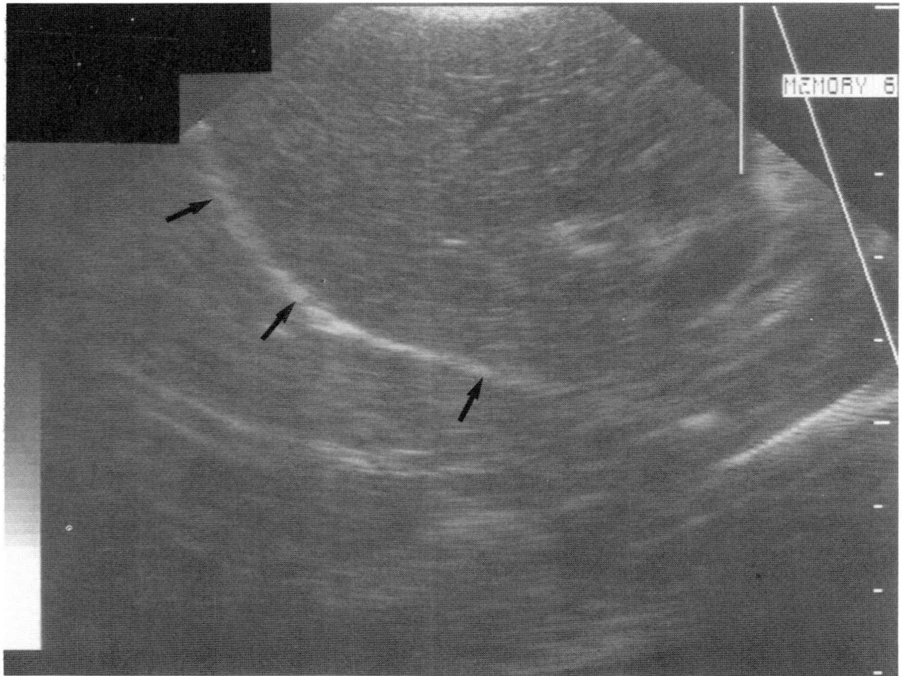

strikes an interface at an angle other than perpendicular, the transmitted sound is refracted. Refraction may cause an object to appear slightly shifted from its real position or create a shadow adjacent to a curved structure (Fig 20).

Range Ambiguity

Range ambiguity artifact is a group of echoic lines within a fluid-filled structure. When the sound is transmitted into a large fluid-filled area, it is reflected off the far wall of the cavity. If the distance is greater than the depth displayed, the sound does not reach the transducer until after the next series of sound pulses has been sent. The computer interprets this as sound that has been reflected by an interface that is much closer to the transducer than it actually is (Fig 21).

Figure 20. Refraction artifact. The white "m" indicates the medulla of the kidney. The refraction artifact created by the curved surface of the cranial and caudal poles of the kidney is identified by the white arrows.

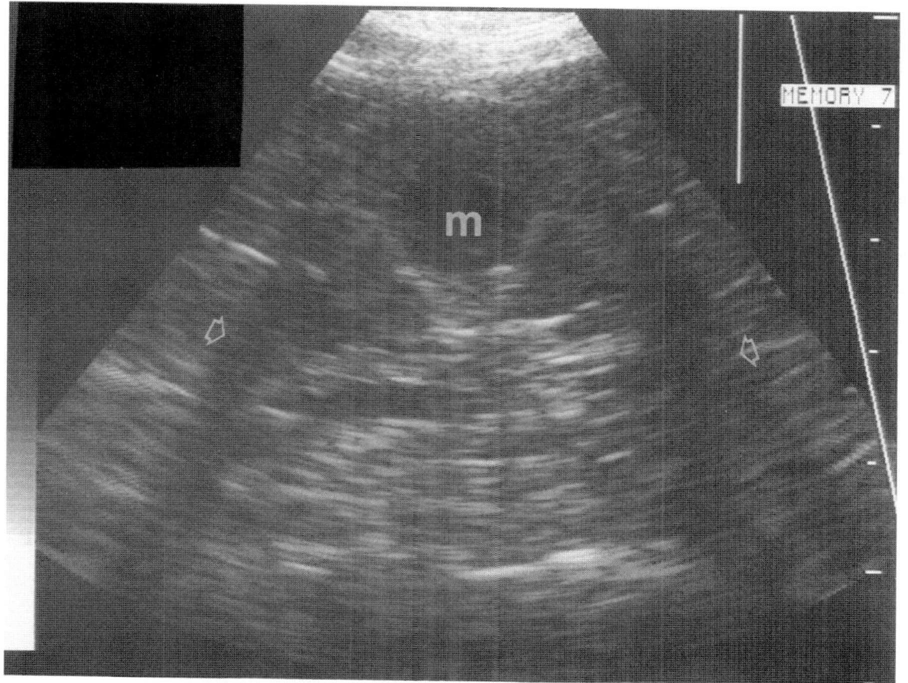

Figure 21. Range ambiguity can be seen as ill-defined echoic lines within this abdominal scan of a dog with ascites.

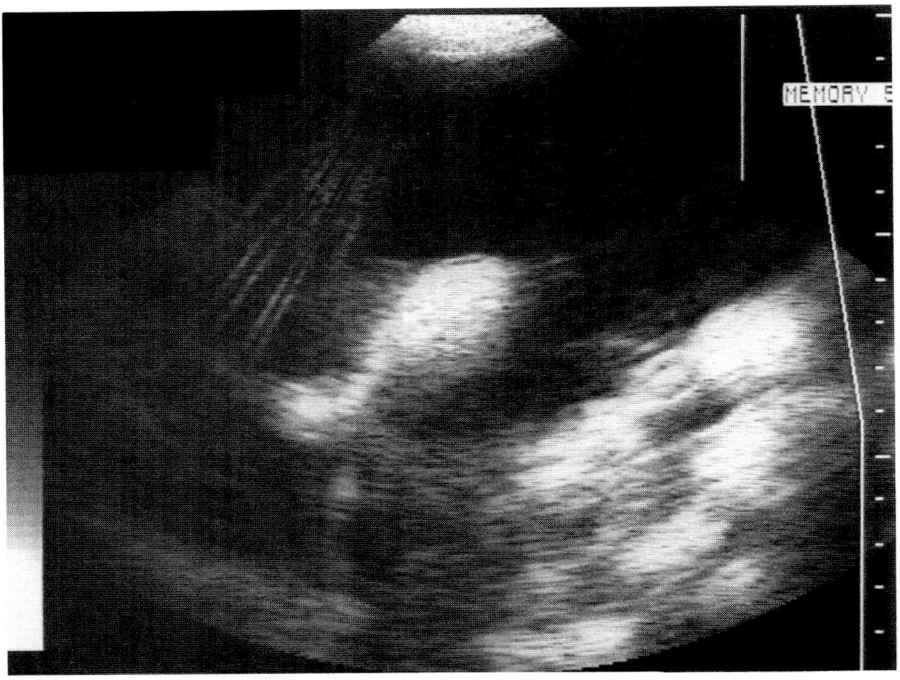

Recommended Reading

Curry TS III *et al: Christensen's Physics of Diagnostic Radiology.* 4th ed. Lea & Febiger, Philadelphia, 1990. pp. 323-371.

Miles KG: Basic principles and clinical applications of diagnostic ultrasonography. *Compend Cont Ed* 11: 609-622, 1989.

Park RD *et al:* B-mode gray-scale ultrasound: imaging artifacts and interpretation principles. *Vet Radiol* 22:204-210, 1981.

Powis RL and Powis WJ: *A Thinker's Guide to Ultrasonic Imaging.* Urban and Schwarenberg, Baltimore, 1984.

Rantanen NW and Ewing RL: Principles of ultrasound applications in animals. *Vet Radiol* 22:196-203, 1981.

Glossary

Acoustic impedance: The ability of living tissue to resist or impede the transmission of sound. Acoustic impedance varies slightly among most tissues, depending upon the density and elasticity of the tissue.

Air-gap technique: One method used to decrease scatter radiation when a grid is not available. The technique uses a 6-foot FFD and a 6-inch OFD. The increased OFD decreases the amount of scatter that reaches the film and the increased FFD decreases the amount of penumbra and magnification created by increasing the OFD.

A-mode: Amplitude mode displays the returning ultrasound echoes as a series of peaks on a graph. The greater the intensity of the returning echo, the higher the peak on the graph.

Anechoic: Describes tissue that transmits all ultrasound waves through to deeper tissues, reflecting none back to the transducer. Anechoic areas appear black on the monitor.

Anode: The site of x-ray generation. It contains a tungsten metal plate on which the electrons are focused.

Arthrography: Introduction of contrast medium into a joint to contrast the articular surface and the joint capsule.

Attenuation: Loss of intensity of ultrasound waves as they travel through tissues, caused by scatter or absorption.

Axial resolution: The ability to differentiate between 2 reflecting interfaces that lie along the axis of a transmitted ultrasound beam.

Barium enema: A radiographic study to contrast the cecum and rectum by administering barium directly into the colon.

B-mode: Brightness mode uses bright pixels or dots on the monitor to represent the intensity of returning ultrasound echoes. The brighter the pixel, the greater its intensity. The image generated is a 2-dimensional slice that is continually updated.

Cathode: Part of an x-ray machine containing a filament consisting of a tightly coiled tungsten wire. As current is applied to the filament, electrons are "boiled off" and become available to be accelerated toward the anode.

Caudal: Situated toward the tail.

Celiography: A radiographic contrast study used to evaluate the abdominal cavity and the integrity of the diaphragm.

Collimator: A device used to restrict the size of the x-ray beam.

Contralateral: Pertaining to the opposite side.

Contrast media: Agents used in radiographic studies to opacify or delineate an organ system against surrounding tissues.

Cranial: Situated toward the head.

Cystography: A radiographic contrast study used to evaluate the urinary bladder.

Developer: The processing chemical that changes the sensitized silver halide crystals into black metallic silver.

Distal: Situated away from the point of attachment.

Dorsal: Situated toward the back or topline of quadrupeds.

Double contrast: A radiographic contrast procedure using both positive- and negative-contrast media.

Echoic: Describes tissue that reflects most ultrasound back to the transducer. Echoic tissue appears white on the monitor. Also referred to as echogenic.

Electron cloud: When current is applied to the cathode filament, electrons are "boiled off," creating an electron cloud.

Esophagography: A radiographic contrast study used to evaluate the esophagus.

Excretory urography: A radiographic contrast study used to evaluate the kidneys, ureters and urinary bladder, and to provide information on renal function.

Exposure latitude: A range of radiographic exposures that produces a film density of diagnostic quality.

Filament: The filament of an x-ray tube is made of a tightly coiled tungsten wire and placed in the focusing cup in the cathode.

Fistulography: A radiographic contrast study that delineates the extent and possibly the origin of fistulous tracts.

Fixer: The processing chemical that removes the remaining silver halide crystals from the film emulsion.

Focal-film distance: The distance from the focal spot to the recording surface (film or cassette).

Focal spot: The site on the anode of the x-ray machine where the electrons are focused. The focal spot is oriented at an 11- to 20-degree angle.

Focal zone: A zone of focused returning ultrasound echoes. The sound beam can be focused by electronic means or by an acoustic lens.

Focusing cup: A device that restricts the diameter of the accelerating electrons to the focal spot on the anode of an x-ray machine.

Fog: A decrease in the differences in radiographic tissue densities between 2 adjacent shadows. Fog can be caused by a low-grade light leak in the darkroom, scatter radiation, high temperatures and improper processing techniques.

Foreshortening: Distortion of the size and length of an object on radiographs when the object is not parallel to the recording surface.

Frequency: The number of complete ultrasound wave forms (cycles) per unit of time.

Gastrography: A radiographic contrast study used to evaluate the stomach.

Grid: A series of thin linear strips made of alternating radiodense and radiolucent interspacers. Grids are used to decrease the amount of scatter radiation and increase the contrast of a radiograph.

Grid cutoff: The absorption of excessive amounts of x-rays caused by improper alignment of the grid to the center of the primary beam or placing the primary beam at an angle other than perpendicular to the grid.

Heel effect: Uneven distribution of x-rays emitted from the x-ray tube.

Hyperechoic: Describes tissues that reflect a large proportion of ultrasound back to the transducer. Hyperechoic tissues appear brighter than surrounding tissues.

Hypoechoic: Describes tissues that reflect a small proportion of ultrasound back to the transducer. Hypoechoic tissues appear darker than surrounding tissues.

Inverse square law: The intensity of the x-ray beam is inversely proportional to the square of the distance between the object and the source of the x-rays.

Isoechoic: Describes tissues with the same echotexture as surrounding tissues.

kVp: The voltage applied between the cathode and the anode of an x-ray machine. Increasing the kVp results in a shorter-wavelength x-ray beam, which is more penetrating.

Latent image: Silver halide crystals in the film emulsion that have been exposed to radiant energy, causing them to become sensitized and susceptible to chemical change.

Lateral: Situated away from the median plane or midline.

Lateral resolution: The ability to differentiate between 2 reflecting interfaces that lie in a plane perpendicular to the transmitted sound beam.

Linear scanners: Ultrasound scanners that produce a rectangular image. They are useful when imaging areas with an unrestricted acoustic window (*eg*, equine tendons).

mA: Milliamperage controls the number of electrons generated at the filament of the cathode of an x-ray machine, increasing the number of x-rays produced.

Medial: Situated toward the median plane or midline.

M-mode: Motion mode of ultrasound is a continuous display of a thin slice of an organ over a time-oriented baseline.

Myelography: A radiographic contrast study used to evaluate the spinal cord for lesions not seen on survey radiographs.

Negative-contrast medium: A radiographic contrast medium with a low atomic number, appearing radiolucent on the radiograph.

Non-selective angiography: A radiographic contrast study used to evaluate cardiac abnormalities.

Object-film distance: The distance from the object being radiographed to the recording surface (film or cassette).

Oblique: A radiographic projection used to delineate an area that would normally be superimposed over another area.

Palmar: Situated on the caudal aspect of the rear limb, distal to the tarsocrural joint.

Pneumoperitoneography: A radiographic contrast study used to evaluate the abdominal organs in animals with decreased abdominal contrast.

Positive-contrast medium: A radiographic contrast medium with a high atomic number, appearing radiodense on the radiograph.

Potter-Bucky diaphragm: A device that sets the grid in motion, blurring the white lines produced by the grid on the finished radiograph.

Proximal: Situated closer to the point of attachment.

Radiodense: Describes an area that absorbs x-rays, appearing white on the finished radiograph.

Radiographic contrast: The differences in radiographic density between adjacent areas on the radiographic image.

Radiographic density: The degree of blackness on a finished radiograph.

Radiographic detail: The degree of delineation of tissues on a finished radiograph. Good radiographic detail shows sharp tissue interfaces with good contrast.

Radiolucent: Describes an area that absorbs fewer x-rays than other areas, appearing darker on the finished radiograph.

REM (roentgen-equivalent-man): A unit of measurement of the absorbed dose of ionizing radiation.

Rostral: On the head, situated toward the nose.

Scatter radiation: X-rays diffused by collision with tissue molecules. Scatter radiation decreases the contrast on the finished radiograph.

Sector scanners: Ultrasound scanners that produce a wedge-shaped image, with a narrow near field and a wide far field. Sector scanners are useful when imaging areas with a restricted acoustic window (*eg*, through an intercostal space).

Sialography: A radiographic contrast study used to evaluate the salivary ducts and glands.

Sonolucent: Describes tissue that transmits most ultrasound waves to deeper tissues, with only a few waves reflected back to the transducer. Sonolucent tissue appears dark on the monitor.

Subject density: The degree to which different tissues absorb x-rays. These differences depend upon the average atomic number and the thickness of the tissue.

Time gain compensation: A series of controls on an ultrasound machine used to make similar tissues look alike.

Transducer: Part of an ultrasound machine that emits a series of ultrasonic pulses and then receives the returning echoes.

Ultrasound: A noninvasive method of imaging soft tissues by sending low-intensity, high-frequency sound waves into tissues and recording the returning echoes.

Upper gastrointestinal series: A radiographic contrast study to evaluate the stomach and small intestines.

Urethrography: A radiographic contrast study to evaluate the urethra.

Vagionography: A radiographic contrast study to evaluate the vagina and urethra.

Velocity: The speed at which sound travels through a medium.

Ventral: Situated toward the underside of quadrupeds.

Wavelength: The length of one complete wave form. With ultrasound it is the distance from one band of compression or rarefaction to the next.

X-rays: A form of electromagnetic radiation, similar to visible light but with a shorter wavelength.

Index

H

humerus, 91, 132, 133

I, J

K

L

M

N

O

P, Q

S

T

U

V

W

X, Y, Z